T0091911

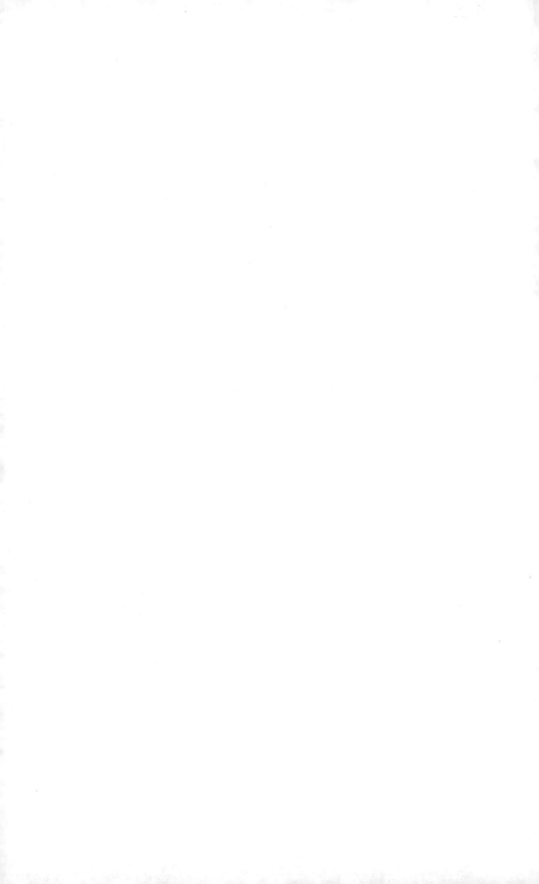

Galen's Treatise Περὶ Ἀλυπίας (*De indolentia*) in Context

Studies in Ancient Medicine

Edited by

John Scarborough (*University of Wisconsin-Madison*)
Philip J. van der Eijk (*Humboldt-Universitat zu Berlin*)
Ann Ellis Hanson (*Yale University*)
Joseph Ziegler (*University of Haifa*)

VOLUME 52

The titles published in this series are listed at *brill.com/sam*

Galen's Treatise Περὶ Ἀλυπίας (*De indolentia*) in Context

A Tale of Resilience

Edited by

Caroline Petit

BRILL

LEIDEN | BOSTON

Cover illustration: 'Mezzotint, Portrait of Galen, bust; by J. Faber, sen.' by Peter Paul Rubens. Credit: Wellcome Collection. CC BY 4.0

The Library of Congress Cataloging-in-Publication Data is available online at http://catalog.loc.gov
LC record available at http://lccn.loc.gov/2018046676

Typeface for the Latin, Greek, and Cyrillic scripts: "Brill". See and download: brill.com/brill-typeface.

ISSN 0925-1421
ISBN 978-90-04-38328-9 (hardback)
ISBN 978-90-04-38330-2 (e-book)

Contents

A Long Lost Text: Galen's Περὶ Ἀλυπίας

Caroline Petit

This volume arises from a one-day conference, the "Galen Day", held at Warwick University on July 1, 2014 and supported by the Faculty of Arts at the University of Warwick, the Department of Classics and Ancient History, and a Wellcome Trust Medical Humanities Small Grant (105153/Z/14/Z). I wish to express my gratitude to those institutions for their support, and to Simon Swain (then chair of the Faculty of Arts) in particular for encouraging and actively backing the project. The chosen theme of the conference was Galen's newly discovered περὶ ἀλυπίας (henceforth: PA), a text that has generated more discussion since its discovery than any other work by the great Galen. Several reasons helped me decide to select the PA as the focus of the conference. A new translation by Vivian Nutton had just appeared, as part of a fine new volume edited by Peter Singer.[1] As a new English translation by the most accomplished Galen scholar alive, it signalled a turning point and marked a significant improvement on what was available to scholars. As such, it was a landmark worth celebrating, and a potential starting point for new discussions around the text. Indeed, the Greek text is available in two main editions (Kotzia/Soutiroudis, and Boudon-Millot/Jouanna/Pietrobelli, henceforth KS and BJP, both published in 2010), which significantly differ from one another; Nutton brings a new take on both, and, with it, new interpretations. No translation is definitive, and neither of the editions cited above is, as recently published conjectures demonstrate;[2] but Nutton's new translation was certainly instrumental in the speakers' preparation, and in finalising the papers presented here. It is certainly a new high for many scholars interested in this vibrant little work. Vivian Nutton was present at the conference, which he accepted to introduce, and chair: this volume is dedicated to him with gratitude, for this and the many other times he has given support and advice.

The inspirational nature of the PA is exemplified by Peter Singer's considerable contribution to this volume, in the form of three different, extensive

---

1 P. N. Singer, *Galen. Psychological Writings*, Cambridge University Press, 2013.

2 For example Polemis, I. 'Διορθωτικά στο Περὶ Ἀλυπίας του Γαληνού', *Ἐπιστημονικὴ Ἐπετηρίδα τῆς Φιλοσοφικῆς Σχολῆς τοῦ Πανεπιστημίου Ἀθηνῶν* 43 (2011), 1–8; Kotzia, P. 'Galen περὶ ἀλυπίας: Title, Genre and Two Cruces'. In *Studi sul De indolentia di Galeno*, ed. D. Manetti, 2012, 69–91.

© CAROLINE PETIT, 2019 | DOI:10.1163/9789004383302_002

pieces, which were originally supposed to make just one chapter. Peter's of-
ferings shed new light on the significance of the manuscript (*Vlat.* 14) and of
the new text, and on Galen's thought as well as his complex compositional
strategies. His contribution far exceeds what any editor would expect from a
collaborator, and I feel humbled in the face of his dedication to this text and, as
a result, to this volume. I owe him very special thanks. I hope readers will feel
equally privileged upon discovering his insights on Galen's *PA*.

Simon Swain has kindly read and corrected the English of non-native speakers' papers (notably mine!), for which I am especially grateful.

Beyond the new English translation, another reason to pick the *PA* among
so many Galenic texts worth studying, was that its sensational discovery succeeded in *finally* bringing together classicists, historians and philosophers
around Galen, well beyond the usual (small) circle of its specialists. The bibliography dedicated to this text demonstrates new, widespread interest in what
Galen has to say about the circulation of texts (medical and not), the Great
Fire of 192, ancient libraries (especially in Rome), and many additional topics
that have little to do with medicine as a technical field. The idea of a "Galen
Day" aimed precisely at bringing together a diverse audience, interested in
the many facets of Galen's *œuvre*, beyond the 'usual suspects'. The *PA*, having
produced so many studies in such a short time by so many different scholars,
thus seemed the ideal focus for such an enterprise. The papers gathered here
embrace multiple aspects of the text, with a purpose to shed as much light as
possible on its various points of interest. It is hoped that they will further the
public's passion for it.

As a recently unearthed treasure, the *PA* has invited us Galen specialists to
cast a retrospective look at what we knew, or thought we knew about Galen,
and how we deal with his texts. The sensational discovery made by Antoine
Pietrobelli more than ten years ago, at the very least reminded scholars that,
against common preconceptions, nothing is definitive about our knowledge
of antiquity: new evidence may resurface any day and invite us to reconsider
some of our assumptions. Finding new material is not the privilege of archae-
ologists. As far as Galen is concerned, it is not impossible that more texts are
found in forgotten manuscripts, not necessarily in Greek, but potentially in
Latin, Syriac or Arabic.[3] There are already many examples of this. Every time a
new text or fragment appears, it might change our notions of Galen's biography

---

3 Examples are found in all three languages, and include the *De virt. cent.* written by a rival
of Galen and edited by Vivian Nutton on the basis of Latin manuscripts; the *Syriac Galen
Palimpsest*, which contains large swathes of Galen's treatise *On simple drugs*; the fragments
from Galen's major work *On demonstration* in Arabic, etc.

and ideas, of his literary production or of his medical practices. But the *PA* has shaken those notions to the core, far much than any other text, from Galen's life at the imperial court and his philosophical opinions, to the contents of his library, and the range of his possessions. Its interest extends to areas of ancient history (such as the location of libraries and storerooms in Rome), literature and philosophy that normally stay untouched by those I am tempted to call "Galenists". Meanwhile, it has ensured that those who didn't read Galen regularly now turn towards him a little more often. The *PA* has brought to Galen a new audience.

In the following pages, I intend to offer a very brief summary of the history and points of interest of this text (all of which have already been extensively and clearly presented by Vivian Nutton[4]), and a presentation of the contents of the present volume.

The existence of Galen's *PA* was known through a handful of quotations in Arabic and Hebrew, but the text was reputed forever lost, until a then-PhD student in Paris, Antoine Pietrobelli, started studying a Greek manuscript in the library of the Vlatades monastery, Thessaloniki, Greece, in 2005. The following examination by Véronique Boudon-Millot led to the 'discovery' of the work in the midst of an impressive collection of Galenic texts, some of which unpublished or previously not available in Greek.[5] This is how the περὶ ἀλυπίας resurfaced among modern scholars. The 15th c. manuscript is poor, and has already generated much debate as to how best to interpret several passages.[6] For that reason, several translations have already appeared, in English, French, Italian and German, with different takes on the difficulties posed by scribal errors and other transmission problems.[7] The papers presented here engage with the various interpretations at hand wherever needed. I will give one example. Although the Budé text by Jouanna and Boudon-Millot is the basis used by the contributors, all contributors in this volume agree on περὶ ἀλυπίας as the best possible title, against the conservative περὶ ἀλυπησίας printed by Jouanna and

---

4 V. Nutton in P. N. Singer (ed.) 2013, 45–76; see also C. Rothschild/T. Thompson 2014, 3–18 and V. Boudon-Millot/J. Jouanna 2010, vii–lxxvi.

5 See A. Pietrobelli, 'Variation autour du Thessalonicensis Vlatadon 14: un manuscrit copié au xenon du Kral, peu avant la chute de Constantinople', *Revue des Études Byzantines* 68, 2010, 95–126.

6 See V. Nutton in P. N. Singer 2013, pp. 100–106; both Garofalo/Lami and Rothschild/Thompson have attempted to provide lists of respective emendations in their editions, and Brodersen offers a list of departure points for his own translation.

7 Available translations include that of Jouanna/Boudon-Millot and Pietrobelli (2010), Rothschild and Thompson (2011), Garofalo and Lami (2012), Vegetti (2013), Nutton (2013) and Brodersen (2015).

Boudon-Millot on the basis of the manuscript.[8] Such disagreements are common with a poorly transmitted text, and chances are that new editions, or at least new conjectures, will appear in the future. Meanwhile, additional examination of the manuscript has led to nuance the importance of *Vlat.* 14 in the textual history of Galenic works generally: the manuscript from Thessaloniki is pivotal in supplementing lacunous texts, such as *Propr. Plac.*, a new edition of which is being prepared by Antoine Pietrobelli; but it is of little interest in the case of other texts with richer, well-established manuscript traditions.[9] Readers will find more information on the contents and significance of the manuscript for Galen's textual history in Peter Singer's adjacent *Note on MS Vlatadon 14*.[10]

Generic definition has been at the heart of discussions around the *PA*: a letter to an anonymous friend, a philosophical treatise on the familiar theme of ἀλυπία (absence of distress, to select but one possible translation), the text has also somehow reminded scholars of the genre of *consolatio* well known through Plutarch and Cicero. A fine *connoisseur* of Greek literature and philosophy, Galen conforms to some well-established literary and argumentative codes and delivers many expected quotations on the topic; Stoic, Epicurean, and other traditions underpin much of his argument. In such respects he may simply be following a trend, or rather, trends. But a large part of the treatise is dedicated to a highly personal account of Galen's own losses, and of the impact of the Fire, as well as Commodus and the plague on life in Rome around 193 AD. Galen thus gives us more than a variation on a common topic. The following papers explore in turn, in great detail, the reasons why this text is an original take on the much-debated topic of ἀλυπία; how it changes, to some extent, our perception of the Galenic corpus and of Galen himself; and how it allows us to think again about such major disasters of that period as the Antonine 'plague' and the reign of Commodus. Following up on previous collective projects,[11] the present studies will hopefully supplement nicely the scholarship already available, raise new questions and bridge some gaps.

The present volume is formed of ten chapters of varying length, and falls into three parts, followed by an epilogue investigating possible engagement of Islamic scholars with the text (Pietrobelli). In the first part, titled *The PA in*

---

8   About the question of the title, see P. Singer in this volume (*Note*) p. 19.

9   See the critical editions of *Libr. Propr.* by V. Boudon-Millot, 2007, pp. 42–49, and of the pseudo-Galenic *Introd. sive medicus* by C. Petit, 2009, p. xciii and n. 137. See also V. Boudon-Millot, 'Un nouveau témoin grec inédit de l'Ars medica de Galien, le Vlatadon 14', 2008.

10   See pp. 10–37.

11   Manetti, D. (ed.) *Studi sul De indolentia di Galeno*, 2012; Rothschild, C. K. and Thompson, T. W. (eds), *Galen's De indolentia*, 2013.

Galen's Œuvre, three chapters explore what precious further insight Galen's PA gives us to understand his monumental, multifaceted *oeuvre*. In *Death, Posterity and the Vulnerable Self: Galen's PA in the context of his later works*, Caroline Petit studies Galen's PA in the context of his later works, looking for new insights into Galen's rhetorical *persona*. Galen's rhetorical mastery, and his concern for public approval appear in most of his works; they especially come through in the autobiographical features of his later writings. The Great Fire of 192 is chosen here as a cut-off date and a turning point in Galen's life. There and then Galen puts the final touches to a character he has created through a lifetime of working and writing, for the sake of his practitioner's reputation, and for posterity. Galen's PA holds no insignificant part in this architecture of words: establishing his own character as one of virtue, resilience and courage, yet not exempt of human frailty, Galen finalises the self-portrait that emerges from the wide-ranging set of works he wrote in his old age. This chapter investigates the evidence scattered in Galen's many later works, in order to emphasise the specific features of PA as an autobiographical and self-characterising effort in the wake of life-changing events.

In the second chapter, *New light and old texts: Galen on his own books*, Peter Singer investigates what PA brings us scholars in terms of new texts (or parts of texts), and explores in some depth new information provided by some passages in PA about Galen's understanding of "publication" (*ekdosis*). Although it is often put forward that Galen distinguishes carefully between works written for his friends or *hetairoi* (in other words, his close circle) and works written *pros ekdosin* (usually translated as 'for publication'), close reading of the passages he devotes to this topic in fact show, Singer argues, that Galen did not necessarily exclude wider circulation of his works as a consequence of writing/dedicating them to friends. Evidence from PA confirms that Galen was content for his work to spread across larger circles, following adjustments and corrections to preliminary versions circulated in private.

In her paper, *Galen and the Language of Old Comedy: glimpses of a lost treatise at PA 23b–28*, Amy Coker focuses on a specific passage of PA, in which Galen provides crucial information on the contents of his lost (and considerable) works on ancient comedy. Based on an extensive review of the available evidence scattered throughout Galen's works and in the PA, Coker reveals the possible range of texts used by Galen in his lost works on comedy, and attempts a reconstruction of the latter. In so doing, Coker hypothesises the possible use by Galen of lexicographers' works and standard plays, and demonstrates the close relationship between Galen and contemporary authors, much in the manner of the "sophists" he tends to vilify. The picture of a medical writer profoundly indebted to, and in phase with Second Sophistic figures, emerges at last. This first part therefore addresses Galen's *PA* as new evidence for our understanding and appreciation of his overall project.

The second and most substantial part of the volume is, understandably, dedicated to Galen's philosophical position in *PA*. All four papers shed light on a particular aspect of Galen's ideas in this text: a long philosophical – not medical – tradition has shaped the ancients' thinking about emotions, especially distress (λυπή). In the first chapter, *Galen's* PA *as philosophical therapy: how coherent is it?*, Christopher Gill explores Galen's new text against the backdrop of long-standing interrogations among Greek philosophers about the possible ways to control our emotions. Galen, although a doctor, deals with those problems in two related surviving works, *Avoiding Distress* (*De Indolentia*, or *Ind.*) and the first book of *The Diagnosis and Treatment of the Affections and Errors Peculiar to Each Person's Soul* (*Aff. Pecc. Dig.*, and *Aff. Dig.* for book I). Here, Gill argues, Galen focuses on *philosophical* therapy, moving away from medical concerns. Issues of structure and coherence are the starting point of Gill's discussion, who goes on to identify patterns of cohesion both internally and between the two works, showing that *PA* offers an original voice among works dedicated to the same topic. Gill concludes, however, with an open question on the therapy apparently adopted and promoted by Galen in this text: suggesting that ἀπληστία must precede ἀλυπία, Galen seems to rule out the therapeutic value of his own life-long (and well-established) medical and literary project. Somehow, Galen seems at odds with the therapy he advocates.

Jim Hankinson's paper focuses on the skeptical background to Galen's *PA*. In fact, for the sake of appropriate contextualisation, he is led to delivering a thorough account of Galen's Stoic, Epicurean and Skeptical background across his many philosophical works. Arguing in favour of Galen's proximity with the Pyrrhonists, with whom he has fundamental disagreements, is bold; but Hankinson points to discrete points of convergence between their ideas and Galen's attempt at tackling distress. Whilst not quite mentioning *metriopatheia*, a sceptic notion, Galen's point of view in *PA* is evocative of similar ideas, and appeals to the powers of reasoning to fight against any invasive emotions, in a way that is not without reminding Sextus Empiricus.

Peter Singer, in *A New Distress: Galen's Ethics in the* PA *and beyond*, argues that *lupè* (distress) is at the crossroads of ethics and medicine. A dangerous emotion if left unchecked and allowed to grow, *lupè* is medical in so far as it has serious physical and mental consequences. More annoyingly for Galen in the context of *PA*, it can develop into a serious obstacle on an individual's moral quest to fortitude. As such, it is pointless to deny the existence of negative emotions or claim they can be superseded – rather acknowledge them, says Galen, but work out the way to control them. Thus Galen's voice is unique among the more trenchant opinions of Stoic as well as other philosophers. *Lupè*, and therefore *alupia*, can be approached through a more acceptant, humbler understanding of emotions. This is what is advocated by Galen.

Finally, Teun Tieleman analyses *PA* against the backdrop of a long tradition of ancient philosophical therapeutics, the roots of which are to be found especially in the Stoic tradition. An ardent admirer of Plato, Galen succeeds in combining his Platonic creed and the Stoic heritage to offer a personal take on the virtue of *apatheia*, which he considers neither wholly attainable nor desirable for vulnerable human beings. Tieleman thus confirms and supplements an important strand of Singer's argument: Galen's undeniably profound engagement with the Stoic tradition.

Part three of the volume delivers new insights into the troubled history of the final years of the Antonines: in *Galen and the Plague*, Rebecca Flemming examines afresh our evidence and recent scholarship about the Antonine 'plague', using Galen's new testimony to show how utterly bewildering and challenging the deadly disease was to Galen and his contemporaries. Whilst attempting to pin down the nature of the disease thanks to ancient and medieval (Arabic) sources, Flemming demonstrates that there is no point in trying to draw too much from imperial writers and other sources: a monstrous fatality imposed on the world, the 'plague' was in no way understood and analysed for what it was, but simply conveyed dread, fear, and resignation. This is true of Galen, too, she argues.

Matthew Nicholls, in *Galen and the Last Days of Commodus*, revisits the dreaded reign of Commodus in the light of Galen's testimony. Galen's letter, he argues, may have arisen from the need to clear himself from any wrongdoing or crime by association, as he remained attached to the Palace throughout Commodus' reign until his assassination. A physician at the service of Marcus Aurelius, and of Commodus since childhood, Galen presumably stood no chance to escape back to Pergamum – but his surviving the reign free of any of the calamities endured by many of his friends may have raised questions, or even malignant suggestions as to his integrity. Whether or not Galen felt compelled to write a somehow apologetic work about his Commodus years, his text remains a highly intriguing testimony about life at court during that period.

Finally, Antoine Pietrobelli's paper stands alone in the final section of the book (*epilogue*), titled *Arabic περὶ ἀλυπίας: Did al-Kindî and Râzî read Galen?* Antoine Pietrobelli's study investigates possible interactions with the text in the Islamic world. Whilst Galen's text was remembered and commemorated, few had a genuine opportunity to engage directly with it: in the Islamic world just like in the West, no known copies of the text survive. According to Pietrobelli however, this may not always have been the case: close reading shows that Râzi most likely read, pondered and imitated Galen's *PA*. Al-Kindi, on the other hand, perhaps for reasons of inter-school rivalry in Baghdad, was almost certainly not able to interact with the Arabic translation of the text. In any case, it is clear that Galen's *PA* haunted medical minds well beyond its production in 193.

A list of the most common abbreviations and editions used in this volume will be found at the end of the following *Note* by Peter Singer.

With regard to the denomination of the text, a flexible approach has been chosen: each contributor favoured either the Greek title (περὶ ἀλυπίας), the abbreviated *PA*, or the Latin title (*De indolentia*, abbr. *Ind.*) – in the footnotes and in the *index locorum*, however, references to the text will be found under *Ind.* (*De indolentia*).

References

Boudon-Millot, V. 'Un nouveau témoin grec inédit de l'Ars medica de Galien, le Vlatadon 14', in *L'Ars medica (Tegni) de Galien: lectures antiques et médiévales*, textes réunis et édités par N. Palmieri, Publications de l'Université de Saint-Etienne, Centre Jean Palerne, Mémoires XXXIII, 2008, 11–29

Kotzia, P. 'Galen περὶ ἀλυπίας: Title, Genre and Two Cruces'. In *Studi sul De indolentia di Galeno*, ed. D. Manetti, 2012, 69–91

Manetti, D. (ed.), *Studi sul De indolentia di Galeno*, Pisa and Rome: Fabrizio Serra Editore, 2012

Pietrobelli, A. 'Variation autour du Thessalonicensis Vlatadon 14: un manuscrit copié au xenon du Kral, peu avant la chute de Constantinople', *Revue des Études Byzantines* 68, 2010, 95–126

Polemis, I. 'Διορθωτικά στο Περί Αλυπίας του Γαληνού', *Επιστημονική Επετηρίδα της Φιλοσοφικής Σχολής του Πανεπιστημίου Αθηνών* 43, 2011, 1–8

Rothschild, C. K. and Thompson, T. W. (eds), *Galen's De indolentia*, Tübingen: Mohr Siebeck, 2013

Editions and Translations of Galen's PA

Boudon-Millot, V. and Jouanna, J. (ed. and trans.), with A. Pietrobelli, *Galien, Oeuvres, tome IV: Ne pas se chagriner.* Paris: Les Belles Lettres, 2010

Brodersen, K., *Die Verbrannte Bibliothek. Peri Alypias (über die Unverdrossenheit)*, Wiesbaden: Marixverlag, 2015

Garofalo, I. and Lami, A. *Galeno: L'anima e il dolore. (De indolentia; De propriis placitis).* Milan: Rizzoli, 2012

Nutton, V. *Avoiding Distress*, in *Galen: Psychological Writings*, ed. P. N. Singer, 43–106. Cambridge: Cambridge University Press, 2013

Rothschild, C. K. and Thompson, T. W. 'Galen: "On the Avoidance of Distress"'. In *Galen's De indolentia*, ed. C. K. Rothschild and T. W. Thompson, 21–36. Tübingen: Mohr Siebeck, 2013

Vegetti, M., *Galeno: nuovi scritti autobiografici.* Rome: Carocci, 2013.

Editions and Translations of Other Galenic Works

Introd. sive medicus =*Introductio sive medicus* (*Introduction; or, the Physician*) [K. XIV] ed. C. Petit, Paris: Les Belles Lettres, 2009

Lib. Prop. = *De libris propriis* (*My Own Books*). [K. XIX]. Ed. V. Boudon-Millot. Paris: Les Belles Lettres, 2007; trans. in Singer, *Galen: Selected Works*

CHAPTER 1

Note on MS Vlatadon 14: a Summary of the Main Findings and Problems

P. N. Singer

The Galenic manuscript fortuitously discovered by Antoine Pietrobelli in a Greek monastery in 2005 contains four items with significant new Galenic material: an entire text which had previously been lost to us, περὶ ἀλυπίας (*Ind.*); the full Greek text of a work which had been available in Greek only in small part, the rest having to be supplied from an Arabo-Latin and a Graeco-Latin translation, *My Own Doctrines* (*Prop. Plac.*);[1] and an additional version of the Greek text of two works which were already extant, but with significant lacunae, in the only previously-known Greek manuscript, *My Own Books* (*Lib. Prop.*) and *The Order of My Own Books* (*Ord. Lib. Prop.*).[2]

In the case of the last two works mentioned, then, the Vlatadon manuscript was able to fill these lacunae. The discovery of the wholly new text, περὶ ἀλυπίας, has given rise to a veritable flurry of international scholarly activity, including both a great deal of philological work on problems in the text and a number of analyses of the new light – and of the questions and puzzles – which the text sheds and raises. Meanwhile, the full Greek version of *My Own Doctrines* has attracted some, though comparatively much less, attention; and discovery of some missing sentences from the two works of auto-bibliography, *My Own Books* and *The Order of My Own Books*, has gone more or less unnoticed. In

---

1 The *editio princeps* of the partial Greek text supplemented by Latin sources was produced by Nutton, V. (1999). *Galen: De propriis placitis*, and that of the full Greek text, with French translation, by Boudon-Millot, V. and Pietrobelli, A. (2005). 'Galien ressuscité: édition princeps du texts grec du *De propriis placitis*', *Revue des Études Grecques* 118, 168–213; the latter scholar is preparing a full critical edition of the text. See Nutton's edition, 14–45 and Pietrobelli, A. (2013). 'Galien agnostique: un texte caviardé par la tradition', *Revue des Études Grecques* 126, 103–35, at 106–9, for further detail on the textual tradition (which also includes a section in Hebrew translation).

2 A peculiarity of the nature of the damage to the single previously known manuscript of these two texts that it gave rise to *lacunae* covering significantly overlapping material in the two texts, which both list Galen's own works. The edition and translation of Boudon-Millot, V. (2007). *Galien, Tome 1*, takes account of the new material; see also Boudon-Millot V. (2014). 'Vlatadon 14 and *Ambrosianus* Q3: Two Twin Manuscripts'. In Rothschild, C. K. and Thompson, T. W. (eds) *Galen's* De indolentia, 41–55.

© P. N. SINGER, 2019 | DOI:10.1163/9789004383302_003

view of the wealth of scholarly publications that have already appeared, in a wide range of different languages, books and journals – and especially in view of the fact that in some cases these have appeared after the publication of the critical editions of περί ἀλυπίας, or at least too late to be fully taken into account by their various editors – it may be helpful to offer an overview both of the new information and fresh insights that have accrued from research on the manuscript thus far, and of the chief problems and areas of dispute. This chapter attempts such an overview, considering both the main research findings and controversies and, in the context of a highly problematic and already much discussed manuscript, the most significant and/or debated textual cruces in the text of περί ἀλυπίας.

1　　　Main Findings

The main gains and research findings arising from the discovery may, I think, be listed under five heads or topics:
(i)　archaeology: the location, and nature, of Roman libraries and storehouses in the imperial period;
(ii)　scholarship and bibliographical practice: specific features of manuscript collection and scholarly traditions in second-century-AD Rome, as well as the nature of book production and book distribution;
(iii)　Galen's practices of book-study and of book-composition;
(iv)　moral philosophy: Galen's contribution to the genre;
(v)　Galen's summation of, and attitude to, his own central philosophical doctrines.

While the text of περί ἀλυπίας sheds new light on topics (i) and (iv) above, both this and the texts of *My Own Books* and *The Order of My Own Books* shed light on topics (ii) and (iii).[3]

A considerable amount of recent scholarship has been devoted to (i), exploring the location and nature of both the public imperial library collections mentioned by Galen and his own private storehouse, as well as the nature and extent of the damage inflicted in this geographical area by the fire of 192. Some clarity has emerged – we seem for example to have a fairly clear idea of the

---

3　But the list is not exhaustive. Another debate re-ignited by the codex concerns the vexed question of Galen's *gentilicium*: is it possible that he was called Claudius after all? See Alexandru, S. (2011). 'Newly Discovered Witness Asserting Galen's Affiliation to the *Gens Claudia*', *Annali della Scuola Normale Superiore di Pisa*, ser. 5, 3/2, 385–433 and Nutton, V. (2015). 'What's in a *Nomen*? Vlatadon 14 and an Old Theory Resuscitated', in Holmes, B. and Fischer, K.-D. (eds), *The Frontiers of Ancient Science: Essays in Honour of Heinrich von Staden*, 451–62.

location of Galen's own storehouse, in the Horrea Pipertaria – but there remain significant uncertainties in relation to library locations, arising from the
highly problematic nature of certain passages of the Greek text. That a library
attached to the Temple of Peace was one of the major ones destroyed in the
fire is clear; a library attached to Tiberius' palace is also mentioned; but a problem arises in the relevant passage (sections 12b–18), as to the precise location,
and number, of the libraries to which Galen is referring when he mentions the
'Palatine' (or 'palace') libraries; and a particularly thorny problem as to the location indicated by Galen's reference to a further set of book losses, not by fire
but by damp and looting (and possibly rodent damage). Is he here referring to
library location in a marshy place in the Forum (and if so, precisely where), or
rather to a library not at Rome at all but in Antium?[4] (See further below for the
problematic passage of text from which this debate arises.)

On topic (ii) – obviously related to (i), but touching on broader questions in
the history of texts and intellectual traditions, as well as the history of the book
as a physical object – there has been even more activity;[5] and here too areas
of clarity are counterbalanced by considerable uncertainties of interpretation.
Among the results that have emerged with clarity we may mention: the existence of a range of texts, most especially but not only in the Aristotelian tradition,[6] that were not previously known to be available to or of interest to Galen;

---

4   A clear overview, of likely geographical situations and of the recent debate and the problems,
    is given by Nutton (2013). *Avoiding Distress*, in Singer, P. N. (ed.) *Galen: Psychological Writings*,
    53–61. See also Dix, T. K. and Houston, G. W. (2006). 'Public Libraries in the City of Rome:
    From the Augustan Age to the Time of Diocletian', *Mélanges de l'École Française de Rome:
    Antiquité* 118:2, 671–717; Houston, G. W. (2008). 'Galen, His Books and the *Horrea Pipertaria* at
    Rome', *Memoirs of the British Academy in Rome* 48 (2008), 45–51; Tucci, P. L. (2008). 'Galen's
    Storeroom, Roman Libraries, and the Fire of AD 192', *JRA* 21, 133–49; id. (2009). 'Antium, the
    Palatium and the Domus Tiberiana Again' *JRA* 22, 398–401; id. (2013). 'Galen and the Library
    at Antium: The State of the Question', *Classical Philology* 108:3, 240–51; Jones, C. P. (2009).
    'Books and Libraries in a Newly-Discovered Treatise of Galen', *JRS* 22, 390–7; Rothschild,
    C. K. and Thompson, T. W. (2011). 'Galen's *On the Avoidance of* Grief: The Question of a Library
    at Antium', *Early Christianity* 2.1, 110–29; cf. Boudon-Millot, V. and Jouanna, J. (2010). *Galien,
    Oeuvres 4: Ne pas se chagriner*, xxii–xxvii and 66; Nicholls, M. 'A Library at Antium?', in
    Rothschild, C. K. and Thompson, T. W. (2013). *Galen's De indolentia*, 65–78.
5   See Nutton, *Avoiding Distress* and Manetti, D. (ed.) (2012). *Studi sul De indolentia di Galeno*;
    further bibliography on specific debates in relation to *cruces* is given below.
6   The focus on and engagement with Aristotle and Aristotelians – and, more specifically, *first-
    generation* Aristotelians – is emphasized by the grouping, 'Theophrastus, Aristotle, Eudemus,
    Clytus and Phaenias' at the beginning of the list of examples of works whose manuscripts
    Galen had carefully corrected to create a new edition, at 15, 6,18–19 BJP. The point is made
    by Rashed, M. (2011). 'Aristote à Rome au IIe siécle: Galien, *De indolentia* §§ 15–18', *Elenchos*
    32, 57–8 (arguing convincingly for following more closely the MS reading κλίτου, against
    Jouanna's emendation Κλειτομάχου). Rashed goes further (73–7), and links the survival of

and the nature of his own use of material from such particular collections, ranging from intensive study and collation to marking up for copying to form new editions. We also gain from this text a far clearer picture than before of the possibilities and realities of scholarly activity amongst intellectuals in imperial Rome, of the nature of library use and of the practices of book-copying, book-editing and book-circulation.[7] Matters that remain debated are: whether or at what points Galen is referring to unique manuscripts from the collection of an illustrious collector (or even, in some cases, the autograph manuscripts of the author himself), as opposed to simply copies deriving from a particular, important manuscript tradition; and, in several cases, the precise identity of the works or authors in question. (On these points again, see the discussion of the problem passages of Greek below.)

The text has also brought new perspectives on broader questions related to the nature of both book production and book distribution in the Graeco-Roman world. One new finding is the apparent existence of an early form of codex or paginated book, at least in the context of collections of drug recipes.[8] A broader area is the (already much discussed) nature or practice of book 'publication' or distribution (*ekdosis*) in the ancient world, and the relationship between texts intended for different persons or uses. The text of περὶ ἀλυπίας certainly provides new evidence on book copying; on book distribution; on the nature of Galen's own intentions and claims in relation to his own works; and, of course, on the extent of his actual losses in the fire – even if the evidence in none of these areas is easy to interpret.[9]

To move to topic (iii): some aspects of Galen's literary and scholarly activity have already been considered under (ii); but as regards his statements on the order, intention and nature of his own compositions, remarks both in Περὶ

---

these Aristotelian works, uniquely in Rome, in the second century AD, with the ancient tradition that Theophrastus' own collection of texts of the school was extant in Athens in the first century BC, from where it was brought to Rome by Sulla after his sack of the city (and subsequently formed the basis of Andronicus' scholarly work).

7   For interpretation of what Galen says in section 13 in relation to specific extant editions, in particular of Plato, see Gourinat, J.-B. (2008). 'Le Platon de Panétius: à propos d'un témoignage inédit de Galien', *Philosophie Antique* 8, 139–51 and Dorandi, T. (2010). '"Editori" antichi di Platone', *Antiquorum philosophia* 4, 161–74.

8   This is the conclusion of Nicholls, M. (2010). 'Parchment Codices in a New Text of Galen', *Greece and Rome* 2:57, 378–86, followed by Nutton, *Avoiding Distress*, 87 n. 67 and BJP ad loc. A 'drug book' of this kind would, then, be a sort of proto-codex, something loosely bound in leather, to which further recipes could be added *ad hoc*. But an alternative interpretation sees the *diphthera* rather simply as a leather folder containing recipes or lists of recipes.

9   These questions are discussed in detail in my chapter 'New Light and Old Books', in this volume.

ἀλυπίας and in the previously missing parts of *Lib. Prop.* and of *Ord. Lib. Prop.*
shed new light. The importance of the latter material, although it is included
by V. Boudon-Millot in her very thorough 2007 edition and commentary on
those works, has not been significantly discussed. It is of considerable interest
in the light it sheds on Galen's own view of the order and relationship between
certain of his central works; and further study is needed to bring these passages in relation to what Galen says about the books in question, and their
place in his oeuvre, elsewhere. But some summary of the 'new' passages may
be of value here.

In *My Own Books*, first: the previous lacuna (at XIX.108 K.) covered the transition from Galen's discussion of his works of anatomy (ch. 4 [3][10]) to that of
his works of disease classification, which thus appeared abruptly, without any
further chapter heading; they now appear some way into ch. 6 [3]; see further
below. Thus, we previously arrived at *De morborum differentiis* (*Morb. Diff.*) in
the middle of a discussion of works of anatomy, without any understanding
of the relationship Galen intended between this work of disease classification
and the immediately preceding, anatomical works. The Vlatadon manuscript
adds a substantial amount of material both to the end of ch. 4 [3] and to the
beginning of ch. 6 [3], while also adding a wholly new chapter 5 – as well as
the chapter titles of both the latter. The new ch. 4 material completes Galen's
account of his epitomes of Marinus', and then Lycus', anatomical works, before
mentioning some more general anatomical works (interestingly including *De
partium homoeomerium differentia*) and summing up by saying that all these
teach the nature of the constitution (*kataskeuē*) of the parts of the body; and
that what follows after these is the discussion of the activities (*energeiai*) and
function (*chreia*) of each part.

Such, indeed, is the heading of ch. 5: 'in which books are contained the activities and functions of those parts which are made apparent in anatomy'. This
is in itself of considerable interest: Galen is essentially isolating a category of
physiological works (those which describe *energeia* and *chreia*), works which
have a distinct position, logically and paedagogically, after anatomical works
but before therapeutic ones – or, to be more precise, before a set of works
which provide a curriculum 'leading up to' the therapeutic works. The chapter starts by listing the lost *The Motion of the Chest and the Lungs, De causis*

---

10   For *My Own Books* I give the new chapter number, resulting from the full text of Vlatadon
      14, followed by the old chapter number in square brackets. The discrepancy that has aris-
      en by ch. 4 [3] is not due to a substantive addition, but simply that of a new chapter title 3,
      'The books written after these', at XIX.17 K., just after the account of his return home, and
      of the reappearance at that stage of certain youthful works, and just before his summons
      to join the imperial party on campaign.

respirationis and the lost *De voce*. Next is *De motu musculorum*. Arresting here is the previously unknown characterization of this work as covering, specifically, the activities of the *soul* – by contrast with *De naturalibus facultatibus*, mentioned next, which covers those of *nature*, as does *Excretion of Urine*. Belonging to the same *theōria*, too (by which is meant, presumably, the overall chapter topic rather than the narrower one 'of nature'), are: *De usu pulsuum, De usu respirationis, An in arteriis sanguis contineatur, De purgantium medicamentorum facultate* and, 'all that has been said on the leading-part[11] of the soul and on the sources that manage us' in *De placitis Hippocratis et Platonis (PHP)*. The reference to *ten* books of *PHP*, here, as opposed to the nine which we now possess, incidentally supports evidence which was already known from the Arabic translation of chapters 3 and 16 of the work, where the work is also mentioned. Indeed, the mention of *PHP* here – alongside those other mentions in *My Own Books*, both in the chronological account and under the heading 'related to the philosophy of Plato – adds to our understanding of Galen's own view of the work within his oeuvre: that is, its status in relation to the teaching of activity and function. Finally, within the new chapter, we have *De usu partium* (*UP*), which is described as 'following from all those mentioned'. This internal self-ordering of Galen's works relevant to anatomy and physiology, and in particular the precise nature of the distinction between discussions of activity (*energeia*) and those of function (*chreia*), are important points to consider in any attempt to understand the status and intention of his various scientific discussions of the human body.[12]

Turning to ch. 6: we are now in a position to understand the proper position of *Morb. Diff.*, and a list of other works related to disease classification, within Galen's suggested order and, more than that, the nature of the whole category to which he claims that these works belong. They are those to be read, or understood, before *The Therapeutic Method* (*MM*). The pivotal, or culminating, place that this gives to *MM* is interesting in itself. We then see how the intellectual ground needed for the understanding of that medical magnum opus is built up, starting from element and mixture theory (*De elementis ex Hippocratis sententia*, the first two books of *De temperamentis* (*Temp.*)), then – though these are optional at this stage – book 3 of *Temp.* and the eleven books of the

---

11   But n.b. that the term *hēgemonikon* here (155 Boudon-Millot) is supplied by Boudon-Millot on the basis of the Arabic.

12   The passage is to be put alongside a similar remark within *UP* itself, at 6.12 (III.463 K. = i.337,22–338,1 Helmreich), where again works on anatomy precede works on *energeia*, which precede discussions of *chreia*.

great pharmacological work, *Simples*; then *De optimo corporis nostri constitu-tione, De bono habitu, De inaequali intemperie.*

The new material thus gives us a much clearer picture than before of an order of instruction which goes from anatomy, through physiology, to element theory and disease classification before reaching therapeutics – as well as of which specific works Galen regards as physiological in this sense (dealing with *energeia* and *chreia*).

That last sequence was, admittedly, already known from *Ord. Lib. Prop.* 2 – where, however, before the discovery of the Vlatadon material, *MM* itself did not make an appearance. It in fact appears, now, right at the beginning of the new material, that is, just after those works just mentioned in the previous paragraph – except that, rather confusingly, it is then followed by a consid-erable list of works which 'precede' it. These, again, to a considerable extent confirm what is now suggested in *Lib. Prop.* 6 [3], mentioning a set of works on disease classification, though the situation is more complex and, one is tempt-ed to say, more rambling, here. The precise order in that other text – ironically, in a work which claims to focus precisely on the question of order – is much harder to follow than that in *My Own Books*. However, the insights which may arise from close study of this text remain unexplored. To take just one example: the text's construction of the category of a 'semiotic' branch of the art of medi-cine, divided into diagnostic and prognostic, and its discussion of a number of texts – in particular on pulse and on crises – in this context, is surely worthy of further consideration.

Topic (iv) has provoked a number of different studies, focussing varyingly on genre and ancient parallels, on social context and on philosophical analysis (or on some combination of these). Christopher Gill's 2010 book gave a seri-ous analysis of aspects of περὶ ἀλυπίας, contextualizing it both within Galen's other ethical work and within the tradition of ethical writing; a number have focussed on questions of genre and socio-literary context; and there has been discussion, too, of the work's position within Galen's philosophical writings.[13] Certain new perspectives on the Galenic concept of *lupē* and his 'practical ethics' are certainly introduced by the work, though again there are passag-es which elude straightforward interpretation. Several chapters in the present book take forward the analysis of Galen's discussion in this ethical area.

Let us turn to topic (v). The discovery of the full Greek text may, arguably, not revolutionize our understanding of the work in question: a considera-ble portion was already extant in Greek, and where there were problems of

---

13   For further details of this bibliography see in this volume my chapter 'A New Distress',
      n. 3.

interpretation with this, the new source does not always resolve them. However, the new complete version of the text in Greek certainly corrects a number of errors, unclarities and distortions in the Arabo-Latin and Hebrew versions; and beyond that, I suggest, it adds fresh material of significant philosophical interest.

Some of this material has already received attention. As shown by Antoine Pietrobelli in his discussion of the opening chapters of the work, relevant passages had been significantly distorted for theological reasons in the 'translations' which were previously our only source for them; there were also some names which were simply garbled in those versions.[14] These passages in fact offer an unambiguous assertion of the gods' direct influence on human affairs, including Galen's own: he has experienced the activity of the Dioscuri at sea, as well as Asclepius' personal interventions (in the latter case, admittedly, there are a couple of similar references elsewhere in the corpus). They also show Galen adopting a distinctive position in relation to religious scepticism and belief. Interesting here is Galen's alignment of his own views with those of Socrates. Although the text is both somewhat elliptical and far from perfectly transmitted, he appears by this to mean that he follows Socrates in his respect for traditional religious observance in general, and in his willingness to obey the specific instructions of Apollo in particular; and moreover that he contrasts this Socratic–Galenic combination of theism on the one hand and professed ignorance of abstract theological–metaphysical questions on the other with the more thoroughgoing agnosticism of Protagoras.[15]

---

14   See Pietrobelli, 'Galien agnostique', esp. 109–20. Apart from the occlusion of individual gods (Asclepius, Dioscuri) for ideological reasons, and the distortion of the argument in relation to Socrates and Protagoras (cf. esp. Pietrobelli's chart laying out the different versions at 109–11), the Arabo-Latin text sometimes just hopelessly distorts names, e.g. that of Empedocles as 'Elumerephilis' (vel sim.) at *Prop. Plac.* 7 (179,23 Boudon-Millot and Pietrobelli), or simply omits them, e.g. those of Plato and Chrysippus in the attribution of arguments on the incorporeal or corporeal nature of the soul at *Prop. Plac.* 7 (179,18 Boudon-Millot and Pietrobelli).

15   For both gods' personal interventions and the argument in relation to Socrates and Protagoras, see *Prop. Plac.* 2 (172,31–173,12 Boudon-Millot and Pietrobelli), with Pietrobelli (cited in the previous note). Pietrobelli's further argument that the text justifies a place for Galen in the history of 'agnosticism' seems to me overstated. Galen is agnostic in specific areas. This is already clear elsewhere in the corpus, although *Prop. Plac.* enriches the picture, elaborating the distinction between unknowable matters which provoke useless discussion and knowable matters, useful for medicine or ethics, with a third category, where arguments of plausibility may be advanced but where secure knowledge claims cannot be made; the last category is further understood as one where secure knowledge would hypothetically be an 'adornment' to the medical and ethical results achieved through things that do admit of precise knowledge (*Prop. Plac.* 14, 188,6–18 Boudon-Millot

Other parts of the text await a more thorough analysis, which may, I suggest, contribute significantly to our analysis of Galen's mature medical–philosophical thought in certain important areas. Those include: his epistemological views on the domain and limits of certainty; his formulation of his own views on certain central doctrinal areas (e.g. element theory, humoral theory, the nature of mixture) in relation to that epistemological framework; his understanding of the relationship of the soul, and of higher-level capacities more generally, to the body.[16]

2   The Cruces

The following is by no means an exhaustive account, either of every locus which has attracted a textual discussion, nor, in the case of those which have, of every individual emendation or interpretive suggestion that has been put forward. It does claim to present the most significant variant readings and interpretations of the most textually problematic passages, and especially for those where the differences are most significant for our understanding on points of substance. Not all of what follows is of equal interpretive significance; but I draw attention especially to points (c), (f) and (g), which address the major – and much-discussed – problems regarding ancient libraries, books and editorial practices; and also points (r), (s) and (t), which are of importance for the understanding of Galen's ethical position, in relation both to Stoicism and to the compromise with 'real life'. The method I follow in presenting these is to print the text which, after consideration, seems to me the most plausible, followed by an apparatus offering the most significant variant options, discussion of these variants and the related interpretations and, where necessary, English translation. (In one particularly complex and debated case, I have in the interests of readability presented two alternative versions of the Greek text, each followed by translation.)

---

and Pietrobelli). In terms of religious agnosticism, while Galen denies that we can know the *substance* of the gods (that is, there is very little we can say about their nature), on their existence and power in the natural world – on the validity of the argument from design – he has no doubt. There is similar agnosticism – again repeated throughout the corpus – on the substance of the soul.

16   A first attempt at such analysis is made in my forthcoming article, 'Galen on his Own Opinions: Textual Questions and Fresh Perspectives from MS Vlatadon 14'.

(a)   The title
       Περὶ ἀλυπίας

ἀλυγισίας MS ἀλυπίας BM ἀλυπησίας BJP

Immediately in the title line we have an indication of the level of the scribal errors in this MS and of the difficulties that will result from them. There
may seem to be little interpretive significance in this case, but BJP argue that
ἀλυπησία (a noun formation paralleled by e.g. ἀοργησία, ἀοχλησία) has a more
active sense and is therefore more appropriate to the context of this work:
while ἀλυπία properly means 'absence of distress', ἀλυπησία would mean 'the
activity of not being distressed'. In favour of BJP's reading is the fact that a
lengthened form (although not the same lengthened form) appears at each of
the four MS occurrences: here; at 69 (21,12 BJP: ἀλυπεισίας); at 79b (24,11 BJP:
ἀλυπισίαν); and in the end line – highly distorted there (ἀλογισίας at 26,4 BJP)
as it is in the title line. Against them is the fact that the emendation involves
the positing of an otherwise unattested Greek word; the fact that the title appears in the more expected form Περὶ ἀλυπίας in its mention in ch. 15 [12] of
Lib. Prop. (XIX.45 K. = 169,17 Boudon-Millot); and evidence for the existence
of a tradition of philosophical works Περὶ ἀλυπίας. The other editors have preferred the less challenging form.

(b)   *Ind.* 4 (3,6–7 BJP)
       πλῆθος ἄλλο τῶν συγγεγραμμένων αὐτοῦ

συγραμένων MS συγγεγραμμένων BM σεσωρευμένων Garofalo

The more obvious emendation, adopted by BJP, seems to make this a reference
to writings made *in situ* ('la masse de mes écrits rédigés ici même'); Nutton,
finding this reference to place odd, follows Garofalo: 'a further mass of things
stored there'. The significance of this latter reading is that if we accept it Galen
is not then mentioning his own writings in this first listing of his losses, but
only comes to them in a subordinate clause some twelve lines later. The notion that Galen is referring to his 'writings composed here' does not seem to
me so problematic as to motivate the emendation to such a distant form, and
I wonder whether in fact αὐτοῦ has to be understood so literally as attached to
συγγεγραμμένων. With regard to the verb σωρεύω, Galen uses this verb on several occasions, usually with a very concrete physical sense of 'pile up', rather than
just 'store'. So, its use here is perhaps not supported by its occurrence a little
later in this same text (where indeed it has that concrete, vivid sense), 10 (5,1–2
BJP): συνέβη κἀκεῖνα πάντα σὺν τοῖς κειμηλίοις ἐκεῖ σωρευθέντα διαφθαρῆναι, 'it

happened that they too [*sc.* the valuables from his own house] had all been piled up with the things stored there, and were destroyed'. If Galen in the second passage is essentially repeating the same information, with a little more detail – that is, referring to the same objects again, those that were added to what was usually in storage in preparation for his departure – this would support the reading σεσωρευμένων; but he may, rather, be adding further information: not only were all these things that I have mentioned already destroyed, but also the valuables I had 'piled on' just recently. (*Pace* Roselli,[17] the adverb αὐτοῦ, given Galen's use of the verb σωρεύω in the concrete physical sense mentioned, rather supports the latter interpretation: the mention of a stock of items 'that I had piled up here' – meaning 'at Rome' would be slightly odd, whereas in the later passage ἐκεῖ σωρευθέντα, 'piled up there', refers to a specific act of adding them to the storeroom.)

(c)   *Ind.* 13 (6,5–7 BJP)
       καὶ γὰρ γραμματικῶν πολλῶν αὐτόγραφα βιβλία τῶν παλαιῶν ἔκειντο καὶ
       ῥητόρων καὶ ἰατρῶν καὶ φιλοσόφων ...

       αὐτόγραφα MS ἀντίγραφα BJP

Here, faced with the apparently implausible claim that there were extant manuscripts *from the hand of* ancient authors, BJP emend αὐτόγραφα to ἀντίγραφα, and their translation thus yields the less challenging claim that there were 'copies' of many ancient grammarians, orators, etc.

Nutton defends the MS reading on the grounds that it there may have been works which were at least *thought* to be from the hand of 'ancient' authors. He translates:

> There were also many autograph copies of ancient grammarians, orators, doctors and philosophers ...

Manetti, however, has a quite different interpretation. Citing parallels on the usage of 'autograph' and similar terms,[18] she offers an alternative translation which seems to remove the implausibility involved in the αὐτόγραφα claim, while preserving the MS reading:

17   Roselli, A. 'Libri e biblioteche a Roma al tempo di Galeno: la testimonianza del *de indolentia*', *Galenos* 4 (2010), 127–48.
18   Manetti, D. 'Galeno περὶ ἀλυπίας e il difficile equilibrismo dei filologi', in Manetti, *Studi*, 15, citing in particular Fronto, *Ad M. Caes.* 1.7.4 (15,13–21 van den Hout).

> There were also the autograph manuscripts of many grammarians, [containing the texts of] ancient authors: orators, doctors and philosophers ...

On this view, the identity of these manuscripts as 'autographs' is indeed being asserted, but not as autographs by those authors. The perceived value of an ancient work could, as she argues, be hugely enhanced by the status of the person who copied it, especially when that was a distinguished scholar or grammarian. She thus separates the two sets of genitives in the above phrase: there are 'many grammarians' and then there are 'the ancients', with 'orators, doctors and philosophers' functioning as a gloss of the latter (an interpretation which perhaps also offers a more natural usage for the three iterations of καί). What is in question, then, is not the rather implausible autograph manuscripts of the ancients, but autograph manuscripts *by* distinguished grammarians *of* the ancients. This seems to me the most convincing solution.

(d) *Ind.* 14 (6,9–10 BJP)

εἰς καθαρὸν ἔδαφος ἐγέγραπτό <μοι> βιβλία τῶν ἀσαφῶς <ἡρμηνευμένων>, ἡμαρτημένων δὲ κατὰ τὰς γραφάς

ἀσαφῶν ἡμαρτημένων δὲ MS ἀσαφῶν μὲν, ἡμαρτημένων δὲ BM ἀσαφῶν ἢ τῶν ἡμαρτημένων [om. δὲ] Roselli ἀσαφῶς ἡρμηνευμένων scripsi

The description is clearly one of manuscripts which contained errors and of which Galen had laboured to produce error-free, 'clean' copies. There is a problem in the syntax, the δὲ seeming to require a previous μέν, which BM supplied; but even then the text reads rather baldly. Roselli points out[19] the relevance to this context of a passage from his commentary on the Hippocratic *Nature of Man*, in which Galen is similarly describing the unclarity that can arise in manuscripts; he attributes it to two causes: poor expression on the part of the writer or error on the part of the transcriber: ἀσαφὲς δέ ἐστιν ἢ μὴ καλῶς ἡρμηνευμένον ὑπὸ τοῦ γράψαντος ἢ διὰ τοὺς μεταγραψαμένους ἡμαρτημένον, HNH (XV.46 K. = 26,2–3 Mewaldt). The fact that Galen seems to have two parallel phenomena in mind here, in conjunction with the similarity of the contexts, leads me tentatively to suggest the above emendation, inserting ἡρμηνευμένων, the omission of which through its similarity to the immediately following ἡμαρτημένων would be a very easy error. It is true that one would prefer a different connection, perhaps reading τε for δέ; but the sense thus provided, that unclarity in the author's expression goes hand in hand with errors that require correction in the MSS, seems the right one.

---

19   Roselli, 'Libri', 141.

(e) *Ind.* 15 (6,19 BJP)
Κλύτου

κλίτου MS Κλειτομάχου BJP

BJP (followed by KS and GL) emend to make this a reference to the second-century-BC Platonist Clitomachus; but as Rashed has shown (see n. 6 above), the context makes Clytus, an Aristotelian of the first generation, a much more likely choice: this also involves a minimal change to the MS reading. (The latter reading is also accepted by Nutton.)

(f) *Ind.* 16–17 (6,21–7,14 BJP)
The problems of this passage have been much discussed. Nutton gives a separate appendix to his translation (101–6); a substantially different interpretation is given by Manetti; Rashed also gives detailed commentary and emendations. In view of the complexities, I print two versions of the Greek text first, that on which Nutton bases his translation (that of BJP with very small changes), then one which adopts the changes suggested by Manetti (2012), followed by an apparatus (with line numbers referring to the first version here printed) and the relevant English translation in each case (mine, in the case of Manetti). Words corresponding to the most important differences in reading and interpretation have been highlighted in bold.

> λυπήσει δέ σε καὶ ταῦτα μάλιστα, ὡς τῶν ἐν τοῖς καλουμένοις πίναξι [τῶν] γεγραμμένων βιβλίων ἔξωθεν εὑρόν τινα κατὰ [τινά] τε τὰς ἐν τῷ Παλατίῳ βιβλιοθήκας καὶ τ<ιν>ὰ[ς] ἐναντίω<ς> ἃ φανερῶς <οὐκ> ἦν οὗπερ ἐπεγέγραπτο, <οὔτε> κατὰ τὴν λέξιν οὔτε κατὰ <τὴν> διάνοιαν ὁμοιούμενα αὐτῷ. καὶ τὰ Θεοφράστου καὶ μάλιστα τὰ κατὰ τὰς ἐπιστημονικὰς πραγματείας – ἔστιν ἄλλα τὰ Περὶ φυτῶν κατὰ δύο πραγματείας ἐκτεταμένας ἡρμηνευμένα πάντες ἔχουσι. ἡ δ᾽ Ἀριστοτέλ<ει> σύναρμος ἀκριβῶς ἦν εὑρεθεῖσά μοι καὶ μεταγραφεῖσα, ἣ καὶ νῦν ἀπολομένη · κατὰ δὲ τὸν αὐτὸν τρόπον καὶ Θεοφράστου καὶ ἄλλων τινῶν ἀνδρῶν παλαιῶν μὴ φαινόμενα κατὰ τοὺς πίνακας, τινὰ δ᾽ ἐν ἐκείνοις γεγραμμένα μέν, μὴ φερόμενα δ᾽αὐτά.

> λυπήσει δέ σε καὶ ταῦτα μάλιστα ὡς τῶν ἐν τοῖς καλουμένοις πίναξι [τῶν] γεγραμμένων βιβλίων ἔξωθεν εὑρόν τινα κατά τε **τὰς** ἐν τῷ Παλατίῳ βιβλιοθήκας καὶ **τὰς ἐν Ἀντίῳ**, ἃ φανερῶς ἦν οὗπερ ἐπεγέγραπτο, κατὰ τὴν λέξιν [ου]τε κατὰ τὴν διάνοιαν ὅμοια. <ἔστι> μὲν αὐτῶν καὶ τὰ Θεοφράστου καὶ μάλιστα τὰ κατὰ τὰς ἐπιστημονικὰς πραγματείας, [ἔστιν] **ἀλλὰ** τὰ Περὶ φυτῶν κατὰ δύο πραγματείας ἐκτεταμένας ἡρμηνευμένα πάντες ἔχουσι, ἡ δ᾽

Ἀριστοτέλ<ους> σύναρμος ἀκριβῶς ἦν εὑρεθεῖσά μοι καὶ μεταγραφεῖσα, ἡ καὶ νῦν ἀπολομένη · κατὰ δὲ τὸν αὐτὸν τρόπον καὶ Θεοφράστου καὶ ἄλλων τινῶν ἀνδρῶν παλαιῶν μὴ **φερόμενα** κατὰ τοὺς πίνακας, τινὰ δ' ἐν ἐκείνοις γεγραμμένα μέν, μὴ **φαινόμενα** δ' αὐτά.

3 τὰ MS τινὰς BJP ἐναντίῳ MS ἐναντίως BJP ἐν Ἀντίῳ Jones οὐκ add. Jones 4 οὔτε add Nutton τε pro οὔτε Manetti 4–5 ὅμοια μὲν αὐτω. καὶ MS ὁμοιούμενα αὐτῷ. καὶ BJP ὅμοια. ἔστι μὲν αὐτῶν καὶ Manetti 6 ἔστιν om. Nutton et Manetti ἀλλα MS ἄλλα BJP ἀλλὰ Manetti 7 Ἀριστοτέλ MS Ἀριστοτέλει BM Ἀριστοτέλους Garofalo σύναρμος MS συνάριθμος Garofalo συνώνυμος vel ὁμώνυμος Nutton 9 φερόμενα MS φαινόμενα Nutton 10 φαινόμενα MS φερόμενα Garofalo, Nutton (Nutton thus transposes the MS φερόμενα and φαινόμενα; Garofalo reads φερόμενα twice.)

Nutton:

> You will be particularly distressed to learn that I had found in the Palatine libraries some books not described in the so-called Catalogues and **some**, that were clearly **not** the work of the author whose name they bore, being similar **neither** in language nor in ideas. **There were also** writings of Theophrastus, and especially his books on science – the other books on plants, explicated in two long treatises, everyone has. There was also a work **of the same name by** Aristotle which I **carefully** found and transcribed but which is now also lost, and likewise works by Theophrastus and other ancient writers that did not **appear** in the Catalogues, as well as others that were mentioned there, but did not **circulate** widely.

Manetti/Singer:

> You will be particularly distressed to learn that, beyond the books described in the so-called Catalogues, I found some, both in the Palatine libraries and **in those in Antium**, which clearly **were** the work of the author whose name they bore, being similar **both** in language **and** in ideas. **Amongst them are** the works of Theophrastus, and especially his books on science; **but** the works on plants, explicated in two long treatises, everyone has, while that of Aristotle was found by me **immediately following on from** that one [sc. that of Theophrastus], and transcribed, but is now lost. And in the same way I found works, both of Theophrastus and of certain other ancient writers which were not contained in the Catalogues, and some which were **mentioned** there, but were **evidently** not those works.

Here there are three key differences: (1) the reading 'in Antium' (proposed by Jones and now widely discussed, but rejected by Nutton and Jouanna); (2) the change of negative to positive propositions in the places noted in bold (note that an emendation is required in either case: other editors have made sense by *adding* the second negative, 'neither'); (3) a different reconstruction of the beginning of the second sentence, and thus of its logical relationship with the first; (4) the interpretation of σύναρμος as 'contiguous', that is to say, 'physically part of the same manuscript' (and of the adverb ἀκριβῶς as qualifying that – i.e. 'immediately' contiguous – rather than referring to Galen's activity).

The question of the reading ἐν Ἀντίῳ (in Antium) arises again in further passages below. Without attempting to address all the arguments, one may point out (a) that a main strength of the reading ἐν Ἀντίῳ is that it provides a linguistically satisfying solution to the problem presented by the MS of three separate occurrences of forms of the word ἐναντίος, none of which admits of an entirely convincing interpretation as such (see further below); (b) that in that case the subsequent discussion of losses due to misappropriation and to water damage would, in both cases, refer to what happened to the collection of this Antium library, rather than to, respectively, a library in Rome and (in a way which is seems difficult to explain) some of Galen's own books; (c) that whatever difficulties the 'Antium' interpretation presents – the main one, of course, is the lack of other evidence for a library in that location – it does thus solve both a linguistic puzzle and a difficulty in understanding the location, as well as explaining what is otherwise an unclear transition to an account of a different cause of damage to books which has nothing to do with fire (see further below).

From that point on, Manetti's readings enable her to reconstruct in a plausible way the connection between the general remark about the books that Galen had found and what follows about Theophrastus and Aristotle. It is some lost works of Theophrastus on science – works which clearly *are* in accord with his views – which he found, in spite of their not being in the 'catalogues'; there follows a parenthetical remark about Theophrastus' work on plants, which by contrast is widely available; and finally we come to the most valuable work lost, that of *Aristotle* on plants (as also accepted by Nutton), which Galen had found in the same manuscript as the equivalent work of Theophrastus. BJP, by contrast, take the reference to be to a work of Theophrastus which was *perfectly in accord with* Aristotle (reading the dative Ἀριστοτέλει), this being their interpretation of the term *sunarmos*; but the exact nature of this book, and its relationship to the previous remark about plants, are then difficult, whereas the interpretation whereby this a lost work *by* Aristotle seems to make much better sense of the sentence as a whole.

The main differences of interpretation, then, are: (a) the identity of the book which Galen describes himself as having discovered and (b) the relationship of the books mentioned here in general to the libraries or their lists,[20] which depends upon whether one adds two additional negatives to the sentence (with BJP and Nutton) or emends (with Manetti) to remove the existing negative. The latter seems to me to give clearly better sense: Galen is talking about works *not* contained in library catalogues, but which *were* evidently authentic works of the authors whose names they bore.

I note here, without going into all its details, the reconstruction of Rashed. This agrees with the above version of Manetti in essentials – the key point is the availability to Galen, before the fire, of works not in the catalogues, which nevertheless were apparently authentic works of ancient authors – but has a more elaborately emended version of the sentence containing the references to Theophrastus, leading however to the same essential conclusion, that Galen had access to and copied Aristotle's *De plantis*, which is now lost. (He emends σύναρμος to συναρμοττοῦσα and takes the word with ἀκριβῶς to mean 'rigoure-sement concordant'.) On the term σύναρμος itself, it seems to me that (a) its usual meaning and (b) its non-appearance elsewhere in Galen argue strongly in favour of the view that it is in this specific context referring to a *physical* feature of a book, and thus in favour of the interpretation of the word as referring here to physical contiguity in a manuscript. The text in question was 'attached to', 'following on from', the other; this thus adds further to the plausibility of Manetti's reconstruction: Galen is here explaining the particular circumstances – attached to a manuscript of Theophrastus – in which he found this otherwise non-extant work of Aristotle.

Finally, on the last part of the passage, after ἀπολομένη. This part is not discussed by Manetti; the main point at issue is the reading and interpretation of the MS words φερόμενα and φαινόμενα. As seen above, Nutton transposes the two terms, to give the sense 'did not appear … did not circulate widely'. BJP have no trouble with φερόμενα in the sense of appearing in a catalogue ('n'étaient pas mentionnés'), and take the latter phrase in the sense 'avaient disparus'.

---

20   We note that Nutton, Manetti and Rashed all take ἔξωθεν prepositionally in relation to the books which appeared in the *pinakes*: 'beyond' or 'not described in'. Manetti takes 'catalogues' (*pinakes*) here to refer simply to the library catalogues, since the famous listing of Andronicus, which has been suggested as the reference here, did, apparently, contain Aristotle's work on plants.

Nutton's transposition seems unnecessary; but there is another point, which is that none of the existing interpretations seems to make good sense of the final word, αὐτά. It seems that Galen is making the additional point that, as well as authentic works which were not in the catalogues (and which he found), there were also some books which *were* in the catalogues, but which were, in fact, 'manifestly not those books' (taking αὐτά as a complement).

(g) *Ind.* 17 (7,14–16 BJP); 18 (8,3–6 BJP)

One should, then, relatedly, consider the two remaining problematic places which give rise to the possible 'Antium' reading:

τούτων οὖν ἐγὼ πολλὰ μὲν ἐν ταῖς κατὰ τὸ Παλάτιον βιβλιοθήκαις εὗρον, τ<ι-ν>ὰ δ᾽ ἐναντίως κατεσεύασα.

τὰ δ᾽ἐναντία MS; τινὰ δ᾽ἐναντίως Jouanna; τὰ δ᾽ἀντίγραφα Leith; τὰ δ᾽ἐν Ἀντίῳ Jones

τ<ιν>ὰ δ᾽ ἐναντίως διὰ τὴν ἀμέλειαν τῶν ἑκάστοτε ἐμπιστευομένων ἐκ διαδο-χῆς αὐτὰ [...] καθ᾽ὃν χρόνον ἐγὼ ἀνέβην εἰς Ῥώμην πρῶτον, ἐγγὺς ἦν τοῦ διεφθάρθαι.

τὰ δ᾽ἐναντίω MS τινὰ δ᾽ἐναντίως Jouanna τὰ δ᾽ἀντίγραφα Leith τὰ δ᾽ἐν Ἀντίῳ Jones ληστευομένων MS πιστευομένων Garofalo ἐμπιστευομένων Manetti In lacuna μυσὶ βεβρωμένα coni. Rashed

If one is not persuaded of Antium, one has a choice of a translation along the lines of 'à l'opposé', with BJP, or Leith's 'copies' – which perhaps works better with the verb, κατεσεύασα, 'I procured' (or 'I had prepared'), at 7,16.[21]

In the second of these two passages, BJP are again forced to expand τὰ to τινὰ; and again Leith's τὰ δ᾽ἀντίγραφα is perhaps the most plausible non-Antium solution: the emendation itself makes much easier Greek than any of the attempts to make sense of some form of the word for 'opposite'; and it provides good sense in these two instances. (It seems to make less good sense in the earlier instance, discussed above at (f), because then the text would seem to say that he found both books in the Palatine libraries *and copies*, when it is precisely the destruction of the Palatine collection that is at stake.) In purely palaeographical terms, the distortion of the fairly common term ἀντίγραφα is harder to explain than that of the unfamiliar place name Antium.

---

21   In this case Nutton presents the problem, but does not actually translate the phrase.

In the remainder of this admittedly corrupt text, one has a choice between the carelessness of a succession of the [librarians] who are being robbed and the carelessness of the [librarians] who were successively entrusted with the books. Rashed's conjecture, based on a consideration of the precise length of the lacuna, as well as the possible discernibility of the letters μ, σ and ι within it, has the manuscripts in question 'eaten by mice' rather than looted. (Rashed also accepts the Antium emendation.) The more fundamental question here remains, whether Galen is now talking about a completely different library, at Antium, or giving further information about depredations at Rome. In the passage immediately following the above, Galen talks specifically of damp (σηπεδόνος, 8,9 BJP) as the cause of the fact that the manuscripts in question are now 'useless': they cannot be opened. This in turn is related to the location: 'marshy' (ἑλῶδες) and 'lying in a hollow' (κοῖλον), which makes it 'stifling' (πνιγηρόν) in summer (8,10–11 BJP). Nutton discusses the archaeological options in detail: it is possible that Galen is talking about some library, or library annex, undamaged by the fire but in a marshy area of the Forum; although it is the easiest emendation of the Greek to accept 'Antium' three times, there is no other evidence for a major library there. The above description of the location as 'marshy, lying in a hollow and stifling in summer' may also seem a major obstacle to the Antium theory: one would expect such a library to have been high up, overlooking the sea. But κοῖλον may mean 'lying between cliffs', as well as 'in a hollow', and ἑλῶδες could perhaps be taken to refer to damp, rather than literally to a 'marshy' environment; and it is, presumably, possible that the specifics of the library's location or construction caused it to be both poorly ventilated ('stifling', πνιγηρόν) and prone to damp.

(h)   *Ind.* 26 (10,10 BJP)

   ... κωμικοῖς, Ἀριστομένει ἢ Ἀριστοφάνει. ἀλλ᾽ ὅσα μὴ σαφῆ ...

   Ἀβυδομὴν ἢ Ἀβυστοκινεῖν. ἀλλ᾽ MS Ἀριστομένει ἢ Ἀριστοφάνει. ἀλλ BM ἀβυδοκόμαν ἢ ἀβυρτάκην, ἀλλ᾽ Polemis

Polemis ends the sentence after κωμικοῖς and starts a new one with ἀβυδοκόμαν ἢ ἀβυρτάκην, which he then connects with the next phrase, reading ἀλλ᾽. The point is that these are obscure lexical items, exemplifying Galen's philological practice: '*Abudokoma* and *aburtakē*, and all other unclear terms, were defined ...' The extreme distortion of the names Aristomenes and Aristophanes in the MS, as well as the particular choice of Aristomenes, seems difficult to explain; and Polemis' ingenious emendation may well be correct.

(i) *Ind.* 28 (10,21–24 BJP)

... ἐν βιβλίοις ὄντα τεσσαράκοντα ὀκτὼ μεγάλοις ὧν ἔνια διελεῖν ἴσως δεήσει
δίχα πλειόνων ἢ τετρακισχιλίων ἐπῶν ἑξαμέτρων ἐχόντων.

ἐξάριθμον MS αμετρον Vlat.γρ ἐξάριθμον ἔχοντα GL ἐξάριθμον Jouanna ἑξαμέτρων
ἐνόντων Puglia 2011, Stramaglia 2011

Galen, speaking of his forty-eight books on the vocabulary of Attic prose authors, adds that some of these may yet have to be divided into further books
because of their length. Jouanna is surely right to prefer a form with rough
breathing: the reference is to a hexameter line, which was used also as a unit
of measurement for prose works, and ἐξάριθμον makes little sense here. But
ἐξάριθμον is a fairly rare term, and the word ἑξαμέτρων – already implied by
the superscript suggestion in the MS – provides a more natural way for Galen
to express this thought, as attested by his use of the very same phrase, ἐπῶν
ἑξαμέτρων (also in the context of line length within a prose work) at *PHP* 8
(v.655 K. = 486,12 De Lacy). (The further emendation of ἐχόντων to ἐνόντων
seems unnecessary: one might prefer it if the grammar more logically (as also
with GL's ἔχοντα) specified the *subset* of these long books, ἔνια, as having this
excessive length – but the sense is clear enough.)

(j)   *Ind.* 32 (11,19 BJP)
ὅσα κατὰ τὴν Ἀσίαν ἦν εὐδοκιμοῦντα παρ᾽ ἑκάστῳ τῶν νῦν ἰατρῶν

οὐσίαν MS Ἀσίαν Garofalo νῦν add. BM

The context is that of a large collection of drugs, in the hands of someone
who, it has been clarified, comes from Asia (τῶν παρ᾽ ἡμῖν, 11,15 BJP). Garofalo's
emendation, adopted by BJP and Nutton, seems plausible, and is printed here;
at the same time, it seems to me not completely obvious that the MS reading
(according to which the drugs were valued 'by virtue of their substance', rather
than 'in Asia') is to be rejected.

(k)   *Ind.* 34 (12,9 BJP) Εὐμενοῦς

Εὐμενοῦς MS Εὐδήμου BM

According to the MS reading, Galen mentions a Pergamene doctor called
Eumenes as the source of a collection of drug recipes which came into his possession, via another fellow Pergamene, Teuthras. The fact that this Eumenes is
otherwise unknown, alongside the fact that Galen elsewhere mentions, in the

specific context of drug recipes, a doctor called Eudemus, who was also from Pergamum, makes BM's emendation tempting; but both BJP and Nutton ad loc. argue against the identity on chronological grounds, and perhaps palaeographic caution should prevail.

(l)   *Ind.* 39 (13,12–15 BJP)
      <ὁ > φιλόσοφος Ἀριστίππος, οὐκ ἀρκούμενος διαίτῃ εὐτελεῖ ἀλλὰ καὶ πολυτε-
      λείαις ὄψων ἑκάστης ἡμέρας διδοὺς ἀργύριον ἑκάστοτε δαψιλὲς ταῖς θερμοτέ-
      ραις τῶν κατ᾽αὐτὸν ἑταιρῶν ...

      φιλότιμος MS φιλήδονος ὢν Kotzia φιλόσοφος prop. Nutton τοῖς θερμοτέροις MS ταῖς
      θερμοτέραις Garofalo εὐμορφοτέραις KS κατ᾽αὐτῶν ἑτέρων MS κατ᾽αὐτὸν ἑταίρων
      BJP κατ᾽αὐτὸν ἑταιρῶν Garofalo

There are further, in particular syntactic, difficulties for the reconstruction of this sentence; but the main points at issue are: with what characterizing noun is Aristippus being introduced, and is he shown lavishing banquets and money on male associates or on courtesans? What is at stake is the precise nature of the example that Aristippus is thought to be offering. BJP defend the MS φιλότιμος, but wish to take it in the sense 'prodigue'; this is an attested sense, but the frequent occurrence of the term and its cognates in Galen, always with reference to a concern for one's own reputation, renders such an interpretation implausible. KS's φιλήδονος ('pleasure-loving', Nutton) certainly makes sense; but on balance the admittedly flat φιλόσοφος, suggested by Nutton (though not adopted in his translation), seems the most likely solution. As for the question of companions (or pupils) versus prostitutes: the use of the adjective θερμός would seem very strange in relation to the former: its usual sense in relation to character is 'hot-headed'. This, in conjunction with the literary tradition on Aristippus' associations with prostitutes, seems – *pace* BJP, and though θερμός as an adjective referring to the *mores* or appearance of women is not very clearly attested – to me to justify Garofalo's emendation, also followed by Nutton. KS's εὐμορφοτέραις would also make good sense, if one accepts the feminine interpretation, but is harder on the basis of the MS.

(m) *Ind.* 50a (16,8–10 BJP)
     οὐδὲ τοῦτο μέγα, μὴ μανῆναι τὴν μανίαν πολλῶν τῶν ἐν αὐλῇ βασιλικῇ
     καταγηρασάντων

     αὐτὴν post τὴν add. Polemis πολλοῖς Polemis κατηγωρισάντων MS κατολιγωρήσα-
     ντα Garofalo apud Nutton καταγορασάντων Jouanna 1 κατηγορησάντων Jouanna 2
     καταγηρασάντων Polemis

Amid many suggestions as to the form of the participle here, Polemis' seems to give the best sense: Galen is commenting on the 'madness' of 'many who have grown old in the imperial court', and this seems in keeping with his remarks elsewhere on the corruption attendant on a life concerned with social or political advancement. (Polemis' other emendations, to give the sense 'the *same* madness *as* many who …', seem to me unnecessary; he is followed by GL on all points.) Jouanna's earlier suggestion, with the sense, 'ceux qui flânent dans la cour du palais', was superseded by that adopted in BJP, whereby the phrase from πολλῶν would be a genitive absolute with the sense 'malgré le nombre des accusateurs à la cour impériale'. Nutton, finally, prefers Garofalo's earlier emendation, and translates 'since I cared little for life at the Imperial court'. But all the suggestions apart from that of Polemis (and Jouanna 1) require τὴν μανίαν to stand alone in an implausible way: it is surely closely dependent on the participle that follows: 'the madness of those who …'. (Nutton translates 'the madness of most people, since …'; but this would require the further insertion of τῶν before πολλῶν.)

(n)   *Ind.* 52 (16,21–2 BJP)
      παιδεύει καὶ θέα πραγμάτων πολιτικῶν ἀναμινμήσκουσα τῶν τῆς τύχης ἔργων
      τέχνης MS τύχης Garofalo

A choice must be made here between two terms which frequently appear as opposites in the philosophical discourse of Galen's time. In spite of BJP's spirited defence of the MS reading, 'observation of the deeds of art' simply does not fit this context, where it is precisely the *praemeditatio malorum*, a consideration of all that may go wrong – focussing here especially on the 'random' nature of political or everyday events – which is recommended to the reader: 'reminding us of the actions of chance' (Nutton) is surely the right sense.

(o)   *Ind.* 52 (17,5 BJP); repeated at 77 (23,8 BJP)
      εἰς φροντίδ᾽ ἀεὶ συμφορᾶς ἐβαλλόμην

      φροντίδα ἐκ συμφορᾶς MS φροντιδ᾽ἀεὶ συμφορᾶς Wyttenbach (cf. BJP)

There are a number of variants in the ancient transmission of this extract from a non-extant play of Euripides, which is cited also by Plutarch and elsewhere by Galen himself at *PHP* 4 (v.418 K. = 282,18–23 De Lacy). The problems are discussed at length by BJP ad loc. But in this particular line, although the ἐκ of the MS is in need of emendation, the genitive singular seems to me to give a preferable sense to the accusative plural elsewhere in the tradition. ἐβαλλόμην should be taken as medio-passive intransitive: 'I used to be thrown/throw myself'; and εἰς φροντίδ' ... συμφορᾶς seems to make perfect sense as 'into worry/concern about disaster'. The alternative, preferred by BJP, takes ἐβαλλόμην as transitive with συμφορὰς as its object: 'I used to throw disasters into my mind'. This seems to me less natural, and φροντίς usually has a sense of sense of 'worry', 'concern' or 'thought', rather than 'mind' as a receptacle for thoughts. (On the other hand, as a further alternative, the text of *PHP* reads εἰς φροντίδας νοῦν συμφορὰς τ' ἐβαλλόμην.)

(p)   *Ind.* 59 (19,4–6 BJP) τὸ μὲν κατὰ τὴν ἀρετήν, τὸ δὲ κατὰ τὴν ἀρχιτεκτονίαν ... ἐν αἷς καὶ αὐτὸς ἐκεῖνος ἦν πρῶτος

οἷς ... αὐτὸ ἐκεινῷ ἦν πρῶτον MS αἷς KS, GL αὐτὸς ἐκεῖνος ... πρῶτος GL

BJP follow the MS, translating: 'domaines dans lesquel la conduite (morale) était aussi, aux yeux de cet homme-là, primordiale', taking αὐτὸ as referring back to τοῦτο, which was used in the previous sentence to stand for a capacity or respect for justice and self-control. But the phrase seems tortured, and it is difficult to see what sense can be made of the conceptual extension of this capacity to the domains of 'virtue and architecture'. GL's emendation – so, 'in which domains that very man, too, was pre-eminent' – seems to be demanded on linguistic grounds, and makes perfect sense in the context of the argument relating both to his own family's virtues and the nature and importance of early nurture and natural endowments.

(q)   *Ind.* 65 (20,15–17) καὶ σχολῇ γ᾽ἂν ἄρμενα καὶ φάρμακα καὶ βιβλία καὶ δόξαν καὶ πλοῦτον ἄξια σπουδῆς ὑποπλάβοιμι.

σχολ καὶ MS σχολῇ γ᾽ἂν GL σχολὴν καὶ BJP post πλοῦτον add. πῶς ἂν BJP, καὶ οὐκ KS

Galen is listing material or social goods which, as a result of his rearing and reasoning, he sets at a low rate. 'Leisure', in such a list as this, seems simply out of place, while σχολῇ in the sense 'hardly' ('figurarsi', GL) seems clearly to provide the required sense: 'I would hardly take instruments, medicines, etc., to be worth the expense of energy.' The reading also obviates the need for BJP's or KS's insertion of further words.

(r)   Ind. 70 (21,13–15 BJP)
      τάχα γὰρ οἴει με, καθάπερ ἔνιοι τῶν φιλοσόφων ὑπέσχοντο μηδέποτε μηδένα λυπηθήσεσθαι τῶν σοφῶν, οὕτως καὶ αὐτὸν ἀποφαίνεσθαι ...

μηδ … μηδὲ νῦν MS μηδέποτε μηδὲ νῦν BJP μηδέποτε μηδένα Garofalo λυπηθήσεσθαι
τῶν φιλοσόφων MS λυπηθήσεσθαι τῶν σοφῶν Garofalo τῶν φιλοσόφων om. BJP λυ-
πήσεσθαι τὸν φιλόσοφον Polemis

The MS repetition of τῶν φιλοσόφων has been universally agreed to be problematic; BJP omit it, giving the sense, 'certain philosophers have promised that
they will not be distressed, even in present circumstances'. But Garofalo's re-
placement of the second occurrence with τῶν σοφῶν, in conjunction with the
easy emendation of μηδὲ νῦν to μηδένα, surely gives the right sense. Galen is, as
throughout this passage (see also the next text, (n) below), casting doubt on
the specific claim made by some philosophers (in particular Stoics) that *the
wise man* (ὁ σοφός) is immune to distress (whereas Nutton follows Polemis:
'that the philosopher will never suffer distress').

(s)   *Ind.* 76 (23,2–4 BJP)
      … μήτε τὸ σῶμα τὴν Ἡρακλέους ῥώμην ἕξειν ἐλπίζω μήτε τὴν ψυχήν, ἣν ἔνιοί
      φασι ὑπάρχειν τοῖς σοφοῖς

      ἐμοί MS secl. Jouanna ἔνιοί Garofalo οἱ σοφοί MS τοῖς σοφοῖς Jouanna

The context is that of adjusting one's aspirations, for both physical and ethical health, to one's own capacities: Galen states that he does not aspire for
his body to have the strength of a Hercules, nor for his soul to have that – on
the MS reading – 'which the wise state that I have'. Both the introduction of
'the wise' as a class of people passing judgement on Galen, and the sense, con-
tradicting the main force of the sentence, seem impossible. Taking Jouanna's
τοῖς σοφοῖς (not in the end adopted by BJP but followed by GL), in conjunction
with Garofalo's ἔνιοί for ἐμοί), we gain the the sense 'which some state that the
wise have', which is surely preferable. On this interpretation Galen is here also
returning to the theme raised by the statement five sections earlier, 'I cannot
say if there is anyone so wise (σοφός) as to be totally unaffected' (71, 21,17–18
BJP), and continuing the tone, anti-Stoic or at least critical of Stoic attitudes
and aspirations, that runs through this whole passage. (Cf. also the previous
passage discussed, (r).)

(t)   *Ind.* 80–81 (25,4–8 BJP)
      … τούτῳ δὲ τῷ μοχθηροτάτῳ βίῳ περιπίπτουσιν οἷς ἄπληστοι ἐπιθυμίαι προσ-
      γίνονται. τίνες οὖν οὐχ ὡς οἱ πολλοὶ λυποῦνται; οἳ μετρίως ἅπτονται τιμῆς καὶ
      πλούτου καὶ δόξης καὶ δυνάμεως πολιτικῆς …

τοῦτο MS τούτῳ KS τούτου δ'ἔτι GL μοχθηροτέρῳ MS μοχθηροτάτῳ KS τοῖς ἀπλήστοις ἐπιθυμίας. προσγίνονταί τινες MS ταῖς ἀπλήστοις ἐπιθυμίαις. προσγίνονταί τινες BJP οἷς ἄπληστοι ἐπιθυμίαι προσγίνονται. τίνες GL οὐχ ὡς οἱ πολλοὶ λυποῦνται om. BJP

Both KS and GL depart from the MS and from BJP (and Nutton), in starting a new sentence after προσγίνονται. (The version of KS is subtly different, and in particular prints τινὲς, starting a new sentence which is not a question.) Such a solution obviates the need to delete the whole phrase οὐχ ὡς οἱ πολλοὶ λυποῦνται, and seems convincing both in the better sense it gives for προσγίνονται and in the clear relationship it presents between non-attachment (or only moderate attachment to worldly goals) and freedom from distress. The sense is thus not: 'they succumb to this wretched form of life through insatiable desires. There then also come some who have a moderate attachment to honour, wealth, reputation and political power', but: ' ... to this most wretched form of life succumb those in whom insatiable desires arise. Who, then, are the ones who do not suffer distress as others? Those who have a moderate attachment to honour, wealth, reputation and political power ...'. On this interpretation Galen is, to be sure, conceding more to the acceptability of attachment to material values than he does usually; but this is perhaps in keeping with the particular rhetorical stance he takes in this text in relation to Stoic views, on the one hand, and practically attainable life goals, on the other.

Acknowledgements

The author gratefully acknowledges the financial support of the Wellcome Trust and the Alexander von Humboldt-Stiftung during the research and writing of this paper. Heartfelt thanks go also to the editor, Caroline Petit, for her invitation to participate in the conference from which this chapter arose, and especially for her very helpful advice and encouragement during its subsequent development. The faults which it retains are, of course, my own.

References

Secondary Literature

Alexandru, S. 'Newly Discovered Witness Asserting Galen's Affiliation to the *Gens Claudia*', *Annali della Scuola Normale Superiore di Pisa*, ser. 5, 3/2 (2011), 385–433.

Boudon-Millot, V. (ed., trans. and notes) *Galien, Tome I*, Paris: Les Belles Lettres, 2007.

Boudon-Millot, V. 'Un traité perdu de Galien miraculeusement retrouvé, le *Sur l'inutilité de se chargriner*: texte grec et traduction française'. In *La science médicale antique: nouveaux regards* (*Études réunies en l'honneur de Jacques Jouanna*), ed. V. Boudon-Millot, A. Guardasole and C. Magdelaine, 73–123. Paris: Éditions Beauchesne, 2007.

Boudon-Millot, V. '*Vlatadon* 14 and *Ambrosianus* Q3: Two Twin Manuscripts'. In *Galen's De indolentia*, ed. C. K. Rothschild and T. W. Thompson, 41–55. Tübingen: Mohr Siebeck, 2014.

Boudon-Millot, V. and Pietrobelli, A. 'Galien ressuscité: édition princeps du texts grec du *De propriis placitis*', *Revue des Études Grecques* 118 (2005), 168–213.

Boudon-Millot, V. and Jouanna, J. (ed. and trans.), with A. Pietrobelli, *Galien, Oeuvres 4: Ne pas se chagriner*. Paris: Les Belles Lettres, 2010.

Dix, T. K. and Houston, G. W. 'Public Libraries in the City of Rome: From the Augustan Age to the Time of Diocletian'. In *Mélanges de l'École Française de Rome. Antiquité* 118:2 (2006), 671–717.

Dorandi, T. '"Editori" antichi di Platone', *Antiquorum philosophia* 4 (2010), 161–74.

Fedeli, P. 'Biblioteche private e pubbliche a Roma e nel mondo romano'. In *Le biblioteche nel mondo antico e medievale*, ed. G. Cavallo, 48–64. Bari: Laterza, 1988.

Gourinat, J.-B. 'Le Platon de Panétius: à propos d'un témoignage inédit de Galien', *Philosophie Antique* 8 (2008), 139–51.

Houston, G. W. 'Galen, His Books and the *Horrea Pipertaria* at Rome', *Memoirs of the British Academy in Rome* 48 (2008), 45–51.

Jones, C. P. 'Books and Libraries in a Newly-Discovered Treatise of Galen', *Journal of Roman Archaeology* 22 (2009), 390–97.

Kotzia, P. 'Galen περὶ ἀλυπίας: Title, Genre and Two Cruces'. In *Studi sul De indolentia di Galeno*, ed. D. Manetti, 69–91. Pisa and Rome: Fabrizio Serra Editore, 2012.

Kotzia, P. and Sotiroudis, P. 'Γαληνοῦ περὶ ἀλυπίας', *Hellenica* 60 (2010), 63–148.

Manetti, D. 'Galeno περὶ ἀλυπίας e il difficile equilibrismo dei filologi'. In *Studi sul De indolentia di Galeno*, ed. D. Manetti, 9–22. Pisa and Rome: Fabrizio Serra Editore, 2012.

Manetti, D. (ed.) *Studi su Galeno: scienza, filosofia, retorica e filologia. Atti del seminario, Firenze, 13 novembre 1998*. Florence: SAMERL, 2000.

Manetti, D. (ed.) *Studi sul De indolentia di Galeno*, Pisa and Rome: Fabrizio Serra Editore, 2012.

Mastro, G. del 'Μέγα βιβλίον: Galeno e la lunghezza dei libri'. In *Studi sul De indolentia di Galeno*, ed. D. Manetti, 33–62. Pisa and Rome: Fabrizio Serra Editore, 2012.

Nicholls, M. 'Parchment Codices in a New Text of Galen', *Greece and Rome* 2:57 (2010), 378–86.

Nicholls, M. 'A Library at Antium?' In *Galen's De indolentia*, ed. C. K. Rothschild and T. W. Thompson, 65–78. Tübingen: Mohr Siebeck, 2013.

Nutton, V. (ed. and trans.) *Galen: De propriis placitis*, Berlin: Akademie Verlag (CMG V 3,2), 1999.

Nutton, V. (trans. with introduction) *Avoiding Distress*, in *Galen: Psychological Writings*, ed. P. N. Singer, 43–106. Cambridge: Cambridge University Press, 2013.

Nutton, V. 'What's in a *Nomen*? Vlatadon 14 and an Old Theory Resuscitated'. In *The Frontiers of Ancient Science: Essays in Honour of Heinrich von Staden*, ed. B. Holmes and K.-D. Fischer, 451–62. Berlin: de Gruyter, 2015.

Pietrobelli, A. 'Variation autour du Thessalonicensis Vlatadon 14: un manuscrit copié au Xénon du Kral, peu avant la chute de Constantinople'. *Revue des Études Byzantines* 68 (2010), 95–126.

Pietrobelli, A. 'Galien agnostique: un texte caviardé par la tradition', *Revue des Études Grecques* 126 (2013), 103–35.

Polemis, I. 'Διορθωτικά στο *Περί Αλυπίας* του Γαληνού', *Επιστημονική Επετηρίδα της Φιλοσοφικής Σχολής του Πανεπιστημίου Αθηνών* 43 (2011), 1–8.

Puglia, E. 'La rovina dei libri di Anzio nel "De indolentia" di Galeno', *Segno e testo* 9 (2011), 55–62.

Rashed, M. 'Aristote à Rome au IIe siècle: Galien, *De indolentia* §§ 15–18.' *Elenchos* 32 (2011), 55–77.

Roselli, A. 'Congetture inedite', *Galenos* 2 (2008), 137–8.

Roselli, A. 'Libri e biblioteche a Roma al tempo di Galeno: la testimonianza del *de indolentia*', *Galenos* 4 (2010), 127–48.

Roselli, A. 'Galeno dopo l'incendio del 192: bilancia di una vita'. In *Studi sul de indolentia di Galeno*, ed. D. Manetti, 93–102. Pisa and Rome: Fabrizio Serra Editore, 2012.

Rothschild, C. K. and Thompson, T. W. 'Galen's *On the Avoidance of* Grief: The Question of a Library at Antium', *Early Christianity* 2.1 (2011), 11–29.

Singer, P. N. *Galen: Selected Works*. Translation with introduction and notes. Oxford: OUP, 1997.

Singer, P. N. (ed.) *Galen: Psychological Writings: Avoiding Distress, The Diagnosis and Treatment of the Affections and Errors Peculiar to Each Person's Soul, Character Traits and The Capacities of the Soul Depend on the Mixtures of the Body*, translated with introduction and notes by V. Nutton, D. Davies and P. N. Singer, with the collaboration of Piero Tassinari. Cambridge: CUP, 2013.

Singer, P. N. 'Galen on his Own Opinions: Textual Questions and Fresh Perspectives from MS Vlatadon 14', forthcoming.

Stramaglia, A. 'Libri perduti per sempre: Galeno, *De indolentia* 13; 16; 17–19'. *Rivista di Filologia e di Istruzione Classica* 139 (2011), 1–30.

Tucci, P. L. 'Galen's Storeroom, Rome's Libraries and the Fire of AD 192.' *Journal of Roman Archaeology* 21 (2008), 133–92.

Tucci, P. L. 'Antium, the Palatium and the *Domus Tiberiana* Again.' *Journal of Roman Archaeology* 22 (2009), 398–401.

Tucci, P. L. 'Galen and the Library at Antium: The State of the Question', *Classical Philology* 108:3 (2013), 240–51.

Vegetti, M. *Galeno: nuovi scritti autobiografici*. Rome: Carocci, 2013.

Texts: Editions, Translations and Abbreviations

Editions and Translations of περὶ ἀλυπίας, with Abbreviation used in this Chapter

Editions

BM: Boudon-Millot, V. 'Un traité perdu de Galien miraculeusement retrouvé, le *Sur l'inutilité de se chagriner*: texte grec et traduction française'. In *La science médicale antique: nouveaux regards (Études réunies en l'honneur de Jacques Jouanna)*, ed. V. Boudon-Millot, A. Guardasole and C. Magdelaine, 73–123. Paris Éditions Beauchesne, 2007.

BJP: Boudon-Millot, V. and Jouanna, J. (ed. and trans.), with A. Pietrobelli, *Galien, Oeuvres 4: Ne pas se chagriner*. Paris: Les Belles Lettres, 2010.

GL: Garofalo, I. and Lami, A. (ed. and trans.) *Galeno: L' anima e il dolore. (De indolentia, De propriis placitis)*. Milan: Rizzoli, 2012.

KS: Kotzia, P and Sotiroudis, P. 'Γαληνοῦ περι ἀλυπίας', *Hellenica* 60 (2010), 63–48.

Translations

Nutton: Nutton, V. *Avoiding Distress*, in *Galen: Psychological Writings*, ed. P. N. Singer, 43–106. Cambridge: Cambridge University Press, 2013.

Rothschild, C. K. and Thompson, T. W. 'Galen: "On the Avoidance of Distress"'. In *Galen's De indolentia*, ed. C. K. Rothschild and T. W. Thompson, 21–36. Tübingen: Mohr Siebeck, 2013.

Editions, Translations and Abbreviations of Other Works of Galen

Texts of Galen are cited by volume and page number in Kühn's edition, followed where available by page and line number in the most recent critical edition.

K. = C. G. Kühn, *Claudii Galeni Opera Omnia*, 22 vols. Leipzig, 1821–1833.

CMG = Corpus Medicorum Graecorum, Leipzig and Berlin, 1908–.

HNH = In Hippocratis De natura hominis. [K. XV]. Ed. J. Mewaldt. Leipzig and Berlin: Teubner, CMG V 9,1, 1914.

Lib. Prop. = De libris propriis (My Own Books). [K. XIX]. Ed. V. Boudon-Millot. Paris: Les Belles Lettres, 2007; trans. in Singer, *Galen: Selected Works*.

MM = De methodo medendi. (The Therapeutic Method). [K. x]. Trans. I. Johnston and
 G. H. R. Horsley. Cambridge, Mass.: Harvard University Press (Loeb), 2011.

Mor. = De moribus (Character Traits). [Not in K.]. Ed. Kraus, 'Kitāb al-Akhlāq', trans.
 D. Davies in Singer, *Galen: Psychological Writings.*

Morb. Diff. = De differentiis morborum. [K. vi].

Ord. Lib. Prop. = De ordine librorum propriorum (The Order of My Own Books). [K. xix].
 Ed. V. Boudon-Millot. Paris: Les Belles Lettres, 2007; trans. in Singer, *Galen: Selected
 Works.*

PHP = De placitis Hippocratis et Platonis (The Doctrines of Hippocrates and Plato). [K.
 v]. Ed. and trans. P. De Lacy, 3 vols. Berlin: Akademie Verlag, CMG V 4,1,2, 1978–84.

Prop. Plac. = De propriis placitis (My Own Doctrines). [Not in K.]. Ed. and trans.
 V. Nutton. Berlin: Akademie Verlag (CMG V 3,2), 1999. Ed. and French trans. of fuller
 text by V. Boudon-Millot and A. Pietrobelli, A., 'Galien ressucité: édition princeps du
 texte grec du *De propriis placitis*', *Revue des Études Grecques* 118 (2005), 168–213. Ed.
 with Italian trans. by I. Garofalo and A. Lami ('GL' above). Ed. with Italian trans. by
 M. Vegetti, *Galeno: nuovi scritti autobiografici.* Rome: Carocci, 2013.

*QAM = Quod animi mores corporis temperamenta sequantur (The Soul's Dependence on
 the Body).* [K. iv]. Ed. I. Müller, in *C. Galeni Scripta Minora*, 2. Leipzig: Teubner, 1891;
 trans. in Singer, *Galen: Psychological Writings.*

Temp. = De temperamentis. (Mixtures). [K. I]. Ed. G. Helmreich. Leipzig: Teubner, 1904.

UP = De usu partium. [K. iii-iv]. Ed. G. Helmreich. Leipzig: Teubner, 2 vols, 1907–9;
 English trans. by M. T. May, *Galen: On the Usefulness of the Parts of the Body.* Ithaca,
 NY: Cornell University Press, 1968.

Abbreviations and editions of other texts
Fronto

Ad M. Caes. = Epistulae ad Marcum Caesarem et invicem. Ed. M. P. J. van den Hout in
 M. Cornelii Frontonis Epistulae. Leiden: Brill, 1954.

PART 1

Περὶ Ἀλυπίας *and Galen's* Œuvre

∴

Death, Posterity and the Vulnerable Self: Galen's *Περὶ Ἀλυπίας* in the Context of His Late Writings

Caroline Petit

The form and contents of Galen's newly recovered letter περὶ ἀλυπίας have come under intense scrutiny, especially since 2010, when both critical editions by Kotzia/Soutiroudis and Boudon-Millot/Jouanna respectively were published. Galen's philosophical mindset, in particular, has attracted considerable interest, since he addresses a number of issues around pain and grief that have concerned philosophers before and after him. Similarly, the additional clues given away by Galen about his own life, possessions and opinions have overall been carefully studied, although some degree of controversy affects the interpretation of the text itself. Most specialists of Galen have come to grips with the meaning of the letter in the context of the rest of his production. But seldom has the text been subject to rhetorical analysis, beyond identifying its main logical articulations and unfolding its overall argument. Galen's words, however, lend themselves quite well to a rhetorical reading: the notion of μεγαλοψυχία ('magnanimity'), prominent in the text,[1] is as typical of a good rhetor's *ēthos* as of a philosopher's. In this chapter, I intend to explore what the περὶ ἀλυπίας brings us in terms of self-characterization by Galen at this point in life. In other words, what does the περὶ ἀλυπίας add to, or transform, in terms of our understanding of Galen's *ēthos*? Is this just a typical old man stance about wisdom and knowledge, or is there more? How does it supplement Galen's other extant texts about himself, especially among the works of his later life?

To answer this question, I will include some thoughts on the evidence about Galen's last few years (a relatively neglected topic) and about the role of old age in his texts, both as a fact and as a literary construct. Indeed, with Galen issues of biography and autobiography and self-portrayal are closely intertwined. Separating the facts of Galen's life from the way he writes about them is near impossible, firstly because he is our only source about himself, and

---

1 As noted by V. Boudon-Millot and J. Jouanna, *Galien. Ne pas se chagriner*, 2010, p. xlvii; see Galen, *Ind.* 50–51. The edition of *De indolentia* I refer to is Boudon-Millot/Jouanna 2010 throughout. About the interpretation of magnanimity as a Stoic virtue, see Tieleman's demonstration in the present volume.

secondly because he is a skilful, conscious author whose every statement must be read in light of his authorial purposes. In other words, Galen's person and *ēthos* intersect largely in his writings – a difficulty that has its benefits for the modern reader, for Galen has left us a particularly vivid portrait of his scholarly and authorial self. I will therefore take the gaps in our knowledge about the last period of his life as a starting point, before turning to the elements of self-portrayal that can be established through his own account. Finally, I will examine the contribution of the newly discovered text to Galen's *ēthos* as we understand it from other works. My point is that Galen, far from simply conforming to the conventional image of a wise old man delving into *otium litterarum*, in fact transforms the traditional *ēthos* of his situation into a powerful intellectual and personal testament that supplements and nuances the self-portrait of his maturity. The path I have chosen is, admittedly, a meandering one, starting from a seemingly remote point towards the actual object of my study through concentric circles; but I hope my combined enquiry of Galen's biography and self-portrayal will show a perceptible shift in Galen's late life and shed some light on the importance of the new text. I am here building on my work on Galen's rhetoric, in which the notion of *ēthos* proves fundamental.[2]

1 Old Age: Facts and Literature

Defining old age, as shown in recent scholarship, is partly a matter of convention (the age of retirement from various duties in Rome was 60, but 70 seems to have been seen as the genuine threshold of old age). To an extent, old age was a subjective matter. Cicero, and, later, Seneca, have provided us with priceless insights into experiencing old age. As Mary Harlow and Ray Lawrence put it:

> There is a host of literary material on the survival into old age, because the elderly used the *otium* or leisure time associated with this period of life as time to write. They wrote as consolation for themselves in old age facing death and it is this format that produces much of what we today associate with a stoic philosophy of survival in adversity. That adversity was old age.[3]

---

2 Petit, C., *Galien ou la rhétorique de la Providence. Médecine, littérature et pouvoir à Rome*, Brill, 2018.

3 Harlow, M. and Lawrence, R., "Viewing the old: recording and respecting the elderly at Rome and in the Empire", in C. Krötzl and K. Mustakallio, *On Old Age. Approaching Death in Antiquity and the Middle Ages*, Brepols, 2011, 3–24. Naturally, not all references to old age in antiquity are negative: Plutarch, *An seni res publica gerenda sit*, offers an upbeat vision of old

Of course, that is not the entire story: writing about old age has developed into a long, complex literary tradition, culminating with highlights such as Petrarch's *Letters of old age*, in which, coincidentally, Galen does play a role next to Cicero and other prominent inspirational authors of the past.[4]

For all the stoicism attached to them, such ancient testimonies about *otium* in old age are not entirely devoid from complacency, as old age becomes the time of reflecting on the past, recording earlier achievements and distributing prizes (to oneself) – Aristotle had long noticed this negative aspect of old age, conveniently opposed to the feelings experienced by the young. Old age, so it seems, is as much a social construction as it is a personal experience. Naturally, it also develops into a rhetorical *topos*. The characters of youth and old age feature prominently in rhetorical theory, starting with Aristotle's *Rhetoric*, with which Galen was familiar. Several Plutarchan works deal with aspects of growing older, such as dealing with the fear of death, and the possibilities of continued public activity beyond retirement (*De tranquillitate animi, An seni respublica gerenda sit*). As suggested by Plutarch, health, not age, should be a criterion for continued activity – the benefits of stable, serene characters of older men are also praised by Cicero. But how does Galen fit in this literature on old age?

Galen's testimony features prominently in recent studies on old age in antiquity, but he is usually quoted as a medical authority: as a physician, Galen has dealt in relatively great detail with old age, especially in his six-book work on hygiene (with the ancient meaning of "preserving health"), *De sanitate tuenda*. He saw aging as the natural process of the human body drying out and withering away over time.[5] Man, of course, mirrors the wider *cosmos*. Like a country, it has seasons. Like a plant, or indeed any living being, the body gradually loses its moisture until its functions fail and it eventually returns to dust. In the process, Galen adds further periodisation to the last part of life: using a rarely found terminology, he highlights three theoretical stages of old age, a feature that singles him out in the extant literature.[6] More importantly, however, he

---

age (*Mor.* 783a–797f). In Plutarch's view, retiring to be a farmer or simply stay at home (like a woman!) are a waste and a shame for the once successful man.

4   Petrarch, *Letters of Old Age* (*Rerum senilium libri*); for an analysis of the theme of old age in Petrarch, see Skenazi, C., *Aging Gracefully in the Renaissance. Stories of Later Life from Petrarch to Montaigne*, Brill, 2013.

5   Galien, *De sanitate tuenda* – now available in a new English translation by Ian Johnston (Loeb, 2 vols., 2018). See also Minois, G., *Histoire de la vieillesse en Occident*, Paris, Fayard, 1987 (chapter on 'la médecine romaine et la vieillesse'); Morand, A. F., '« Chimie » de la vieillesse. Explications galéniques de cet âge de la vie', In L. Mathilde Cambron-Goulet and Laetitia Monteils-Laeng (ed.), *La Vieillesse dans l'Antiquité, entre déchéance et sagesse, Cahiers des études anciennes* 55, 2018, pp. 125–143.

6   Galen, *San. Tu.* V, 12 p. 167 Koch.

analyses aging in the context of nutrition and lifestyle, and provides advice and cures to live longer, and in better health – thus answering widespread anxiety in Roman society about the vicissitudes of the last part of life, as witnessed by Pliny the Younger, whose account of the old age of Spurrina exemplifies the desirable outcome of a well-managed life in the Roman upper classes.[7] According to Galen, regimen, appropriate exercise, bathing and massage all contribute to aging gracefully: his own health history, he claims, demonstrates the quality and the validity of his lifestyle choices and should incite others to follow. Naturally, he also illustrates his point by recording a number of cases of old men thriving under his care, the most famous being Marcus Aurelius.[8] Galen's insight as a physician is therefore priceless, but his contribution on experiencing old age and facing death has been overlooked. In the περὶ ἀλυπίας, written in 193 AD or slightly later, a 63-ish Galen advocates patience and courage in the face of loss and grief; he writes to his anonymous friend in a posture that is, to some extent, similar to that of Cicero writing to Atticus in their early sixties (*Att.* VI, 14, 21, 3),[9] or to that of Seneca writing to Lucilius in his late sixties (*Ep.* 24). He is thus framing his thoughts in a literary and philosophical context.

Indeed, Galen could not ignore the rich literary background to writing on old age: Cicero's *De senectute* and Seneca's *Letters to Lucilius* are only the most famous ancient texts on aging. Countless aphorisms and maxims about the elderly appear in tragedy, comedy and poetry; aging was also a rich philosophical theme even before Plato. Either pictured as epitomes of wisdom or laughing stock for the younger ones, educated elderly men were not always comfortable with their situation, as demonstrated in their texts (again, consider Plutarch's *An seni resp. gerend. sit*); those who provided a personal testimony on old age postured as wise old men (the archetypal wise old man being the Homeric Nestor), whilst acknowledging debilitating conditions (such as Seneca's asthma) or moodiness and irritability (Cicero). Between philosophical posturing and genuine confession, aging *litterati* made old age a matter for discussion. Galen's medical representation of old age is not just the objective stance of a doctor; it is combined with a subjective account in his later works, some of which he penned in his sixties and maybe later. The two areas conflate when

---

7   Pliny *Ep.* 3, 1, the old age of Spurrina – "the ideal old age for the upper class Roman male" (see Harlow, M. and Lawrence, R., *Growing up and Growing old in ancient Rome: A Lifecourse Approach*, Routledge, 2001, pp. 123–124). About the (three) stages of old age, see Galen *San. Tu.* V, 12 = p. 167 Koch and for a survey of similar notions in ancient Greek texts, see Parkin, T. G., *Old Age in the Roman World: A Cultural and Social History*, Johns Hopkins University Press, 2003 (Appendix C., pp. 299–301).

8   Galen, *De praen.* 11 Nutton.

9   See his *De senectute*, written when Cicero was 62 and dedicated to a 65-year old Atticus.

Galen shows off his own excellent health in the above-mentioned *De sanitate tuenda* (he was then in his early fifties[10]), a work in which his own healthy state serves as a selling point for his general method. But the promotional dimension seems to fade in the later hints at his weakening body and faltering convictions. As we will see, Galen no less chisels his own aging self-portrait than others do in the same period; and he no less cares for his own image than he did as a younger, ambitious doctor eager to promote his skills and methodology. I am interested in tracing this shift in Galen's writing, looking for clues in his extant later works, before turning to the περὶ ἀλυπίας.

2   Can the Enigma of Galen's Last Years be Solved? Looking for a 'testament'

Galen's later years have been left out of most accounts on his life, partly due to the lack of evidence. In the penultimate chapter of her authoritative biography of Galen, Véronique Boudon-Millot explores the available evidence on the "diseases and death of a doctor".[11] While Galen is comparatively loquacious among ancient doctors about his own ailments, he is less and less inclined to record such personal information in his later works.[12] As for the date of his death, accumulated evidence from Byzantine (beyond the *Souda*) and Arabic sources points to the later part of Caracalla's reign, hence the now commonly accepted date of 216 instead of 199.[13] Of course, issues regarding the authenticity of late works[14] cast a shadow on Galen's last years: but it seems safe to assume that Galen lived for another twenty to twenty-three years after he wrote his *De indolentia* in 193; this fits well with the picture of a still-prolific author, who penned *inter alia* the best part of thousands of pages of pharmacological works. Nonetheless, it is impossible to establish with certainty when Galen actually stopped thinking and writing, for his testimony does not hint at any significant late life impairment.[15] In this hazy context, Galen's mentions of health

---

10   Written shortly after the death of Marcus Aurelius (c. 180) according to Heiberg, followed by Koch.

11   Boudon-Millot, V., *Galien de Pergame. Un médecin grec à Rome*, Paris, Les Belles Lettres, 2012, pp. 225–245.

12   *Ibid.* pp. 225–226.

13   *Ibid.* pp. 241–244.

14   Especially in the case of the *Theriac to Piso*, of disputed authorship.

15   *Pace* V. Boudon-Millot, *Galien de Pergame*, 2012, p. 233. Hearing a book read aloud was considered a soothing form of entertainment in old age, not a sign of physical decline, as shown by Pliny the Younger's famous description of Spurrina's perfect regimen; *Cf.* Pliny the Younger, *Ep.* III, 1.

problems linked with aging are rare: a recurring issue seems to have been the state of his teeth, since he comments on his difficulties as early as *Alim. fac.* (written before Marcus Aurelius died in 180), when he couldn't chew on lettuce any more, and as late as *Comp. med. sec. locos* (written after 193), where he comments on the nature and location of toothache, in the gum or in the tooth itself (without quite referring to an actual pain at the very time of writing).[16] Allusions to disease in *Character Traits* (cf. P. N. Singer, *Galen's Psychological writings*) are tricky, because the date of the treatise is uncertain, although recent scholarship points to a post-192 date as plausible. More to the point, it is an epitome, surviving in Arabic: it is therefore relatively delicate to use. What we have, then, in Galen's later works, is a body of indications of another nature. He is focussing on his legacy.

Galen famously has relatively few explicit mentions among writers in his lifetime;[17] later biographers often sought to re-write his life in a colourful way, following new agendas.[18] Therefore we have to rely on internal evidence in the Galenic corpus to understand how the Pergamene dealt with his physical decline – if it is at all represented or even hinted at. As 192 AD marks a shift in his priorities, namely the recording and preserving of his own works in the form of his catalogue (*Libr. Propr.*; *Ord. libr. propr.*) and of additional copies of his own works, it is perhaps useful to use this date as the conventional beginning of Galen's old age – at the very least, the devastation caused by the great fire made the preservation of his works a pressing matter such as he never felt before, trusting the safety of the Palatine storage rooms. This is a turning point in Galen's life, seemingly shifting his priorities. In order to gather the evidence given by Galen himself about his later years (roughly after the fire of 192), it is necessary to focus on the extant works clearly written after the event.[19] Those include the last seven books (VII–XIV) of the *De methodo medendi*, the last three books (IX–XI) of *De simpl. med. fac. ac temp.*, and the bulk of his other

---

16   Galen, *Alim. fac.* II, 40 (K. VI, 626); *Comp. med. sec. locos*, V, 4 (K. XII, 848). Cf. V. Boudon-Millot, *Galien de Pergame*, pp. 232–233; D. Gourevitch & M. Grmek, 1986, 45–64 (p. 58–59).

17   See, however, Nutton, V., 'Galen in the eyes of his contemporaries', *BHM* 58, 1984, pp. 315–324 (Nutton refers especially to Athenaeus I, 1).

18   Illuminated by Swain, S. C. R., 'Beyond the Limits of Greek Biography: Galen from Alexandria to the Arabs', in B. McGing and J. Mossman (eds), *The Limits of Ancient Biography*, The Classical Press of Wales, 2006, pp. 395–433. To my knowledge, the first 'biography' of Galen based on his own account is given by Symphorien Champier in his *Speculum Galeni*, 1517 (about which see Petit, C. 'Symphorien Champier (1471–1539) et Galien: Médecine et littérature à la Renaissance', to appear in C. La Charité & R. Menini eds., *La médecine au temps de Rabelais*).

19   *Cf.* V. Boudon-Millot, *Galien de Pergame*, 2012, pp. 220–224.

pharmacological works (*Comp. med. sec. locos; Comp. med. sec. gen.; Antid.*[20]).
The last book of *De sanitate tuenda* should be added, together with the brief *De bonis malisque sucis*; the *De foet. formatione*, and the last four books (preserved only in Arabic) of *De anatomicis administrationibus*. Last but not least, Galen's *De propriis placitis*, dubbed "Galen's philosophical testament", highlights the issues that really matter to him now that his life has reached its course and his work is completed. Several psychological writings, including the περὶ ἀλυπίας, are also thought to belong to the later period of Galen's life (again, post-192 AD): the evidence is, however, slightly more contentious for some of them and in all cases, one should bear in mind Peter Singer's cautious remarks on Galen's compositional style.[21] Indeed, there are reasons to envisage multiple layers of writing in many, if not most, Galenic works. Supposed dates of composition are thus relative, and one should be mindful of the fact that Galen may have more or less constantly altered his own writings. All in all, though, those works represent a considerable amount of text (thousands of pages in the standard edition of Kühn) and must have been written over many years in the aftermath of 192–193, although it is difficult to be more accurate than that, and to pin down the moment when Galen stopped writing (just as it is impossible to establish the date of his passing). Just like many of his predecessors and literary models, Galen may have enjoyed enhanced *otium* in his old age, perhaps retiring from everyday medical practice in order to dedicate his time to writing; he may also, we can speculate, have appreciated a loosening of the imperial grip over the Palace in the wake of Commodus' death. Still, such a considerable volume of work could not have been achieved without exceptional personal abilities and outstanding material support, in the form of personnel, books, and other resources.

Galen gives us hints about his working priorities: by his own account in *De simpl. med. fac. ac temp.*, it sounds like he is on a mission to complete a large section of his oeuvre, namely his pharmacological project, covering simple and compound drugs, as well as the so-called εὐπόριστα (easy to procure remedies), purgatives and antidotes. Galen is not without expressing a certain sense of urgency. In one of the later books, Galen indeed makes the following statement:

ταῦτα καίτοι τῆς προκειμένης οὐκ ὄντα πραγματείας, ἔγραψα διὰ τὸ θαρρεῖν τῷ φαρμάκῳ, μηδενὸς μηδέποτε ἀποθανόντος τῶν ὡς εἴρηται χρησαμένων αὐτῷ.

---

20   It is unclear whether any of the three books of the *Euporista* currently preserved in the Kühn edition is authentic.

21   P. N. Singer, *Galen. Psychological Writings*, 2013, pp. 34–41; see also his contribution 'New light and old texts' in this volume.

ποιήσομαι δὲ καὶ κατὰ μόνας ἑτέραν πραγματείαν περὶ τῶν ἰδιότητι τῆς ὅλης
οὐσίας ἐνεργούντων, ἐν οἷς ἐστι καὶ τὰ τοιαῦτα πάντα. συγγινώσκειν οὖν χρὴ τῷ
τῆς γραφῆς ἀκαίρῳ καὶ νῦν καὶ κατ' ἄλλα χωρία τῆσδε τῆς πραγματείας ἐνίοτε
γεγονότι, διὰ τὴν ἐκ τῶν λεγομένων ὠφέλειαν μεγίστην οὖσαν, ἣν διασώζεσθαι
βούλομαι τοῖς μεθ' ἡμᾶς ἀνθρώποις, εἰ καὶ μεταξὺ θάνατος γενόμενος
ἀποκωλύσει με γράψαι τὰς ἐφεξῆς τῆσδε τῆς πραγματείας.[22]

Even though such details do not belong to the present work, my faith in
this medicine[23] leads me to record it, for no one who has used it according to the prescription has ever died. I shall write a particular treatise
about medicines that work as a result of the specific character of their
general composition, including all such remedies as this one. You will
need to forgive me for passages that are beside the point both here and
occasionally elsewhere in this book, because the information is extremely valuable and I wish to preserve it for the sake of posterity, in case death
should prevent me from writing treatises following this one.

A few pages away from completing his major work on simple drugs, then,
Galen hints neatly at his age and the lurking possibility of death, with dramatic effect – and potentially dramatic consequences for posterity, he suggests:
Galen is so worried that he may not finish his work, that some exceptionally
useful remedies might be lost forever if he doesn't record them at once. This
explains, Galen says, why his treatise *On simple drugs* includes material that
should not be there.[24] This sense of urgency (and fear?) is not found anywhere
else in Galen's works. But it is not the first time Galen attributes a change in his
text to a particular circumstance in his life: in book x of the *De usu partium*,
he explains that he was persuaded by a divine warning in a dream to include
a development on the eye at this point in his work, against the plan he had
initially formed.[25] Contemplating imminent death seems to have prompted
Galen to alter his plan in a similar way. In both cases, the urgency is compel-
ling. At any rate, the evidence of the many pages that were subsequently added
to his work *On simple drugs* in the form of additional treatises shows that
Galen was blessed to continue writing for quite a while, and his fears, if genuine, unfounded. Had Galen not been in his late sixties when he wrote those

---

22   Galen, *Simpl. med. temp. ac fac.*, XI, 34 (K. XII, 357–358).

23   Galen has just discussed the usefulness of burnt crab powder in rabies cases.

24   Another passage in the same work echoes this sense of urgency, when Galen apologises
      for inserting a digression on the preparation of theriac, for fear of not completing the rest
      of his pharmacological works (chapter XI, 1 on vipers' flesh, K. XII, 319).

25   Galen, *Usu part.* X, 12 (Helmreich vol. II, 92–93).

lines, there may have been a case for a rhetorical device here. But, given his age and the scale of the remaining books to be written to fulfil his publication plans, it should be stressed that Galen's concerns are plausible – just as when he was persuaded in a dream to add this piece about the eye in book x of the *De usu partium*. Whilst he apparently brushes aside any considerations about his health at this point, age and the possibility of sudden death clearly are on his mind. This, in fact, fits well with the conspicuous haste affecting many of his late writings; as already observed by Vivian Nutton, "several of the books he wrote in old age end abruptly", especially the final section of the *Method of healing*.[26]

A debated question is whether or not Galen stayed in Rome until he died: could he have travelled back to Pergamum, his native city, as suggested by some? Or did he enjoy the comfort of his home (in one of his several houses) to complete his work in the best possible conditions, instead of risking an exhausting, potentially fatal journey home? Again, later sources cannot be relied on, and there are hardly any clues to be gleaned from Galen's own words about a change of scenery; but why would a court physician who stayed through Commodus' horrendous reign depart at any point following the relief brought by his death? Galen must have had either good reasons to stay, or no choice at all. In order to return to Pergamum permanently, Galen may have needed imperial permission, indeed to be granted a favour. We know, however, that apart from his special relationship with Marcus Aurelius, with whom he was able to negotiate to an extent, there is no evidence of similarly relaxed relationships with later emperors such as Septimius Severus: as noted by Alain Billault, Galen may have been part of Julia Domna's circle – but we have no evidence.[27] In any case, this is pure speculation.

I am tempted to interpret (even more tentatively) some features of his later works as signs that he may have stayed on in Rome. For example, in one of his last works, *De antidotis* I, 1 (K. XIV, 3–5), Galen recalls at some length the effects of theriac on Marcus Aurelius' health, which might hint at a Roman readership; in *Comp. med. sec. genera* III, 2 (K. XIII, 603), he also evokes briefly his disciples' disciples (in other words, a second generation of students) now reading anatomy (through *his* books on anatomy), hinting at an educational context. Many additional references to his dedicated audience, his ἑταῖροι, appear in his later pharmacological works, especially *Comp. med. sec. locos* and *Comp. med. sec. genera* (in the latter, he often addresses them in the second

26   Nutton, V., 'Galen's Philosophical Testament', in J. Wiesner ed., *Aristoteles. Werk und Wirkung, Paul Moraux gewidmet* Berlin/New York, vol. II, 1987, 27–51 (p. 44).

27   Billault, A., *L'univers de Philostrate*, Bruxelles, 2000, p. 6.

person).[28] Where better than Rome could this have taken place, a city in which he has almost entirely built his career, reputation and network?

A "philosophical testament" does survive among Galen's later works: his *De propris placitis* (On my own opinions), a work in which the physician's customary references to time and circumstances are absent. It is thus difficult to date, but definitely belongs to Galen's late production. As pointed out by its first editor Vivian Nutton before the discovery of a full Greek text in ms. *Vlatadon* 14, this work does not aim at promoting new ideas, or firm conclusions about any philosophical issue; rather, it states Galen's final opinions on debated questions (notably the role of the soul) for the sake of posterity. Just like his *De libr. propr.* and *Ord. libr. propr.* aim at excluding any inauthentic work from his oeuvre, similarly his *On my own opinions* aims at dissipating any misunderstanding about his actual opinions, in order to disprove forgeries and avoid misguided criticism.[29] Thus in this work and others from the same period, Galen emphasises his concern to see his own, authentic voice echoing through ages: posterity is as central to this work, as the actual contents of his own opinions about the covered topics. This genuine concern contrasts with the old man's frailty, as the work lacks the hallmarks of Galen's previous rhetorical mastery. Vivian Nutton notes about the book's abrupt ending:

> The old man's powers to control the overall structure of his investigations are noticeably weaker, his judgment less forceful, his criticisms less vigorous. Whether death, or simply reaching the end of his secretary's book roll, caused Galen to break off here is a matter only for sad conjecture.[30]

Whether Galen intended the apparent lack of order and completeness of his work is unclear. It may hint at Galen's decline, or haste, or it could be a draft which he could not complete or rework for whatever reason. In any case, as we shall see, this sheer concern for posterity is central to Galen's late *ēthos*.

But what Galen lets us know is certainly not the whole story; there are gaps in our information. Those are essentially due to accidents, such as works missing: either they were lost, or simply were not deemed authentic or worth copying.

---

28   The dozens of mentions of ἑταῖροι in Galen's later pharmacological works are only matched by his *Anat. adm.*, also aimed at a students readership. I echo Peter Singer's remarks in 'New Light and Old Texts', note 14.

29   Galen, *Propr. Plac.* 1 Nutton. *Cf.* Nutton, V., 'Galen's Philosophical Testament', in J. Wiesner ed., *Aristoteles. Werk und Wirkung, Paul Moraux gewidmet* Berlin/New York, vol. II, 1987, 27–51 (p. 51); *eiusd., Galen. De propriis placitis*, CMG V, 3, 2, 1999, introd. pp. 45–47; comm. p. 127.

30   V. Nutton, *Galen. De propriis placitis*, CMG V, 3, 2, 1999, comm. p. 218.

Among lost works from his later life, we could mention a work κατ᾽ Ἐπικοῦρον mentioned in the περὶ ἀλυπίας (*Ind.* 68); a brief work περὶ τῶν φιλοχρημάτων πλουσίων, also mentioned in the same work (*Ind.* 84); and probably a work in two books *On medicine in Homer* (περὶ τῆς κατ᾽Ὅμηρον ἰατρικῆς), mentioned by Alexander of Tralles and Hunayn ibn Isḥaq alike. Gaps thus occasionally get filled by later sources, although their credibility has been questioned. In the case of the latter work, *On medicine in Homer,* authenticity has been dismissed on account of Galen's 'rationalist' approach to medicine; Hunayn himself was unconvinced by the contents of the work.[31] If we follow Alexander, however, Galen recognised the power of amulets and other magical remedies late in life, a fact that was reflected explicitly in the lost treatise. In fact, a simple comparison between the contents (as described, and quoted by Alexander) and Galen's statements in the last three books of *On simple drugs* shows remarkable agreement, and demonstrates a change in Galen's opinions, or at least, enlarged views.[32] As argued by Alexander of Tralles, Galen held more pragmatic, inclusive views about remedies in his later life. It is therefore necessary to acknowledge this additional evidence in assessing Galen's final viewpoint on the medical art. More importantly, in all likeliness this episode shows that we are missing part of the picture: Galen's exact feelings and thoughts may only come through partially, a limitation we must acknowledge.

3   *Self-characterization in Galen's Later Works: a* Moraliste[33]

A distinctive tone creeps into Galen's later works, away from the boisterousness of some of his earlier works. Galen appears as a *moraliste*, displays revised (in a more sceptical fashion) views on the soul, shows off his experience and, finally, his detachment from the more materialistic aspects of life. Galen's moralistic statements seem to echo the Plutarchan preoccupations[34] showed by his later works (see above, Galen's lost περὶ τῶν φιλοχρημάτων πλουσίων) as well

---

31   Kudlien, F., "Zum Thema 'Homer und die Medizin'", *Rheinisches Museum* 108, 1965, 293–299.

32   See Petit, C., 'Galen, Pharmacology and the Boundaries of Medicine: A Reassessment', in M. Martelli and L. Lehmhaus eds., *Collecting Recipes: Byzantine and Jewish Pharmacology in Dialogue,* De Gruyter, 2017, 50–80 (p. 77–80).

33   In the following pages, I understand the French *moraliste* in the acceptation of an author describing the mores and ills of the society he lives in, in order to offer a reflection on human nature and condition. As there is no English equivalent to the best of my knowledge, I am using the French term.

34   See Plutarch, *De cupiditate divitiarum.*

as his long-standing interest in ethical philosophy.[35] One such text appears at the beginning of book x of *Simple drugs*.[36] In a long preface to the book, which is dedicated to animal parts in medicine, Galen provides precious information about past scholarship on the topic; faithful to his sharp and critical mind, he exposes others' lack of dignity and lawfulness. One victim of this charge is Xenocrates of Aphrodisias, the author of a comprehensive study about the use of animal parts. Animal parts famously include *human* body parts and fluids; Galen stresses his disgust (as expected from an educated Greek, and a Roman citizen) at the ingestion of bodily secretions such as earwax and menstrual blood. This statement is important in providing finishing touches to his self-portrait: by criticising Xenocrates and his followers, he distances himself from dubious medical practices and presents himself as an enlightened practitioner (and somehow a καλός κἀγαθός). Undoubtedly, Galen is aware that slander could affect him as a medical practitioner in a hardly-regulated field,[37] and aims at diverting them through a clear statement; whether or not he is genuinely disgusted by the very thought of drinking menstrual blood does not really matter here. Prefatory rhetoric is instrumental in his authorial and medical posture.

Ultimately, however, this statement comes at a defining self-characterization moment in the context of his later works: a supremely experienced physician, Galen dominates the field and its turpitudes and stresses the usefulness of *some* animal-based remedies. In the last two books, Galen accepts a number of them, including those involving animal, even human excrements. But displaying a moral condemnation of the remedies closest to black magic gives him the higher ground; it conveniently puts him in a *moraliste*'s position. The tone of this very preface sounds distinctive, if compared with another preface in the same work, namely the preface to book VI, written much earlier in his life (before 180): in book VI, Galen simply ridicules Pamphilus as an incompetent writer, whereas in book x Galen directs his criticism towards an apparently similar target, Xenocrates, only to turn his attention and indignation towards more dangerous prescriptions. Let us read indeed the last section of the preface to book x. Galen's stance turns bitter as he accuses rogue practitioners of writing down harmful, even lethal recipes:

---

35   Galen, *Libr. Propr.* 15; the extant works of this category appear in P. N. Singer's *Galen. Psychological Writings*, 2013.

36   For a study of this preface (*Simpl. med. temp. ac fac.* x, 1) in the context of Galen's work *On simple drugs*, see my article cited n. 24.

37   As demonstrated in subsequent statements, for example dismissing crocodile blood for eye diseases, "because slanderers are swift to condemn physicians as sorcerers" (*Simpl. med.. temp. ac fac.* x, 6 = K. XII, 263).

As far as I am concerned, I will not mention basilisks, elephants, hippo-
potamuses or any other animal of which I have no personal experience;
as for the so-called philtres and charms to generate love, dreams or ha-
tred (I am deliberately using their very words), I would not mention them
in writing even if I had sufficient experience in them, just as I would not
record deadly poisons or those they call disease-makers. Their alleged
properties are ridiculous: binding adversaries, for example, so they cannot speak in court, causing a pregnant woman to miscarry, or preventing
a woman from conceiving, and other similar stupidities. Experience has
shown that most such charms are ineffective, and a few of them, albeit effective, are harmful to human life, which makes me wonder, by the gods,
by what line of reasoning they came to write them down. For how could
they believe that the knowledge that brings them infamy in life would
bring them fame after death? If they were kings who tested these things
on people sentenced to death, they would not be doing anything wrong.
But since they had the arrogance to write these things down as laymen,
over their entire life, then it can be only one of two explanations: either
they write about things they have neither tested nor know, or, if they have
tested them, then they are the most impious of all men, giving deadly
poisons to people who have done no wrong, sometimes even to excellent
men, for the sake of experimenting. A man noticed two physicians next
to some hawkers and approached them to sell them some honey, as it
seemed. Upon tasting it, they discussed the price, and, since they offered
little, he quickly vanished, but neither physician survived. In sum, it is
just to hate those who have written <about such poisons> more, not less,
than those who commit all such poisonings, insofar as it is a lesser crime
to do evil alone than it is to do so with the help of many others. And the
knowledge of one's evil deeds dies with the perpetrator, while knowledge
of all the writers is immortal, providing weapons to criminals to perform
their evil deeds. Let us now discuss things that are useful to men to the
best of our knowledge.[38]

Here Galen gradually moves beyond the realm of the use of dubious (or magical) remedies and practices; this passage is about authorial responsibility and
the very core of medical deontology: *to help, or to do no harm.* From the wide
embracing look that he casts upon the field of medicine, Galen castigates
criminals and the lack of law enforcement against them. He is asking strong
questions from his professional field, but also, indirectly, from the Empire he

---

38   Galen, *Simpl. med. temp. ac fac.* x, 1 (K. xii, 251–252). As per my article cited above.

lives in. A *moraliste* he definitely is in those late-life pages. His 'virtuous' self, whilst befitting a good orator's posture in general, is of course part of a more complex project of characterization: Galen offers an authorial perspective on the dangers of medical practice, especially of pharmacology. Galen's insistence here on the lasting power of his writings and the responsibility that comes with authorship is also essential to his self-definition – as a scholar concerned with his legacy.

The posture of a righteous, Hippocratic doctor is ideally supplemented by Galen's life-long experience and concern for patients outside his usual elite practice. In a small work, *De bonis malisque succis*, Galen begins with an illustrative tale about the direct effects of poor nutrition on health: his long opening paragraph describes the effects of imperial economy on the health patterns of the countryside, which he links with hunger and emergency alimentation practices triggered by the cities, which absorb most or all of the good crops, leaving nothing but alternative roots and herbs for countryside people. This detailed description of the ever-increasing symptoms of malnutrition and rise of diseases can be read, at some level, as criticism of imperial policy, but Galen is careful not to explicitly condemn his rulers. What Galen is clear about, however, is how his life-long experience helps him identify and correct such patterns, to the best of his knowledge. His description plays as a demonstration of his experience and talent for observation, which he stresses in the final sentence of this paragraph.[39] It also potentially demonstrates a caring personality, a doctor who is interested in the welfare of people generally beyond the small Roman elite that he is supposed to work with exclusively. The catastrophic fate of those poor people at the other end of the Empire resonates through Galen's words. It is unlikely that his intention was primarily to draw attention to their plight; rather, his extremely accurate description is a display of competence and knowledge, of observational powers and experience. At no point does Galen describe the facts in a way to arouse *pathos*. In my view, however, this description echoes Thucydides' description of the plague of Athens, and thus contains more than facts. It is, once again, arising from a *moraliste*'s gaze, beyond its medical theme. A keen observer of Roman society, Galen is eager to transfer his experience into an informed, perceptive narrative, conveying authorial prowess and superior insight.

In the above mentioned "testament" of his *De propriis placitis*, Galen adds some finishing touches to the parts of his oeuvre that confine to philosophy. As pointed out by Vivian Nutton, not all topics broached by Galen through a lifetime of work are present in the text. Rather, this is a selection of particularly

---

39   Galen, *Bon. Mal. Succ.* 1, 14 (CMG V, 4, 2, p. 392= K. VI, 755).

sensitive topics about which his views could easily come under fire or be mis-represented. In terms of contents, what is striking is the lack of firm answers to some questions, such as the role of the soul or its exact relationship with the body. In stark contrast to the 'rhetoric of certainty' that pervades his earlier works,[40] his final texts exude intellectual prudence. This openly stated uncer-tainty is no carelessness on Galen's part. Rather, the relative scepticism that comes through this testamental work is emphasised, so as to lay bare an old man's humility. By finally saying "I don't know", Galen chisels a more humane portrait of himself as a scholar and physician; perhaps, even, the portrait of a vulnerable old scholar. As we will see, this emphasis on uncertainty is no slip. On the contrary, it finalises Galen's self-portrayal as a honest intellectual and gentleman. This "philosophical testament", together with the revised approach to borderline remedies that he expresses towards the end of *On simple drugs*, give the reader an impression of a non-dogmatic scholar: a firmly grounded physician, whose knowledge is essentially down to experience and hard work. Another late work, *De dubiis motibus* (*On unclear movements*), also projects the image of a pragmatist.

A moraliste, a humble scholar, an old, experienced physician who has seen it all and understands the very mechanisms of Nature in and around the body, Galen is also deprived of greed, or any of the common human flaws chastised by philosophers. He is not accessible to sorrow or desire, to anger or envy. His famous pages about his education and values, if they are as late as is often sug-gested (they are echoed in *De bonis malisque succis* and in the περὶ ἀλυπίας any-way), show off in retrospect a good natured young man, keen to imitate only the virtues around him, namely those displayed by his father. Discussing prob-lems of character and temper among his peers, Galen is keen to dismiss anger as a particularly degrading flaw. Galen's self-characterization is thus finalised with reference to philosophical ideals of peace, self-control and ἀπάθεια. As we shall see, the newly discovered treatise adequately completes this self-portrait of humble wisdom – by contrast with the more confident texts of his youth, such as the self-promotional *On prognosis* (*De praecogn*).

4 Galen's περὶ ἀλυπίας: *Finalising a Scholar's Self-portrait?*

It is now time to go back to Galen's περὶ ἀλυπίας and our proposed investiga-tion. Much of the treatise (about half of it) revolves around Galen's personal

---

40   See Nutton, V., 'Galen and the Rhetoric of Certainty' in J. Coste/D. Jacquart/J.Pigeaud (eds.), *La rhétorique médicale à travers les siècles*, Genève, Droz, 2012, 39–49.

experience and losses in the Great Fire of 192 AD. It is worth examining how Galen talks about himself, in a highly codified literary context. *Periautologia* or 'discourse about oneself' has its pitfalls, and Galen more than anyone else is aware of the way he should (or should not) present himself to his chosen audience.[41] The virtues of the orator correspond to a great extent to the philosophical virtues commonly extolled in the imperial period (and hailed by Galen himself). The same virtuous conduct is expected of physicians in particular, who, at least in principle, model their lifestyle onto high moral standards.[42] Galen is one of the most vocal promoters of the "doctor-philosopher" in ancient literature.[43] Thus in his ethical discussions, Galen demonstrates awareness of the character he should be displaying and promoting; in displaying and promoting it, he certainly shows his abilities to play on the social and literary codes of moral excellence. Yet, how original is his self-characterization, in the light of this newly discovered text? What special character, exactly, is Galen constructing here? Do we get a new picture of the great Galen?

It is not my purpose here to describe the περὶ ἀλυπίας in terms of rhetorical devices and strategies: this would require extensive space. In the wake of my previous remarks on Galen's later works, I want to examine a limited aspect of Galen's rhetoric in this text: the way he constructs his own *ēthos* here, and how this echoes his other late works. Among the many features that invite a rhetorical reading in the περὶ ἀλυπίας, the theme of moral strength (or resilience) is of particular relevance. It is not by chance that μεγαλοψυχία (usually translated by 'magnanimity' but clearly revealing a form of strength, of resistence in this context, hence the term of 'resilience' I have chosen here) features at the turning point of the treatise, when Galen moves from exposing and narrating the facts to his moral stance on detachment from material goods. The term has a deep background in rhetoric and philosophy, as one of the chief components of ἀρετή;[44] μεγαλοψυχία is rarely used by Galen, but always in contexts of stark

---

41   Pernot, L., '*Periautologia*. Problèmes et méthodes de l'éloge de soi-même dans la tradition éthique et rhétorique gréco-romaine', *Revue des Etudes grecques* 111–1, 1998, pp. 101–124; Rutherford, I., 'The poetics of the *Paraphthegma*: Aelius Aristides and the Decorum of self-praise', in D. Innes/H. Hine/C. Pelling (eds), *Ethics and Rhetoric. Classical essays for Donald Russell on his Seventy-Fifth Birthday*, Oxford, 1995, pp. 193–204. Both studies explore in depth the precious hints provided by Plutarch in *De laude sui ipsius*.

42   *Cf.* Von Staden, H., 'Character and competence. Personal and professional conduct in Greek medicine', in H. Flashar/J. Jouanna (eds), *Médecine et morale dans l'antiquité. Entretiens de la Fondation Hardt vol. 43*, Genève, Droz, 1997, 157–195.

43   Galen, *The best doctor is also a philosopher*; see edition with tr. and commentary by V. Boudon-Millot, *Galien. Oeuvres, Tome I*, 2007.

44   See Aristotle, *Rhet.* I, 6; I, 9; II, 12. Cf. Woerther, F., *L'èthos aristotélicien. Genèse d'une notion rhétorique*, Paris, 2007, pp. 222–223. According to Aristotle, μεγαλοψυχία belongs to young

admiration (talking about Chrysippus, *PHP* III, 2, 18, 1; Hippocrates, *Dieb. crit.* II, 12 = K. IX, 894) or as a virtue enabling the soul to overcome grief (λυπή): in *Loc. Affect.*, V, 1 (K. VIII, 302) quoted below, Galen identifies those with a strong "tension" (τόνος) in the soul as the most resilient and less vulnerable patients. Others, weak in their souls and lacking education, are more likely to die from sudden, violent causes of distress.

> ὅσοις γὰρ ἀσθενής ἐστιν ὁ ζωτικὸς τόνος, ἰσχυρά τε πάθη ψυχικὰ πάσχουσιν ἐξ ἀπαιδευσίας, εὐδιάλυτος τούτοις ἐστὶν ἡ τῆς ψυχῆς οὐσία· τῶν τοιούτων ἔνιοι καὶ διὰ λύπην ἀπέθανον, οὐ μὴν εὐθέως ὥσπερ ἐν τοῖς προειρημένοις· ἀνὴρ δ' οὐδεὶς **μεγαλόψυχος** οὔτ' ἐπὶ λύπαις οὔτ' ἐπὶ τοῖς ἄλλοις ὅσα λύπης ἰσχυρότερα θανάτῳ περιέπεσον· ὅ τε γὰρ τόνος τῆς ψυχῆς αὐτοῖς ἰσχυρός ἐστι τά τε παθήματα σμικρά.

In all those whose vital tension is weak and who are afflicted by grave psychological ailments as a result of their lack of education, the substance of the soul is readily dissolved. Some of these even died of distress (λύπη), though not always instantly as in the cases I mentioned before; but no high-minded (μεγαλόψυχος) man ever died as a result of distressing experiences or of any other affliction stronger than distress. With them the tension of the soul is strong, the ailments are small.

This passage clearly foreshadows Galen's argument in the περὶ ἀλυπίας, in which resilience naturally accompanies a strong (masculine) soul, just like Galen's, which was shaped and strengthened through generations of instilled virtue, as he carefully and pointedly explains (*Ind.* 58–60). It is thus most appropriate to find μεγαλοψυχία twice within a couple of lines in the very centre of a work dedicated to ἀλυπία (*Ind.* 50–51); it is also a self-conscious assessment of Galen's own moral accomplishment and, consequently, of his reliability as an «orator», or author.[45] The intertwining of moral strength and authorial *kudos* is essential to our understanding of Galen's *ēthos*. As we have seen above, Galen's sharp authorial self-awareness is one of the defining features of the last period of his life, after 192 and the destruction of a great part of his library; his μεγαλοψυχία, in turn, allows him to move on and complete his authorial

---

men rather than old. Galen is certainly playing on the expectations of his audience here. See also Teun Tieleman's contribution in this volume.

45 As demonstrated in great detail by F. Woerther, the notion of *èthos* or character is consistent and coherent throughout Aristotle's works on ethics and rhetoric. Cf. Woerther, F., *L'èthos aristotélicien. Genèse d'une notion rhétorique*, Paris, 2007.

destiny by gathering scattered copies of his works and rewriting whatever can be rewritten, and completing the works he has intended to write, such as his pharmacological texts.

There is no connotation of arrogance in μεγαλοψυχία; rather, as suggested by Galen, it represents the core of human resilience in front of adversity. The detailed, precise account of his losses in the first part of the letter serves, of course, as a proof of his μεγαλοψυχία; the various echoes to his other ethical and psychological works (such as the reference to cultivating his family virtues, *inter alia*) not only strengthen his case: they confirm the authenticity of his *ēthos* as a virtuous, resilient individual. In this sense, Galen's περὶ ἀλυπίας definitely fills a gap in his production: this is the work where he best combines proofs of his superior nature, of his moral awareness, and of his drive towards posterity. If Galen's concern for his legacy is apparent in many works of his later period, as shown above, only the περὶ ἀλυπίας brings together with such intensity and effectiveness all the strings of Galen's last push towards immortality. The factual details of a defining event, the 192 catastrophe that struck him and so many of his contemporaries, help build a truly resilient figure and a towering moral individual.

Others have rightly stressed Galen's apparent humility in the περὶ ἀλυπίας: far from boasting of his resilience, Galen emphasises the limits of his powers of resistance, both physical and psychological.[46] Under Commodus, Galen was not exempt from fear (*Ind.* 54–55); and he would not want to undergo the tortures of the Phalaris bull (*Ind.* 71). His core aspiration, in this later period of his life, is health (*Ind.* 74). In confessing his vulnerability in the wake of this proof of resilience, Galen probably scores higher than a standard, heroic Stoic. Galen's περὶ ἀλυπίας thus portrays him in a special light, that of a humble creature eager to outlive Commodean terror, to enjoy his home and to finish his job as a medical author. In so doing, is Galen not distancing himself from the standard old man posture of imperial literature? Is he not giving us more than the strength of character involved in μεγαλοψυχία? While he plays on a number of commonplaces and standard *exempla* in his argument, and uses well-known literary quoting liberally, Galen, through a sincere self-assessment, succeeds in portraying himself as the quintessentially honest and strong gentleman he has always advocated for others.

Galen's confessed vulnerability in the περὶ ἀλυπίας should not be downplayed. In confessing fear during the reign of Commodus, for himself and for his friends, fear at the prospect of exile or excessive physical pain; in reporting

---

46   See for instance V. Boudon-Millot and J. Jouanna, *Galien. Ne pas se chagriner*, intr. pp. liii–lv.

others' collapse through similar experiences (for example the grammarian who lost everything to the great fire and died of sorrow, *Ind.* 7), Galen displays a facet of his personality that is, as far as I am aware, hardly ever highlighted: he offsets his tale of μεγαλοψυχία with expression of natural human feelings. This chimes with rare passages highlighted above, such as his indignant stance against rogue practitioners in *Simple drugs*; or the prospect of death in the same work, and the fear that he will unable to complete his project. Thus Galen's vulnerability may not be due simply to the familiar context of a letter; according to me, it is deliberately underscored as part of Galen's finishing strokes to his self-portrait, as the necessary counterpart to his moral and intellectual excellence. Humbly affirming his uncertainties and emotions, though downplaying them for the sake of rhetorical and social conventions, Galen may seem no exception in the light of recent scholarship.[47] But it must be stressed that Galen does so consciously, and purposefully: indeed, the last section of the treatise is a personal comment following up on what he thinks is an accurate answer to his addressee's question (how does he avoid distress, in the face of such adversity?): in *Ind.* 70–78 in particular, Galen insists that he is not inaccessible to the feelings of fear and sorrow that he has seemingly beaten. As a precise qualification (διορισμός) offseting the narrative of resilience that has dominated his treatise, this section builds on hints Galen gave his reader earlier on about the draining circumstances of living at court under a tyrant. It also mentions health and disease as essential components, not of happiness, but simply of "absence of distress" (ἀλυπία). Galen does not want to come across as this infallible, invincible human citadel he has been describing all along. He lists all the circumstances that could break him, and he prays to the gods to spare him such events that he may not overcome. He therefore deliberately brings in humility and vulnerability as the finishing touches to his self-portrait. The importance of this last twist to his argument is underpinned by the very phrasing of *Ind.* 70, in which he uses his signature coordinating device ἀτὰρ οὖν καί, which he seldom uses, perhaps once per work, but always with a view to emphasise an important moment in his argument.[48] Prayer (εὔχομαι), too, is an unusual word in Galen's texts, highlighting his loathing and fear of any unnecessary toils. He is thus offering an original take on the characteristic old man of rhetorical treatises – and cunningly playing on his reader's expectations in this respect.

---

47   Cf. Harris, G. W., *Dignity and Vulnerability. Strength and Quality of Character*, University of California Press, 1997; McCoy, M., *Wounded Heroes. Vulnerability as a Virtue in Ancient Greek Literature and Philosophy*, Oxford, OUP, 2013.

48   C. Petit, 'Greek particles in Galen's *Œuvre*' (forthcoming).

5   Conclusion

Galen's self-characterisation is an ongoing, long-term process that starts off in his earlier works and becomes finalised, quite logically, in the works of his old age. It is an important component of his diverse compositional strategies, aiming at presenting himself under the best possible light to his educated audience of students and *philiatroi*. In so doing, Galen demonstrates his sound rhetorical training and his acute awareness of the power of words. The image conveyed by Galen's later works exudes humility and detachment, whilst also highlighting his exceptional experience and intellectual honesty. A gentleman unafraid of displaying his vulnerabilities, Galen bares his profound nature to his readers, taking the last opportunities offered by his remarkable longevity to bring essential finishing touches to his self-portrait. Whilst this self-portrait will never be really complete for us, due to the loss of part of his works, characteristically the περὶ ἀλυπίας brings added insight into Galen's psyche and self-assessment. It chimes with other extant works, hinting at a humble, authentic and vulnerable scholar whose chief purpose and desire is to finish the immense task he has set for himself, and whose core values remain *philanthropia*, friendship, a simple life, and self-respect. Galen's περὶ ἀλυπίας may convey the views of a philosopher;[49] it may reflect the concerns of a man potentially compromised by his status as court physician to a despicable, recently assassinated emperor;[50] it certainly completes Galen's conscious self-portrait in view of posterity. Galen's concern for his intellectual and practical legacy comes through in many of his later works; in the περὶ ἀλυπίας it revolves around his moral fortitude as well as his lack of heroism in the face of adversity. Combined with his conscious, repeatedly asserted authorial project and the strong sense of responsibility that accompanies it, this display of authenticity creates a powerful intellectual and personal testament.

There is no easy way to untangle the real from the fictional Galen, especially in this later part of his life, when his authorial voice seemed shaped by urgency and anxiety (of influence, at least). There is nevertheless a case to be made for an enquiry into Galen's last years: however speculative, such investigations are unseparable from the analysis for his post-192 production. If Galen, as an author, wears a mask, this was, for his learned readers, a transparent one; his conscious play on the literary and philosophical codes of his time could only delight his *hetairoi* (not fool them). It is important to bear in mind

---

49   As shown in the thorough analyses of this text by Peter Singer, Christopher Gill, Jim Hankinson and Teun Tieleman in this volume.

50   A path explored by Matthew Nicholls in this volume.

Galen's essentially artificial *persona*. But, like his advisory dreams and his patient encounters, Galen's allusions to imminent death, tyranny, or unsavoury practices in his later years are all rooted in his personal experience. By all accounts, his περὶ ἀλυπίας is the most troubling testimony about his life to date; it shines back, in turn, on other later works and illuminates their significance and urgency.

Acknowledgements

I am grateful to Simon Swain and the anonymous referee for their helpful comments on earlier versions of this paper.

References

Billault, A., *L'univers de Philostrate*, Bruxelles, 2000.

Boudon-Millot, V., *Galien de Pergame. Un médecin grec à Rome*, Paris, Les Belles Lettres, 2012.

Boudon-Millot, V. and Jouanna, J., *Galien. Ne pas se chagriner*, Paris, Les Belles Lettres (avec la collaboration d'A. Pietrobelli), 2010.

Boudon-Millot, V., *Galien. Œuvres, Tome I*. Paris, Les Belles Lettres, 2007.

Gourevitch D. & Grmek, M. D., '*Medice, cura te ipsum*. Les maladies de Galien', *Etudes de Lettres*, 1986, 45–64.

Harlow, M. and Lawrence, R., "Viewing the old: recording and respecting the elderly at Rome and in the Empire", in C. Krötzl and K. Mustakallio, *On Old Age. Approaching Death in Antiquity and the Middle Ages*, Brepols, 2011, 3–24.

Harlow, M. and Lawrence, R., *Growing up and Growing old in ancient Rome: A Lifecourse Approach*, Routledge, 2001.

Harris, G. W., *Dignity and Vulnerability. Strength and Quality of Character*, University of California Press, 1997.

Kudlien, F., "Zum Thema 'Homer und die Medizin'", *Rheinisches Museum* 108, 1965, 293–299.

McCoy, M., *Wounded Heroes. Vulnerability as a Virtue in Ancient Greek Literature and Philosophy*, Oxford, OUP, 2013.

Minois, G., *Histoire de la vieillesse en Occident*, Paris, Fayard, 1987.

Morand, A. F., '« Chimie » de la vieillesse. Explications galéniques de cet âge de la vie', In L. Mathilde Cambron-Goulet and Laetitia Monteils-Laeng (ed.), *La Vieillesse dans l'Antiquité, entre déchéance et sagesse, Cahiers des études anciennes* 55, 2018, pp. 125–143.

Nutton, V., 'Galen and the Rhetoric of Certainty' in J. Coste/D. Jacquart/J.Pigeaud (eds.), *La rhétorique médicale à travers les siècles*, Genève, Droz, 2012, 39–49.

Nutton, V., 'Galen's Philosophical Testament', in J. Wiesner ed., *Aristoteles. Werk und Wirkung, Paul Moraux gewidmet* Berlin/New York, vol. II, 1987, 27–51.

Nutton, V., 'Galen in the eyes of his contemporaries', *BHM* 58, 1984, 315–324.

Parkin, T. G., *Old Age in the Roman World: A Cultural and Social History*, Johns Hopkins University Press, 2003.

Pernot, L., '*Periautologia*. Problèmes et méthodes de l'éloge de soi-même dans la tradition éthique et rhétorique gréco-romaine', *Revue des Etudes grecques* 111–1, 1998, pp. 101–124.

Petit, C., 'Galen, Pharmacology and the Boundaries of Medicine: A Reassessment', in M. Martelli and L. Lehmhaus eds., *Collecting Recipes: Byzantine and Jewish Pharmacology in Dialogue*, De Gruyter, 2017, 50–80.

Petit, C. 'Symphorien Champier (1471–1539) et Galien: Médecine et littérature à la Renaissance', to appear in C. La Charité & R. Menini eds., *La médecine au temps de Rabelais*, forthcoming.

Petit, C., 'Greek particles in Galen's *Oeuvre*', forthcoming.

Petit, C., *Galien ou la rhétorique de la Providence. Médecine, littérature et pouvoir à Rome*, Brill, 2018.

Rutherford, I., 'The poetics of the *Paraphthegma*: Aelius Aristides and the Decorum of self-praise', in D. Innes/H. Hine/ C. Pelling (eds), *Ethics and Rhetoric. Classical essays for Donald Russell on his Seventy-Fifth Birthday*, Oxford, 1995, pp. 193–204.

Singer, P. N., *Galen. Psychological Writings*, Cambridge, CUP, 2013.

Skenazi, C., *Aging Gracefully in the Renaissance. Stories of Later Life from Petrarch to Montaigne*, Brill, 2013.

Swain, S. C. R., 'Beyond the Limits of Greek Biography: Galen from Alexandria to the Arabs', in B. McGing and J. Mossman (eds), *The Limits of Ancient Biography*, The Classical Press of Wales, 2006, pp. 395–433.

Von Staden, H., 'Character and competence. Personal and professional conduct in Greek medicine', in H. Flashar/J. Jouanna (eds), *Médecine et morale dans l'antiquité. Entretiens de la Fondation Hardt vol. 43*, Genève, Droz, 1997, 157–195.

Woerther, F., *L'èthos aristotélicien. Genèse d'une notion rhétorique*, Paris, 2007.

CHAPTER 3

Galen and the Language of Old Comedy: Glimpses of a Lost Treatise at *Ind.* 23b–28

Amy Coker

Towards the middle of the περὶ ἀλυπίας, Galen singles out as a particular loss in the fire of AD 192 a treatise he had produced on the vocabulary of Old Comedy (*Ind.* 20–28). Galen describes this work in some detail at 23b–28, as follows:[1]

> But Fate ambushed me, by destroying, along with many other of my books, most especially my work on the vocabulary of the entire of Old Comedy [τὴν τῶν ὀνομάτων πραγματείαν …τῆς παλαιᾶς κωμῳδίας ὅλης], (24a) of which, as you know, Didymus had already made a study, both the everyday words and those requiring explanation [τὰ πολιτικὰ …τά τε γλωττηματικὰ πάντα], in fifty books, of which I made an epitome in 6,000 lines. (24b) Such a procedure seemed to be of some value for orators and grammarians, or in general for anyone who might want to use an Attic idiom [ἢ οἵτινες ὅλως ἀττικίζειν βούλοιντο], (25) or words that have a significant bearing on practicalities, like the question that arose recently in Rome when a respected doctor announced that groats were not yet in use [οὔπω τὴν χρῆσιν εἶναι τοῦ χόνδρου] in the time of Hippocrates, and that that was why in *Regimen in Acute Diseases* he advocated barley gruel [πτισάνην] over all other cereal foodstuffs; for if groats had been known to the Greeks, he would not have chosen anything else in preference. (26) But groats are mentioned particularly in *Regimen for Health*, which some ascribe to him but others to Philistion or Ariston, both very early doctors [ἀνδρῶν παλαιοτάτων], and also in the writers of Old Comedy [ἀλλὰ καὶ παρὰ τοῖς παλαιοῖς κωμικοῖς]. Words like *abudokomas* or *aburtakē*[2]

---

1 Trans. Nutton in Singer, *Galen. Psychological Writings*, 2013, pp. 85–6; the Greek text follows Boudon-Millot *et al.*, *Galien. Ne pas se chagriner* (2010) (= BJP), with the exception of the emendation at the end of 26 by Polemis, see n. 2.

2 BJP print here Ἀριστομένει ἢ Ἀριστοφάνει, understanding the difficult sequence of letters in the manuscript as concealing the names of comic poets; Polemis (2011) 3–4 instead conjectures – I believe correctly – two obscure words in the Accusative Singular ἀβυδοκόμαν ἢ ἀβυρτάκην, and is followed by Nutton (2013). The significance of these two words is discussed below. Polemis (2011) 4 also suggests a change in punctuation in the passage, and that the

<and> (27) whatever else was unclear to the audience were defined in our treatise – and was anticipated nicely in Didymus' exposition – as follows: emmer, chick peas, vetch, groats and the other cereals, vegetables and late-summer fruits, wines made from the marc of grapes, with or without the addition of water, bushes, fruits, plants, animals, instruments, equipment, tools, and everything else in daily life, and their names. (28) My selection of such words in Old Comedy [τὰ μὲν οὖν (λοιπὰ) ἐκ τῆς παλαιᾶς κωμῳδίας ἐξειλεγμένα τῶν τοιούτων ὀνομάτων] had not yet been transferred to Campania, but luckily my selection from prose authors already had, in forty-eight large books, of which those with the equivalent of more than 4,000 hexameter lines will perhaps have to be divided in two.

It is clear from the detailed exposition in this passage, and comments elsewhere in the Galenic corpus, that the language of Old Comedy was important for Galen, valuable as both a model of clarity of expression, and because of its practical utility in solving questions about the text of Hippocrates. None of Galen's works on Old Comedy have however survived. Rather than focussing on how Galen frames these losses listed here within the broader rhetorical strategy of the *Peri alupias*,[3] this chapter takes this passage as a starting point for discussion of what Galen's monumental treatise on the vocabulary of Old Comedy lost in the fire would have looked like, using clues from both the *Peri alupias*, and mentions of comedy scattered throughout the rest of the Galenic corpus. In doing so, this chapter raises questions about the place of Galen within the wider literary culture of second-century AD Rome, rather than considering him solely as a physician or philosopher.

Firstly, after discussing in brief the place of Old Comedy within Galen's view of language,[4] quotations from comic texts in the works of Galen extant in Greek are collected in order to allow an overview of his preferred authors, suggesting perhaps the range of authors included in the lost work. Secondly, a close reading of the final part *Ind.* 23b–28 allows further speculation about the source-texts and format of Galen's work on Old Comedy, as well as about

---

words ἀλλὰ καὶ παρὰ τοῖς παλαιοῖς κωμικοῖς should be taken with what follows them, not with what proceeds. On this basis, with a full stop after 'doctors' in Nutton's version, an English translation might read 'But also from the playwrights of Old Comedy, the words *Abudokomēs* or *aburtakē*, and/or <ἤ> others not clear to the audience were defined in our treatise – and was anticipated nicely in Didymus' exposition – as follows'. Sense-wise, it is difficult to chose between either version, although see the comments in n. ooo, this chapter.

3 On which see Rosen (2014).

4 A study of the use of the vocabulary of Old Comedy itself within Galen's Greek is beyond the scope of this chapter, and a desideratum of future work.

his working practices more broadly. As will be shown, Galen's *oeuvre* has more in common with lexicographically-informed works of the second century AD, and Galen with their authors whom he pejoratively labels 'sophists', than his scathing remarks about their linguistic endeavours sometimes suggest.[5]

1   Galen's Atticism & Galen's Comedy

Despite writing at a period of fervent interest in the revival of Attic Greek as the aspirational standard of the educated man,[6] it is well known that Galen is criti-cal of those who seek to reproduce apparent Attic norms for their own sake, especially if this is at the expense of clarity.[7] For Galen, it is precision above all which should dictate matters of linguistic expression. Adherence to strict antiquarian norms are not useful *per se*, but some words from the *sunētheia* of the Classical past – if used correctly – can be tools for maintaining clarity: this is explicit in Galen's own words at the end of his treatise *The Order of My Own Books*:[8]

> It was because of the number of doctors and philosophers who lay down new meanings for Greek words [...] for this reason I made this commen-tary on the words which I collected in forty-six books from the Attic prose-writers (and some others from the comic poets [καθάπερ ἐκ τῶν κωμικῶν ἄλλα]).[9] The work is, as I have explained, written for the sake of the actual objects signified; at the same time, the reader gains a knowledge of Attic vocabulary, **though this is of no great value in itself** [σὺν τούτῳ δ' εὐθέως ὑπάρχει τοῖς ἀναγνωσομένοις αὐτὰ καὶ ἡ τῶν Ἀττικῶν ὀνομάτων γνῶσις οὐδὲν αὐτὴ καθ' ἑαυτὴν ἄξιον ἔχουσα μεγάλης σπουδῆς]. Because of those who

---

5   Nutton (2009) 34 highlights this as a distinct – albeit perhaps controversial – possibility, cf. Kollesch (1981). As Zadorojnyi (2013) 389 puts it, "Notwithstanding his dislike of 'sophistry', Galen is a dextrous (if grouchy) self-promoter well-versed in the challenges and strategems of the Second Sophistic."

6   See Kim (2010) for a recent state-of-the-art account of linguistic archaism in the first two centuries AD, which stresses the internal variety of Atticism; Swain (1996) and Schmitz (1997) are now classic works on the topic.

7   See for example von Staden (1995) 516 with further references, and Sluiter (1995); Hankinson (1994), esp. 171–180, dicusses Galen's principles of naming, as does Morison (2008); Barnes (1997) explores Galen's apparently "schizophrenic" attitude to language, ambivalence mixed with strictness.

8   *Ord. Lib. Prop.* 5.4–6 (= XIX.61 K.) ed. Boudon-Millot, trans. Singer (1997) 28–9.

9   The same work on prose mentioned at *Ind.* 28, and listed by Galen in *Lib. Prop.* 20.1 (see below n. 17), as being in 48 books.

use words badly, however, I composed another work, on their correctness [πραγματεία περὶ τῆς ὀρθότητος αὐτῶν] – a work, in fact, which would be best read first of all.

Here it can be seen that it is the misuse of vocabulary with novel meanings which riles Galen – a concern he held in common with the Atticist lexicographers – and it is for this reason that he produced a work for the specific purpose of elucidating the proper meaning of words.[10] These works are not catalogues of philological ornaments, as the efforts of those who 'hyper-Atticise' were sometimes characterised by the more satirical commentators of the period.[11] Such works are associated in particular with Phrynichus and his ilk, a kind of scholarly enterprise from which Galen seeks to distance himself, despite sharing much common ground.

The most overt indication that it is words from Attic Comedy, as opposed to those from other varieties of the Classical language, which for Galen are the most useful in maintaining his principle of clarity, is found in the first book of the Περὶ τῶν ἰατρικῶν ὀνομάτων, or De nominibus medicis 'On Medical Names' (Med. Nom.), a text which survives only in Arabic translation.[12] Here Galen tells us it is Aristophanes' usage of words which should be followed as a model because of the intelligibility of the language of the comic theatre for the populace in general.[13] This explains in part why in Galen's other catalogue of his works, On My Own Books, no fewer than five treatises on comedy and comic playwrights are listed (Lib. Prop. 20.1 = XIX.48 K.). Going by their titles which, notwithstanding any new discoveries is all that survives of these works, there is one on the vocabulary of each of the 'big three' playwrights of Old Comedy (Cratinus, Aristophanes and Eupolis),[14] and two more general works, one on

---

10   Perhaps to be identified with the work entitled Ἀττικῶν παράσημα listed at Lib. Prop. 20.2, see n. 17, but otherwise unknown.

11   See for example the figure of the teacher of rhetoric in Lucian's Praeceptor rhetorum, esp. 17; compare Galen's own comments at PHP 5.7.42.

12   Meyerhof & Schacht (1931) gives the Arabic text and translation into German; a brief history of its transmission in Arabic and Syriac is given at (1931) 4; Deichgräber (1957) discusses the text and its significance for Galen's principles of naming. On comedy and clarity see von Staden (1995) 81–2.

13   Meyerhof & Schacht (1931) 31–3 (= 103v–104v).

14   On vocabulary current at the time of Eupolis, three books (τῶν παρ' Εὐπόλιδι πολιτικῶν ὀνομάτων τρία), On vocabulary current at the time of Aristophanes, five books (τῶν παρὰ Ἀριστοφάνει πολιτικῶν ὀνομάτων πέντε), On vocabulary current at the time of Cratinus, two books (τῶν παρὰ Κρατίνῳ πολιτικῶν ὀνομάτων δύο). πολιτικά is taken to mean 'everyday', as for example Nutton (2009) 30 n. 76 and Rosen (2014) 168, against other translations as

vocabulary found only in comic plays,[15] and one on the utility of Old Comedy as reading for students.[16] A number of other works on language are also listed in this final section of *On My Own Books* under τὰ τοῖς γραμματικοῖς καὶ ῥήτορσι κοινά,[17] but not the 6,000 line epitome of Didymus on Old Comedy mentioned in the *Peri alupias*.[18] Presumably after the destruction of this work in AD 192 Galen did not (or could not, through the loss of his source texts) reproduce it or, if he did, he reworked or rearranged the material so that it could be called by a different name, and it lurks behind one of the titles Galen lists in catalogues of his own works.

The loss of all of Galen's works on Old Comedy necessitates an alternative approach to the matter of which comic texts or comic playwrights he is using or reading. The list below stands as a first pass at capturing mentions of comedy and comic playwrights in Galen's extant works, assembled through electronically searching the online *Thesaurus Linguae Graecae* (*TLG*).[19] This is an admittedly crude approach and does not claim to provide a comprehensive account of Comedy in Galen, yet produces a larger amount of material than hitherto collected, and allows some positive statements to be made about the

---

'political'. Sluiter (1995) 524 suggests an opposition in Galen of language which is normal or proper (πολιτικός), and that which is rhetorical.

15   *Examples of words peculiar to comedy, one book* (τῶν ἰδίων κωμικῶν ὀνομάτων παραδείγματα ἕν).

16   *If old comedy is useful reading for students* (εἰ χρήσιμον ἀνάγνωσμα τοῖς παιδευομένοις ἡ παλαιὰ κωμῳδία), perhaps reminiscent of Plutarch's earlier *Comparison of Aristophanes and Menander* (*Mor.* 853a–854d).

17   At 20.1 is listed τῶν παρὰ τοῖς Ἀττικοῖς συγγραφεῦσιν ὀνομάτων ὀκτὼ καὶ τεσσαράκοντα (*On the vocabulary of Attic writers, forty eight books*), and at 20.2 πρὸς τοὺς ἐπιτιμῶντας τοῖς σολοικίζουσι τῇ φωνῇ ἑπτά (*Against those who are critical of the authors of solecisms in their language, seven books*); Ἀττικῶν παράσημα ἕν (*Improprieties in Attic, one book*); περὶ σαφηνείας καὶ ἀσαφείας (*On clarity and obscurity*); εἰ δύναταί τις εἶναι κριτικὸς καὶ γραμματικός ἕν (*If one can be at the same time critic and grammarian, one book*). Morison (2008) 116–7 gives a convenient list of Galen's works on language, Skoda (2001) a sketch of his lexicographical interests; she dubs Galen "un amateur de lexicologie et de linguistique" (p. 194).

18   At *Ind.* 28 Galen tells us that 4000 hexameter lines is around the upper limit for the length of a single book, suggesting perhaps that Galen's epitome was in two books. On ancient book lengths see *BJP* ad loc (pp. 94–5), and especially Johnson (2004) 87–8, 143–60, who stresses the complexity of identifying a standard length for a papyrus bookroll.

19   http://stephanus.tlg.uci.edu/. Searches took place in June 2014, and were checked again in May 2015. The initial search strings were κωμικ, κωμῳδ (to catch general references), ἀριστοφ, κρατιν, εὐπολ, μενανδ (for playwrights) and λυσιστρ, θεσμοφ, βατραχο, εκκλησι, πλουτο, αχαρν, ιππε, νεφελα, σφηκ, ειρην, ορνιθ (as a sample for finding plays, based around the eleven extant complete plays of Aristophanes). All texts listed in the *TLG* under "Galen" and "Ps-Galen" were searched, with "Ps-Galen" yielding no results.

extent of Galen's knowledge of ancient comic texts.[20] Quotations are listed first (1.1), with the quoted text in footnotes, followed by additional mentions of names of plays, playwrights, or 'a comic poet' divided into those which make linguistic comment (1.2) and those which are more general (1.3).[21]

1.1 Quotations from Comic Plays in Galen

Hipp. Art. XVIIIa.340 K.	Eupolis, *fr.* 60 K-A (Αὐτόλυκος α' β', *Autolycus*)[22]
Aff. Dig. 7.10 (*CMG* V 4.1.1) (= v.38 K.)	Eupolis, *fr.* *105 K-A (Δῆμοι, *Demes*)[23]
Diff. Puls. VIII.653 K.	Eupolis, *fr.* *116 K-A (Δῆμοι, *Demes*)[24]
Dig. Puls. VIII.943 K.	Eupolis, *fr.* *116 K-A (Δῆμοι, *Demes*) (= *previous note*)
SMT 11.37 (= XII. 360 K.)	Aristophanes, *Birds* 471 (Ὄρνιθες, *Birds*)[25]
Gloss. XIX.113 K.	Aristophanes, *Acharnians* 872 (Ἀχαρνῆς, *Acharnians*)[26]
Gloss. XIX.66–7 K.	Aristophanes, *fr.* 205 K-A (Δαιταλῆς, *Banqueters*)[27]

---

20   Some quotes from Comedy in Galen are listed in Nutton (2009) 29–31, who also considers Galen's reading of classical literature more broadly; compare too the collection by von Staden (1998) 81–2, n. 56. As a check, all the citations given under Galen in the index to Rusten (2011) 740 are captured by this method: the true test will be when the volume of *Indices* to *Poetae Comici Graeci* appears. De Lacy (1966) is more limited than its title suggests.

21   Excluded are examples of κωμῳδ found in a doublet τραγῳδία καὶ κωμῳδία *vel sim.* where these refer to comic competition or performance, e.g. *Comp. Med. Loc.* XIII.6 K., *UP* IV.356 K., *Hipp. Epid.* XVIIa.507 K.; there is also κωμικοὶ καὶ τραγικοὶ ποιηταί at *PHP* 5.7.43, and *HNH* XV.24 K. (= *comm.* 1.2, on which see n. 58), cf. also von Staden (1998) 68 n. 12, 70 n. 25. Examples of the search words in *Lib. Prop.* and *Ord. Lib. Prop.* are also excluded.

22   Eupolis, *fr.* 60 K-A: (A.) ἐπὶ καινοτέρας ἰδέας ἀσεβῆ βίον, ὦ μοχθηρός, ἔτριβες. (B) πῶς ὧ πολλῶν ἤδη λοπάδων τοὺς ἄμβωνας περιλείξας; Galen quotes the second half of the second line: "καὶ τις τῶν κωμικῶν ἐπεῖπειν ἐπισκώπτων τινὰ δὴ τῶν λοπάδων τοὺς ἄμβωνας περιλείχειν". The quotation in Galen is identified in Manetti (2009) 165.

23   Eupolis, *fr.* *105 K-A: (A.) † ἡτίας ὢν † ἐγένου δίκαιος οὕτω διαπρεπῶς; | (Ἀρ.) ἡ μὲν φύσις τὸ μέγιστον <ἦν>, ἔπειτα δὲ | κἀγὼ προθύμως τῆι φύσει συνελάμβανον.

24   Eupolis, *fr.* *116 K-A: λαλεῖν ἄριστος, ἀδυνατώτατος λέγειν. Also probably quoted at *Med. Nom.* (Meyerhof-Schacht 1931, 31 = 102v).

25   Aristophanes, *Birds* 471: ἀμαθὴς γὰρ ἔφυς κοὺ πολυμπράγμων, οὐδ' Αἴσωπον πεπάτηκας. Kühn's text of Galen has μεμάθηκας as the final word.

26   *Gloss* XIX.313 K.: κόλλικας· τοὺς τροχίσκους· καὶ τὸ ἐν Ἀχαρνεῦσι, κολλικοφάγε βοιώτιε, ἐπὶ τῶν σμικρῶν ἀρτίσκων εἴρηται; *Acharnians* 872 (OCT) ὦ χαῖρε, κολλικοφάγε Βοιωτίδιον.

27   Aristophanes, *fr.* 205 K-A: (A.) ἀλλ' εἰ σορέλλη καὶ μύρον καὶ ταινίαι. | (B.) ἰδοὺ σορέλλη· τοῦτο παρὰ Λυσιστράτου. | (A.) ἦ μὴν ἴσως σὺ καταπλιγήσηι τῶι χρόνωι. | (B.) τὸ καταπλιγήσηι τοῦτο

Gloss. XIX.65 K.	Aristophanes, *fr.* 233 K-A
	(*Δαιταλῆς, Banqueters*)[28]
Alim. Fac. 1.27.1 (*CMG* V 4.2)	Aristophanes, *fr.* 428 K-A
(=VI.541 K.)	(*Ὁλκάδες, Merchant Ships*)[29]
Hipp. Aph. XVIIIa.148 K.	Aristophanes, *fr.* 526 K-A
	(*Ταγηνισταί, Fry Cooks*)[30]
Hipp. Fract. XVIIIb.347 K.	Aristophanes, *fr.* 630 K-A
	(*incerta fabula*)[31]
Med. Nom (Reconstructed from	Aristophanes, *fr.* 346 K-A
Arabic, see Deichgräber 1957)	(*Θεσμοφοριάζουσαι β'*)
Hipp. Aph. 7.149 (*CMG* V 4.1.2)	Plato (= Plato comicus) *fr.* 200 K-A
(= XVIIIa.149 K.)	(*incerta fabula*)[32]
Qual. Incorp. XIX.467 K.	Menander, *fr.* 477 K-A
	(*incerta fabula*)[33]
PHP 4.6.34 (= V.412 K.)	Menander, *fr.* 476 K-A
	(*incerta fabula*)[34]
Diff. Puls. VIII.656 K.	*Adespota fr.* 229 K-A[35]
Hipp. Art. XVIIIa.531 K.	"Aristophanes", according to Galen[36]
Di. Dec. IX.814–5 K.	'The Comic'[37]

παρὰ τῶν ῥητόρων. | (A.) ἀποβήσεταί σοι ταῦτά ποι τὰ ῥήματα. | (B.) παρ' Ἀλκιβιάδου τοῦτο τἀ-ποβήσεται. | (A.) τί ὑποτεκμαίρηι καὶ κακῶς ἄνδρας λέγεις | καλοκἀγαθίαν ἀσκοῦντας; (B.) οἴμ' ὦ Θρασύμαχε, | τίς τοῦτο τῶν ξυνηγόρων τερατεύεται; There are a large number of differences between Kühn's text of Galen and the fragment reconstructed in *PCG*.

28 Aristophanes, *fr.* 233 K-A: πρὸς ταύτας δ' αὖ λέξον Ὁμήρου γλώττας· τί καλοῦσι κόρυμβα; | ˘ ˘˘-˘˘-˘˘-˘˘- τί καλοῦσ' ἀμενηνὰ κάρηνα; | (B.) ὁ μὲν οὖν σός, ἐμὸς δ' οὗτος ἀδελφὸς φρασάτω· τί καλοῦσιν ἰδύους; | ˘˘-˘˘-˘˘-˘˘-˘˘- τί ποτ' ἐστὶν ὀπύειν;

29 Aristophanes, *fr.* 428 K-A: ἀράκους, πυρούς, πτισάνην, χόνδρον, ζείας, αἴρας, σεμίδαλιν.

30 Aristophanes, *fr.* 526 K-A: κατὰ δὲ τὸν αὐτὸν τρόπον ἀμφαριστερὸν Ἀριστοφάνης εἶπεν ἐν Ταγηνίταις [*sic*] ἄνθρωπον ἀμφοτέρωθεν ἀριστερόν.

31 Aristophanes, *fr.* 630 K-A: χωρεῖ πὶ γραμμὴν λορδὸς ὡς <εἰς> ἐμβολήν.

32 Plato comicus, *fr.* 200 K-A: μετὰ ταῦτα δὲ | † Εὐαγόρου ὁ παῖς ἐκ πλευρίτιδος Κινησίας † | σκελετός, ἄπυγος, καλάμινα σκέλη φορῶν, | φθόης προφήτης, ἐσχάρας κεκαυμένος | πλείστας ὑπ' Εὐρυφῶντος ἐν τῶι σώματι.

33 Menander, *fr.* 477 K-A: ταῦτα σ' ἀπολώλεκ', ὦ πονηρέ; as with *fr.* 476, introduced as τὸ Μενάνδρειον.

34 Menander, *fr.* 476 K-A: [˘/- - - ˘ -] τὸν νοῦν ἔχων ὑποχείριον | εἰς τὸν πίθον δέδωκα (δέδυκα Cobet).

35 *Adespota fr.* 229 K-A: οὔτε στρεβλὸν ὀρθοῦται ξύλον | † οὔτε γεράνδρυον † μετατεθὲν μοσχεύεται.

36 εἴπερ δὴ κρανέω γε καὶ εἰ τετελεσμένον ἔσται given as a quotation; see below, p. 72.

37 καὶ σπάνιόν ἐστ' ἄνθρωπος ὅτ' ἄνθρωπος given as a quotation; see below, p. 72.

1.2   Additional 'Linguistic' Observations without Quotation

SMT XI.450 K.	On spelling (χυλός/χυμός)
HVA XV.455 K.	Comic poets using the word χόνδρος
(= comm. 1.17 CMG V 9.1)	
Alim. Fac. 3.15.11 (CMG V 4.2)	Comic poets using the word πυριάτη
(= VI.694 K.)	
Hipp. Art. XVIIIa.385 K.	Explanation of τιμωρεούσας using the title of a play by Menander (Αὐτὸν τιμωρούμενος test. ii K-A)

1.3   Reports of Jokes and Other Observations without Quotation

Hipp. Epid. XVIIb.263 K.	Mockery of Socrates in Aristophanes' *Clouds*
(= comm. VI, 5.11 CMG V 10.2.2)	
Hipp. Epid. XVIIa.819 K.	Comic poets joking about the size of Pericles' head
(= comm. VI, 1.3 CMG V 10.2.2)	
QAM IV.784 K.	Hippocrates' sons as exemplars of foolishness
HVA XV. 424 K.	Example from Eupolis, Αὐτόλυκος β
(=comm. 1.4 CMG V 9.1)	(Eupolis, *Autolycus* test. ii K-A)
Nat. Fac. II.67 K.	Menander as a writer of comedy (Menander test. 115 K-A) (passage below, pp. 74–5)

The most immediate feature of this collection is its paucity; even if one allows for citations which have not been captured by these electronic searches, such as those labelled with playwright names or play titles not searched for, relative to the size of the Galenic corpus this collection of examples is very small. Perhaps this indicates that Galen restricted his discussion of comedy relatively strictly to those treatises explicitly on comedy, or rather that Galen just does not give a reference for quotations when used: this may be the case with the as yet unidentified line from *On Critical Days* (*Di. Dec.* IX.814–5 K., last item of [1.11]) which has at least the benefit of being tagged as "comic".[38]

As can be seen, comic material is used widely in the commentaries on Hippocrates,[39] echoing Nutton's comments on Galen's use of Classical litera-

---

38   This suggests the tantalising possibility that there are other unidentified snippets of ancient literature still hidden in the Galenic corpus.

39   As well as several times in *Diff. Puls.*, a work in which according to Hankinson (2008) 173, "irritations over language are a constant refrain"; metaphor is also discussed at length in this work, see von Staden (1995), esp. 500–13. On the commentaries in general, see

ture in general to elucidate Hippocratic texts.[40] Note too that in the *Peri alu-pias* passage, the problem given as an example of what Galen's work on Old Comedy could help solve is also Hippocratic in nature: were groats (χόνδρος, whole grains) in use in Hippocrates (the answer being yes, so the 'respected doctor in Rome' is wrong).[41]

In the Hippocratic commentaries, and elsewhere, comic material is some-times used to make points about language, but not always. As can be seen from the lists of citations which do not include quotations (1.2, 1.3), some do talk about language but many have rather an anecdotal quality, and refer to an-cient jokes or sayings as opposed to commenting on any philological content. Likewise, many of the direct quotations are given by Galen for their encyclope-dic or gnomic quality: we find for example Menander cited as part of a discus-sion on the loss of reason (*PHP* 4.6.34), Plato (the comic playwright) alongside the cautery of abscesses (*Hipp. Aph.* XVIII a.149 K), and Aristophanes' *Birds* in a discussion on larks (*SMT* XII.360 K., Περὶ κορύδων).[42] When it comes to linguistic matters, we find texts quoted to illustrate matters of spelling (*Alim. Fac.* 1.27.1 on the spelling of the name of ἄραχος, 'wild chickling'), vocabulary (words for left-handedness at *Hipp. Aph.* XVIIIa.148 K., the difference between λαλεῖν and λέγειν at *Diff. Puls.* VIII.653 K.) and on the invention of new words (*Gloss.* XIX.65–7 K.); at *Hipp. Art.* XVIIIa.385 K., the title of a play by Menander is adduced to explain the meaning of a tricky participle in Hippocrates (on which more shortly).

As to the material from which Galen was drawing these examples, the state-ment in *Med. Nom.* that Aristophanes is the best model is corroborated by the predominance of quotations from, and references to, this playwright in the ex-tant works. We could expect from the preservation of the titles of lost works by Galen on Cratinus, Aristophanes and Eupolis (see n. 14) that the first and last of these playwrights would also figure, and we do indeed find three quotations from Eupolis – but three only – and none from Cratinus. There is one quotation from Plato (comicus). Two of the Eupolis quotations are from Δῆμοι (*Demes*),

---

Manetti & Roselli (1994), esp. 1571–1575, and Hanson (1998) *passim* on what they reveal about Galen's attitude to authorship.

40   Nutton (2009) 29.

41   In the edition of *BJP*, and Nutton's translation as reproduced here, Galen gives the use of χόνδρος in Old Comedy as a witness to this problem; Polemis' repunctuation (see p. 63, n. 2) on the contrary construes 'from Old Comedy' with the description of the treatise which follows. Either way, Galen mentions this word as used in comedy (again) at *HVA* XV.455 K.

42   In a similar vein we have an Αἰσώπειος μῦθος at *Hipp. Prorrh.* XVI.614 K. and an Αἰσώπου λόγος at *Adv. Jul.* XVIIIa.291 K.; stories from Aesop also appear alongside the quotation from Aristophanes' *Birds*.

and while one of these is attached to the name of Eupolis (*fr.* *105 K-A), the other is introduced only by ὁ Κωμικός (*fr.* *116 K-A).[43] Does this suggest that for Galen Eupolis had a kind of pre-eminence, the same way that Homer is often simply "The Poet"? If this is the case, does this in turn imply that the line quoted at *Diff. Puls.* VIII.656 K. (= *Adespota fr.* 229 K-A) and introduced by "the Comic" should also be attributed to Eupolis? Even more speculatively, does it follow that there is an unseen quotation of Eupolis in the passage from *On Critical Days* (*Di. Dec.* IX.814–5 K.)?:

> ἔστι δ' ὅτε καὶ ἐξόχως καθ' ὑπεροχὴν ἔνια τὴν τοῦ γένους ὅλου προσηγορίαν σφετερίζεται, ὥσπερ καὶ παρὰ τῷ ποιητῇ λέγεσθαί φαμεν τόδε τι, οὐκ ἂν οὐ-δενὸς | ἄλλου παρὰ τὸν Ὅμηρον ἀκουομένου, καίτοι μυρίοι γ' εἰσὶν ἄλλοι ποι-ηταί. τοιοῦτον δ' ἐστὶ καὶ τὸ παρὰ τῷ Κωμικῷ· καὶ σπάνιόν ἐστ' ἄνθρωπος ὅτ' ἄνθρωπος.

> Sometimes a thing appropriates through its prominence the name of a whole class, just as when we say that something is said in the work of 'a poet', we understand only that it is in Homer and no-one else, even though there are countless other poets. This sort of thing is found in the Comic: '*a man who is just a man is a rare thing*'.

If the final words of this passage are indeed a quotation, as printed in Kühn they are almost a trimeter, with one syllable missing. Alternatively – and more likely – is that "The Comic" in this passage of *On Critical Days* is in fact Aristophanes, which would seem more likely on the basis of the prestige given him elsewhere by Galen, meaning that *fr.* *116 from Δῆμοι (*Demes*) is misattrib-uted by Galen, if we assume that he uses the label ὁ Κωμικός with any consis-tency. Have we caught Galen making a mistake? So too, Galen quotes a line he attributes to Aristophanes at *Hipp. Art.* XVIIIa. 530–1 K.:

> [...] τελευτῶσι δέ τοι οὗτοι δεσμοί, καθάπερ καὶ αὐτὸς ὁ νωτιαῖος ἄχρι τοῦ κατὰ τὴν | ῥάχιν πέρατος. ὠνόμασε δὲ αὐτὸς ὁ Ἱπποκράτης τὸ τελευτῶσιν ὁμοίως τῷ ποιητῇ Ἀριστοφάνει
> εἴπερ δὴ κρανέω γε καὶ εἰ τετελεσμένον ἔσται.[44]

---

43   Capital as Kühn. Both Plutarch (*Alcib.* 13.2) and Aulus Gellius (1.15.12) attribute the words of this fragment (*fr.* *116) to Eupolis.

44   The closest parallels I have been able to find is found are the Homeric line ὧδε γὰρ ἐξερέω, τὸ δὲ καὶ τετελεσμένον ἔσται 'for thus will I speak, and this thing shall be brought to pass' (found several times, with some initial variation e.g. *Iliad* 1.212, 8.401, 23.410, etc.) and a

This line does not appear among the fragments of Aristophanes in *PCG*, but nonetheless Galen thought it was Aristophanic. If there is misattribution in Galen in either of these examples (especially Eupolis, *fr.* *116), is this Galen slipping up, or his source? Or, more simply, does the use of the tag κωμικός imply Galen does not know from which poet this quotation comes? (And did he ever know?) This raises the question of the nature of Galen's sources for these quotations, and whether he is reading plays in full, or drawing only from compilations or lexica, as his reference to Didymus in the *Peri alupias* suggests.[45] There are similar examples of such misattribution in Latin texts of the late Republican and Imperial period which appear to indicate the use of anthologies, or similar sources, of ancient Greek comic plays, rather than engagement with complete texts.[46] It should be noted that most of the quotations are not introduced by Galen with anything approaching a modern-style reference, and in some examples are not obviously quotations: play names are given rarely,[47] and as we have seen poets are not always named in association with quoted words or lines.[48] Similarly, sometimes we find simply phrases such as παρὰ τοῖς παλαιοῖς κωμικοῖς οὕτως εὑρίσκεται (*SMT* XI.450 K.) or καλεῖν δ᾽ ἐοίκασιν οἱ παλαιοὶ κωμικοί (*Alim. Fac.* VI.694 K.), which apparently draw on Galen's knowledge of Old Comedy, but yet are unsubstantiated by examples. Galen's characteristically confident statements about wide reading of Classical texts should be treated with some considerable caution.[49] Before moving on to these questions of sources, a few words on Menander.

---

quotation at Plutarch *Mor.* 62e (*How to tell a flatterer from a friend*) εἰ δύναμαι τελέσαι γε καὶ εἰ τετελεσμένον ἐστί.

45   von Staden (1998) 68 n. 12 notes for example that some of Galen's quotations are probably at second hand.

46   See for example the misattributions collected by Ruffell (2014) 304 from Cicero, Valerius Maximus and Vitruvius; in Cicero (*Att.* 12.6a), a quotation from Eupolis mistakenly attributed to Aristophanes' *Acharnians* is corrected, see ibid p. 292, n. 64 on this example.

47   I found only *Gloss.* XIX.66 K. *Banqueters* (*twice*) and at 113 *Acharnians*; *SMT* XII.360 K. *Birds; Hipp. Aph.* XVIIIa.148 K. *Fry Cooks; Alim. Fac.* VI.541 K. *Merchant Ships; Hipp. Epid.* XVIIb.263 K. *Clouds*; and *HVA* XV.424 K. *Autolycus*. None of these play names recur elsewhere in Galen.

48   The names of playwrights are associated with quotations for example at *Aff. Dig.* V.38 K. (Eupolis), *Hipp. Fract.* XVIIIb.347 K. (Aristophanes) and *Hipp. Aph.* XVIIIa.149 K. (Plato comicus). Excluding Galen's catalogues of his own works, Aristophanes is named eight times in the extant Greek works, Eupolis twice.

49   We find such confidence in the rhetoric of control over his material at for example *Med. Nom.* (Meyerhof-Schacht 1931, 33 = 103r–104v): "Ich könnte dir nachweisen, daß alle Komödiendichter den Namen"Fieber" | in ihrer Redeweise ebenso anwenden, mit zahlreichen zum Beweise dienenden Belegstellen aus ihren Worten, mit denen man,

So far the discussion has centred around Old Comedy, since this makes up the bulk of the material in Galen, and indeed it is a work on ἡ παλαιά κωμῳδία specifically which Galen talks about in the *Peri alupias*.[50] However, there are a few references to Menander, a playwright of New Comedy.[51] This is perhaps surprising, especially the philological point on the meaning of τιμωρεούσας noted at *Hipp. Art.* xviiia.385 K since Menander's Greek was not universally accepted as a model for 'good Attic' in the first few centuries AD.[52] For Galen, Menander perhaps still represented a Greek usage which was widely intelligible – because of its use in mass entertainment – and thus preferable to other forms. Whatever Galen's view of Menander's Greek, the significance of this Μενάνδρειον lies in the fact that it is the title of a play 'Self-Tormentor' which is quoted, rather than anything from the text of the play itself. Given that verbal voice was a concern in Greek lexicographers[53] (on whom more shortly), what we have here is a solid and eminently quotable – and perhaps thus even widely used? – authoritative example of a verb in the middle (τιμωρέομαι) taking an accusative. The inclusion of the play name in Galen is not then indicative of a close attachment to Menader's language as such, but rather can only be interpreted as a superficial nod to his plays. This is not to say that Galen did not know – and indeed enjoy – Menander; assuming the tone of the following passage is sincere, Galen himself displays a degree of fondness for Menander in *On the Natural Faculties*, even if he does not speak as an advocate for his works as models of good style:[54]

> Now such of the younger men as have dignified themselves with the
> names of these two authorities by taking the appellations 'Erasistrateans'

wenn man wollte, dickere Bücher füllen könnte als die Bücher des Menedotos und des Menemachos."

50   ἡ παλαιά κωμῳδία in Galen is taken in this chapter to mean 'Old Comedy' in the sense of the plays ancient Athens broadly termed, not in the modern technical sense which often differentiates strictly between Old and Middle Comedy; the fact that the labels Old, Middle and New were not used in antiquity consistently does not alter the conclusions reached in this chapter. A note on the terminology is conveniently found at Nervegna (2014) 388–89.

51   The title of a recipe given as 'an enema against dysentery from Nicostratus, which Menander employed' (ἔνεμα πρὸς δυσεντερικοὺς ὡς Νικόστρατος, ᾧ Μένανδρος ἐχρήσατο) at *SMT* xiii.299 K. is unlikely (I think) to refer to the comic playwright. Karavas & Vix 2014, 184–185 also collect and discuss references to Menander in Galen.

52   On which see Tribulato (2014), who rehabilitates Menander's authoritative status for some lexicographers of the period.

53   Tribulato (2014) 208–209.

54   *Nat.Fac.* ii.67 K., trans. Brock (1916).

or 'Asclepiadeans' are like the *Davi* and *Getae* – the slaves introduced by the **excellent Menander** (τοῦ βελτίστου Μενάνδρου) into his comedies.

2   Sources, Working Practices & Format

The questions of Galen's choices of what to use of Old Comedy rest partly upon which texts were extant in his lifetime, and available at Rome, Pergamum or other centres of Classical learning.[55] What this section argues is that the body of material to which Galen had access when it comes to Comedy was shared with his contemporaries – as was the attitude he took to that material.

It is reasonably safe to assume that, in contrast to the more popular New Comedy, a relatively small number of complete plays of Old Comedy from fifth century BC Athens had been preserved, alongside compilatory texts with a basis in Alexandrian scholarship.[56] By Galen's time at least, and most likely substantially earlier, the extant canon of Old Comedy had shrunk almost entirely to works by Cratinus, Aristophanes and Eupolis, and of these Aristophanes was pre-eminent.[57] Galen himself in fact notes that texts written by well-known comic (and tragic) playwrights have been lost by his day, implying that he had knowledge of the names of playwrights, but no access to the texts of their plays.[58] In Latin poets of the late Republic and first two centuries AD, this triad

55 As posed by Nutton (2009) 33–34. See Nicholls (2011) for libraries in Rome in Galen's lifetime, based on the new evidence of the *Ind.*, and König et al. for libraries in general, esp. Zadorojnyi's contribution, pp. 389–398; Hanson (1998) 39 notes that if Galen did visit the library at Alexandria during his time in the city, he makes no mention of it.

56 Wilson (2014) gives a short introductory sketch of the afterlife of the texts of the plays of Old Comedy, and Quadlbauer (1960) the detail of comedy in literary criticism, covering some similar ground to Ruffell (2014); Le Guen (2014) considers the evidence for performance in the Hellenistic East and West, see esp. 369 on the choice of plays. It seems likely that only a few manuscripts of the plays of Old Comedy made it even to Alexandria – if a large number of plays did survive intact in Rome or in the Greek East, it seems likely their readership was very limited.

57 See Pfeiffer (1968) 160, 204–5 on the selection of the canonical poets. Rusten (2011) 81–2 collects some sources on the triad, Plato comicus sometimes being added, see e.g. Storey (2003) 40–41. On the basis of papyrus fragments, Sommerstein (2010) 410f. suggests a dramatic change around 300 BC whereby Eupolis, Cratinus and other comic dramatists stop being read. For Eupolis' reception in antiquity, see Storey (2003) chapter 1, esp. 34–40, who notes that knowledge of Eupolis exists primarily in the scholarly tradition (p. 34). Bakola (2010) 4 claims Cratinus was read until at least the second or mid third century AD, on the basis of the likely date of the papyrus hypothesis of *Dionysalexandros*.

58 *HNH* XV.24 K. (= *comm.* 1.2): καὶ τί θαυμαστὸν ἀπολέσθαι τὰ βιβλία τῶν ἀλλοκότους δόξας γραψάντων, ὅπου γε καὶ παρὰ τοῖς Ἀθηναίοις εὑρίσκονταί τινες εὐδοκίμως ἠγωνισμένοι κωμικοί τε καὶ τραγικοὶ ποιηταὶ δράμασιν οὐκέτι διασῳζομένοις; Trans. Hanson 1998, 38: 'So why is it

stands for the genre as a whole (for example as expressed at the beginning of Horace, *Sat.* 1.4.1–2),[59] and the same pattern of quotation, in its paucity and preferences, appears to obtain for many Greek authors of this period, although with some obvious exceptions, such as Athenaeus.[60] Even those few who may be experiencing complete plays directly are almost certainly doing so through reading, rather than performance.[61]

The scattered statements in the extant Galenic corpus, and Galen's catalogue of his own treatises on the subject, suggest therefore that the familiar 'big three' playwrights of Old Comedy for Galen appear to have been what broadly speaking constituted "the entire of Old Comedy" (*Ind.* 23b), as in many of his contemporaries. The collection of quotations and mentions of comic texts presented above shows us that Galen's preferences above all were for Aristophanes: Eupolis barely features, and Cratinus not at all.[62] Galen tells us that his work on Cratinus comprised only two books, as opposed to five on Aristophanes. This suggests that Cratinus' works were already by the second century AD less-well known, or less well-preserved, than those of Aristophanes.[63] If we compare for example the scant material in Galen with the vast collection of comic fragments in Athenaeus' *Deipnosophistae*, the tale of a fictional symposium at which a fictionalised Galen in fact appears as a guest (he speaks about types of wine at 1.26c–27d, and bread at 3.115c–116a) and which is most likely almost contemporaneous with the *Peri alupias*, Galen's range of comic material looks

---

surprising that the books of those who wrote down their various opinions perish, when even at Athens well-reputed comic and tragic playwrights are found with their dramas no longer surviving?'.

59   *Eupolis atque Cratinus Aristophanesque poetae | atque alii, quorum comoedia prisca virorum est*; see also Quintilian, *Inst.* 10.1.66.

60   This is a central concern in the essays collected by Marshall & Hawkins (2016), which stands as a state-of-the-art report. On collections of quotations of Old Comedy in particular, see Sidwell (2000) 142–152 (in Athenaeus, and Lucian) and Bowie (2007) (in Dio of Prusa *fl.* c. 70–120 AD; Aelius Aristides ?117–181 AD, and Maximus of Tyre *fl.* c. 180–192 AD, and others), also including Menander. Lucian (*fl.* c. AD 120–180) seems to display deeper knowledge, see the more extended studies by Storey (2016), esp. 163–164 and Rosen (2016). On quotations of Menander across a range of Imperial authors, see Karavas & Vix (2014). Nutton (2009) 24 also notes some overlap between Galen's reading and Gellius'.

61   Evidence for performance remains sketchy, although there may have been some private revivals at Rome under Hadrian, perhaps involving the the artist known as 'Attic Partridge' (Ἀττικοπέρδιξ); see Jones (1993) for discussion.

62   Notwithstanding any unnoticed quotations, given our own paucity of knowledge about Eupolis and Cratinus.

63   This echoes Ruffell's observation (2014) 303 on Latin authors that "(k)nowledge of Cratinus in particular seems less than that of his younger rivals".

very limited indeed, and is rather on the slighter end of the scale.[64] My impression is that the same can most probably also be said of the Atticist lexicographers of this period, with a focus on the canonical triad, rather than other playwrights.[65] We know from literature written in Latin that, with rare exceptions and perhaps only Aulus Gellius, any engagement with Old Comedy appears to be through anecdotes in the biographical tradition or through Hellenistic scholarship, rather than first-hand knowledge.[66]

All this suggests that Galen is basing his work only on pre-existing compendia and lexica, and can be supported by strong echoes of quotations used by him in common with other authors.[67] Eupolis' *Demes*, from which Galen quotes, was likely one of the best known non-Aristophanic play of Old Comedy in antiquity,[68] again pointing to Galen as a more average reader of Old Comedy than we might think from his magisterial self portrayal. Storey suggests that the inclusion of the name of the speaker of the quotation of *fr.* *105 in *Aff. Dig.* relies upon direct consultation of the play text – but concedes that this may be by Galen's source;[69] Nutton likewise notes that the long quotation from Plato comicus indicates Galen likely had a copy in his own library, but similarly there is no reason to think that these lines did not already exist as an excerpt.[70] Vegetti also observes that while in *PHP* Galen is working directly from a large number of texts of the works of philosophers and doctors, many of the quotations from poetry come via Chrysippus, i.e. an intermediary source.[71]

All this is not to say that Galen never read a play of Aristophanes in full, but that such reading may be more limited than it would appear at first sight. This is perhaps as a result of what was available as a full play text, but also

---

64   Even though Athenaeus is more important as a source for Middle Comedy, this work still preserves a great range of material from Old Comedy.

65   Searching the texts of Aelius Dionysius, Phrynichus, Pollux and Pausanias (Att.) via the *TLG* shows 461 examples of the name Aristophanes, 128 Cratinus and 112 Eupolis (again echoing Galen's 5 books on the first of these poets, versus 2 and 3 for the other two respectively); in contrast, in these same authors there are for example only 11 examples of Philippides and 12 of Amipsias (two other comic playwrights), neither of whom are found in Galen.

66   Ruffell (2014) 302–4, in line with an interest in Old Comedy for its historical, not philological, interest; Cucchiarelli (2006) covers a slightly different range of Latin authors, and is more sympathetic as to the depth of familiarity with Aristophanes granted to some.

67   As intimated by Ruffell (2014) 304.

68   Storey (2003) 34 and 111. Eupolis, *fr.* *116 is quoted by Gellius and Galen (and by Plutarch), and both also quote from Aristophanes, *Merchant Ships*, although different lines (Gell. 19.13.3 = *fr.* 447)

69   Storey (2003) 37.

70   Nutton (2009) 30.

71   Vegetti (1999) 339–340.

perhaps because alternative sources were available – it is after all easier to recycle an existing lexical collection than it is to start from scratch. Galen is indeed clear about his working practices on this point, telling us upfront that he has produced an epitome of Didymus on Old Comedy, and is therefore using just such a pre-existing source.[72] Examples of misattribution – if these are misattributions – do also support the case that he is working with anthologies or lexica, in which excerpted lines have already gone astray from their original author. We can only say for certain how far Galen was reading the complete plays of Old Comedy, and excerpting what he thought was useful, through a study of the notes and vocabulary he employs which do *not* feature in the lexicographical works of his near contemporaries, and through better knowledge of which plays were likely wholly extant in this period, both desiderata of future work.[73] For the time being, what follows flags Galen's reuse of earlier material, albeit perhaps at the expense of downplaying his own contribution which remains to some extent unknown. It should be noted that this is not a negative judgement of Galen's work, nor anything of which he himself was ashamed. Wilkins' words ring just as true for Galen's lexicography as of his medical works: 'Compiling is not a term of abuse (as it is often applied to Athenaeus), in the mind of Galen at least, since he, the cataloguer with utility in mind, clearly sees it as vital for medical practice.'[74]

Despite the scorn which Galen often pours on those Atticisers who are concerned with linguistic 'quibbling', it is striking that there is a small but significant overlap between Galen's own works and the surviving contemporary Atticising lexica,[75] particularly in the choice of words discussed.[76] This includes a number of words which are very rarely found in the extant corpus

72   As Galen similarly relied on digests of some medical and other materials, used at secondhand, see e.g. Roselli (1999) on medical digests and Hanson (1998) 35–7 for collected bibliography on earlier commentaries and lexica relating to Hippocrates.

73   Manetti (2009) 161–1 indeed argues that the lack lexicographical analogue to the fragment of Aristophanes quoted at *Hipp. Fract.* indicates Galen's own 'careful studies' of the language of comic poets.

74   Wilkins (2007) 85.

75   Strobel (2009) is a convenient introduction to some of the major Atticist lexica.

76   Both this scorn for Atticists, and engagement with their material, can be seen for example in *Alim. Fac.* 2.29.3 (= VI.612 K.; trans. Powell 2003, 94 adapted): "Some of those who call themselves Atticisers, who have practiced no skill of value for life, think it right to refer to this fruit in the feminine *amygdalē* (ἀμυγδάλη) 'almond', but others of them in the neuter *amygdalon* (ἀμύγδαλον), not realizing about this very matter that they take so seriously, that the Athenians wrote both names". This word and its gender also features in Moeris (*Lexicon Atticum* α 15) and Athenaeus 2.52f (= 2.39–40 Kaibel); other such examples of comments on the gender of Classical words which co-occur across different lexica from this period, and in Galen, are collected in Appendix A of Coker (2010).

of Greek texts up to and including Galen, but yet feature frequently – sometimes more frequently – in the lexicographical tradition. To give just two examples for starters, πυριάτη given by LSJ (s.v.) as 'beestings curdled by heating
over embers'[77] and its synonym πυρίεφθον, are found only a handful of times
in texts from Classical antiquity (Eubulus *fr.* 74 (K-A) (᾿Ολβία), Aristophanes,
Wasps 710, Cratinus *fr.* 149 (K-A) (᾿Οδυσσῆς), Philippides *fr.* 10 KA (Αὐλοί)), but appear in Aelius Dionysius π 77 (Erbse),[78] Pausanias π 43 (Erbse),[79] Pollux 1.248
(Bethe),[80] Galen, *Alim. Fac.* VI.694 K.,[81] and elsewhere in the later lexicographical tradition, all in relatively similar formulations. This strongly suggests that
Galen is reading and replying to one or more live lexicographical traditions
(represented here by Aelius Dionysius et al.) which draw at least indirectly on
Hellenistic and Alexandrian scholarship. Put differently – and more pejoratively – we might say that Galen has a close connection with contemporary
'sophistical' work.

This is supported further by the mention of a work by Didymus at *Ind.*
24a. Assuming Galen's Didymus is the famous Alexandrian scholar Didymus
Chalcenterus ("bronze-guts") of the first century BC,[82] then the work from
which Galen composed his own epitome is one of the 3,500–4,000 works he allegedly composed, or a version of one of them. Writing almost at the end of the
great Alexandrian tradition of scholarship, Chalcenterus' works are generally
characterised as derivative, based in turn mostly on the works of earlier lexicographers and commentators such as Aristophanes of Byzantium.[83] Pfeiffer

---

77 Meaning a type of cheese made from cow colostrum; such a cheese is made in Tamil Nadu
    and Ukraine.

78 πυριάτη· θηλυκῶς τὸ πυρίεφθον· οὐχὶ πυρίατος οὐδὲ πυριατὴ ὀξυτόνως οὐδὲ πυρίεφθος. "Puriatē:
    Feminine, and means *puriephthon*. There is no word *puriatos* or *puriatē* (accented on the
    final syllable), nor *puriephthos*."

79 πυόν· τὸ πυρίεφθον· τινὲς δὲ πᾶν γάλα νέον ἢ ὃ ἂν μετὰ γάλακτος ἑψηθῇ χθεσινοῦ. "*puon* ('co-
    lostrum'): (means) *puriephthon*. Some people use this to mean any milk, either fresh or
    whatever is boiled with yesterday's milk."

80 πυριάτη τὸ ὑπὸ τῶν πολλῶν λεγόμενον πυρίεφθον. "*puriatē*, called *puriephthon* by many peo-
    ple." πυριάτη is also found at Pollux 6.54, where Philippides is quoted.

81 καλεῖν δ' ἐοίκασιν οἱ παλαιοὶ κωμικοὶ τὸ οὕτω παγὲν γάλα πυριάτην· οἱ δὲ παρ' ἡμῖν ἐν Ἀσίᾳ
    πυρίεφθον ὀνομάζουσιν αὐτό. "Writers of Old Comedy were accustomed to call milk curdled
    in this way *puriatē*; we in Asia name the same thing *puriephthon*."

82 *BJP* ad *Ind.* 24a (= p. 81) identifies this Didymus as Chalcenterus, but there are other can-
    didates, notably a Δίδυμος ὁ νεώτερος, placed at Rome in the 1st century AD. The *Suda*
    lists three Didymi as grammarians (δ 872–4), who may not all be discrete individuals. See
    Dickey (2007) 7, n. 18 as an entry into the debate.

83 West (1970) has a rather poor view of the quality of Didymus' historical and philological
    scholarship; Pfeiffer (1968) 279 is altogether more positive, seeing Didymus' vast output
    as only possible (he was only "enabled to become the most efficient servant of an ancient

notes that after Homer, this scholar's prime focus was Attic comedy: he collected a vast amount of information on "literary, historical, biographical and
prosopographical" matters, and we know he compiled a work on comic words
(sometimes labelled Λέξεις κωμικαί).[84]

If Galen is indeed using a text circulating under the name of Didymus'
Comic Words, it is just possible that there are traces of this work at the end
of the passage from the περὶ ἀλυπίας with which this chapter started (26–7).
A convincing emendation by Polemis (above p. 63, n. 2) conjectures two words
given by Galen as examples of the sorts of unclear vocabulary items which
his treatise helped to explicate: ἀβυδοκόμης and ἀβυρτάκη. The first of these
appears a handful of times in the lexicographical tradition – and only in this
tradition – as a nickname for a sycophant[85] and the second, only marginally
more common, is a type of sauce (LSJ *s.v.* "*sour sauce of leeks, cress, and pome-
granate-seeds*").[86] Nutton has already suggested that these two words, both beginning with αβ-, may well have stood at the beginning of Galen's own treatise
on Old Comedy – if it was arranged alphabetically.[87] Some evidence however
for both words as coming directly from a pre-existing lexicographical tradition
is also found in Pausanias' lexicon, (mid/late 2nd century AD), which in its surviving form (ed. Erbse 1950) contains Ἄβυδος (another name for a sycophant,
with ἀβυδοκόμης in the lemma) and ἀβυρτάκη as the third and fourth words of
Alpha.[88] It seems unlikely that such organisational similarities would appear
across different texts if both Galen and Pausanias were independently alpha-
betising a non-alphabetical source, or were using no source text at all.

---

intellectual community", in Pfeiffer's own words) because of the peace brought about by
Augustus. Manetti (2009) 165 flags the role played by work by Aristophanes of Byzantium
in some of Galen's lexicographical material: Didmyus may thus be the intermediary
source.

84   Pfeiffer (1968) 276. Scant fragments of a work given the title Λέξις κωμική are collected at
Schmidt (1854/1964) 27–82; Didymus also compiled a Λέξις Ἱπποκράτους (pp. 24–27), but
whether this was available to Galen must remain speculation.

85   e.g. Hesychius α 225 (Latte): ἀβυδοκόμας· ὁ ἐπὶ τῷ συκοφαντεῖν κομῶν.

86   Found for example at Pherecrates, *fr.* 185 K-A, Theopompus *fr.* 18 (Θησεύς) K-A, Antiphanes
fr. 140 (Λευκάδιος) K-A, Alexis *fr.* 145 (Μανδραγοριζομένη) K-A.

87   Nutton (2013) 86 n. 57.

88   α 3 Ἄβυδος· ἐπὶ συκοφάντου τάττεται ἡ λέξις διὰ τὸ δοκεῖν συκοφάντας εἶναι τοὺς Ἀβυδηνούς·
καὶ Ἀβυδοκόμαι οἱ ἐπὶ τῷ συκοφαντεῖν κομῶντες. τίθεται δὲ καὶ ἐπὶ τοῦ εἰκαίου καὶ μηδενὸς
ἀξίου. κωμῳδοῦνται δὲ <οἱ> Ἀβυδηνοὶ καὶ εἰς ἀκολασίαν, καὶ [ἡ] παροιμία· 'μὴ εἰκῆ τὴν Ἄβυδον',
ᾗ ἐχρῶντο ἐπὶ τῶν εἰκαίων καὶ οὐδαμινῶν.

α 4 ἀβυρτάκη· ὑπότριμμα βαρβαρικὸν ἐκ δριμέων σκευαζόμενον, ἐκ καρδάμων καὶ σκορόδων
καὶ σινάπεως καὶ σταφίδων, ᾧ πρὸς κοιλιολυσίαν ἐχρῶντο.

For the use of the town name Abydos as an abusive epithet, see Kajava (2007) 25–28.

It is not unreasonable to assume that Galen maintained this alphabetical order in his own work, which is why these two words appear as they do in the *Peri alupias*, standing as the first two of his now-lost epitome, and recalled from memory. Galen is often in favour of alphabetisation (order κατὰ στοιχεῖον), although he also used other arrangements of material.[89] Alphabetical order is used for example in some of the books of *SMT* (e.g. 6, 7 and 8, all on plants), where Galen explicitly tells his reader he is imitating the order of an earlier work by Pamphilus, *On Plants* (6, proem = XI.793–4 K.);[90] the *Glossary of Hippocratic Terms (Gloss.)* is in addition fully alphabetical, in contrast to other contemporary lexica which are only broadly so.[91] It seems likely too that Galen's forty-eight book work on Attic prose was also alphabetical: just before the passage from *Lib. Prop.* quoted earlier in this chapter on p. 65 Galen tells us about another πραγματεία of his, identified with this work on prose, ἐν ᾗ τὰ παρὰ τοῖς Ἀττικοῖς συγγραφεῦσιν ὀνόματα κατὰ τὴν τῶν πρώτων ἐν αὐτοῖς γραμμάτων ἤθροισται τάξιν.[92]

There are however traces of an alternative, thematic pattern of arrangement in this passage from the *Ind.*. If lexical collections such as that by Didymus, or versions of it, represent one body of knowledge from which Galen was drawing (in common with Atticist lexicographers, Pollux, Lucian etc.) there may be an additional body of work also evident. At *Ind.* 27 (repeated below from the beginning of this chapter), Galen gives what looks like a list of contents, although it is not immediately clear whether this list refers to the mentioned work by Didymus, or to Galen's own epitome:

ὄλυραι καὶ λάθυροι καὶ ὄροβοι καὶ χόνδρος τά τε ἄλλα **Δημήτρια σπέρματα** καὶ λάχανα καὶ ὀπῶραι καὶ **θάμναι** καὶ **δευτερίαι** καὶ θάμνοι καὶ καρποὶ καὶ βοτάνοι καὶ ζῷα καὶ ἄρμενα καὶ σκεύη καὶ ὄργανα καὶ τἄλλα πολιτικὰ πράγματα καὶ ὀνόματα πάντα.

---

89 On the various methods of presentation of material used by Galen, see Flemming (2007) 247–58, and *passim*, and the comments below.

90 Wilkins (2007) 81: 'Galen appears to find Pamphilus to be a bad botanist, but a good lexicographer.' Does *Ind.* 27 Δίδυμος ἔφθασεν ἐξηγήσασθαι καλῶς suggest Galen passes the same judgement on Didymus? This Pamphilus and his 95 volume Περὶ γλωσσῶν καὶ ὀνομάτων of the 1st century AD is sometimes seen as an intermediary between Didymus' work and grammarians of the second century AD.

91 Dickey (2007) 45. Purely alphabetical arrangements of material was not the rule, although there were for example earlier texts of medical interest arranged κατὰ στοιχεῖον, see Flemming (2007) 254; compare Pollux' *Onomasticon* as an example of the encyclopedic or thesaurus format, as Tosi (2007) 3–5. On alphabetisation in antiquity, see Daly (1967) 9–69.

92 *Ord. Lib. Prop* 5.1–2 (= XIX.60 K.).

emmer, chick peas, vetch, groats and the other **cereals**, vegetables and late-summer fruits, **wines made from the marc of grapes, with or without the addition of water**, bushes, fruits, plants, animals, instruments, equipment, tools, and everything else in daily life, and their names.

Rosen sees this list as an allusion to catalogues of foodstuffs in Old Comedy,[93] but two strong echoes are found much closer to lexicographical home. The list – and in particular the order in which items appear – bears more than a passing resemblance to a passage in Pollux 1.247–8 (the text is untranslated because of the large number of synonyms):

καὶ ἀπὸ μὲν κριθῶν πτισάνη καὶ ἄλφιτα, ἀπὸ δὲ σίτου χόνδρος καὶ σε|μίδαλις. ζειαί, σήσαμα, κέγχροι, μήκων, λίνος. ἄμυλος ἄρτος, καχρυδίας ἄρτος, κεγχρίας, ὀβελίας ἄρτος καὶ ὀβελίτης. καὶ ἄρτους κολλάβους. ἀθάρη ἐκ καγχρυδίου, πανοσπρία, πῦος, πυριάτη τὸ ὑπὸ τῶν πολλῶν λεγόμενον πυρίεφθον. εἶτα κρίμνα, μᾶζα, κόλλυρα, στέμφυλα, κυρήβια· τὰ γὰρ φαυλότερα τῶν πυρῶν κυρήβια καλεῖται. οἶνος γλυκύς, ἡδύς, ἐπαγωγός, πότιμος, ἀνθοσμίας· ὁ δ' ἄλλος **δευτερίας**, ἐξεστηκώς, τροπίας, ἐκτροπίας, ὀξίνης.

First in Pollux are listed grains and cereals (including χόνδρος, the word used by the 'respected doctor' whose opinion Galen debunks in *Ind.* 26) – equivalent to the Δημήτρια σπέρματα of *Ind.* 27 – and then wines of various kinds, including δευτερίας in both passages. To find this rare word for a type of wine (see *BJP ad Ind.* 27, = pp. 90–2) reinforces the idea that the similarities between these two passages are more than chance. πυριάτη – given above as an example of the strength of grammatical tradition – also appears here. The second passage for comparison is from Galen's *Med. Nom.*:[94]

Nun haben jene Leute, wenn sie dies behaupten, doch nicht nur keine Kenntnis von der Natur und dem Wesen des Blutes oder vom Wesen der heißen Schwellung, welche auf griechisch φλεγμονή heißt, oder vom Wesen der Augenentzündung (Ophthalmie), sondern es entgeht ihnen die Kenntnis **vom Wesen des Weizens, von dem Wesen der Gerste, dem Wesen der Kichererbse, dem Wesen der Pferdebohne, dem Wesen des Öls und dem Wesen des Weines:** außerdem kennen sie ja auch nicht richtig das Wesen von irgendwelchen **Pflanzen** oder **Tieren**, wie sie (selbst) ihr eigenes Wesen nicht kennen.

---

93   Rosen (2014) 169.
94   Meyerhof & Schacht (1931) 27 = 99v.

Now those people, when they say this, are not only unaware of the nature and the essence of blood or of the nature of the hot swelling which is called φλεγμονή in Greek, or of the nature of inflammation of the eye (ophthalmia), but they are also lacking in knowledge of the nature of **wheat, barley, chickpea, horsebean,** oil and **wine**: in addition they do not really know about the nature of any **plants** or **animals**, just as they do not even know their own nature.

Even though we are several stages here removed from Galen's Greek (through the German translation of the Arabic text, which is in turn a translation of the Greek), again we have a list (corresponding to the emboldened words) comprised of wheat, barley, chickpea, horsebean (= *Ind.* τὰ Δημήτρια σπέρματα), and wine (= *Ind.* θάμναι καὶ δευτερίαι), followed up by plants and animals (= *Ind.* βοτάνοι καὶ ζῷα).

This arrangement of substances – and in the order *grains, plants* and *animals* is also used by Galen in *Alim. Fac.*, and indeed specifically outlined there as a ranking of the relative values of foodstuffs.[95] There were various ways of organising edible substances and their subsets in dietetic treatises in antiquity, often sophisticated and complex, but some sets of similar principles appear to have operated.[96] More work needs to be done on outlining such organisational principles before Galen, but it seems likely that the lists we find here are in some way a reflection of an earlier tradition.

There are also echoes of the vocabulary in *Alim. Fac.* of this list in *Ind.*: the Δημήτρια σπέρματα again appear (*Alim. Fac.* 2.1 = VI.554–5 K., and elsewhere in Galen), as does δευτερίας (*Alim. Fac.* 2.9 = VI.580 K.) to give just two examples. The only places that this latter word appears in Galen are here in the *Alim. Fac.*, and in the *Ind.*. It may be significant that in the first of these treatises Galen gives it as a word used specifically by οἱ Ἀττικίζοντες – yet still choses to use it.

There are a number of possible explanations of these two sets of correspondences, none of which however can be proved conclusively. It is on the face of it impossible to posit a single source text for Galen's treatise on Old Comedy which is both alphabetical and thematic: are there then rather multiple texts from which Galen is compiling his new work, one alphabetical collection of words also used by some Atticist lexica, and one thematic used by Galen and

---

95   Book 1 is the grains, with legumes and pulses; Book 2 vegetables and fruits and Book 3 animal products. See Wilkins' foreword (p. ix) to Powell's translation (2003); Galen outlines and justifies his order at *Alim. Fac.* 2.1 (= VI.554–5 K.).

96   For plants, for example, either based around appearance, or effect on the body. Hardy & Totelin (2016) 63–92 sketch some of the wider taxonomic landscape, with pp. 75–88 on various ancient systems of classification.

Pollux? Or, does the correspondence with Pollux indicate only a close relationship between these two authors, and Pollux is influenced by Galen, rather than any prior text which both share?[97] On balance – and however Pollux fits into this picture – it seems more likely on the basis of the limited evidence presented here that Galen's own text on Old Comedy was arranged alphabetically, and that the list of topics given at *Ind.* 27 represented his own ideas about arrangement, perhaps a list which automatically came to mind at the very mention of foodstuffs. If a written text with thematic arrangement does however lie behind the list – and even goes back to some work of Didymus, if the list at *Ind.* 27 does indeed outline ἃ Δίδυμος ἔφθασεν ἐξηγήσασθαι καλῶς – then the alphabetical coincidences highlighted above must however still be accounted for.

3   Galen the Sophist?

This chapter has sought to think in more concrete terms about the shape and contents of a lost work of Galen described in the περὶ ἀλυπίας, and in doing so to place Galen within the literary and lexicographical culture of the Roman empire of the late second century AD.

In structural terms, Galen's epitome of Didymus on Comedy may have been alphabetical (starting with *abudokomas* and *aburtakē*), but there are also striking indications of the presence of a thematic organisational principle: it remains unclear however whether Galen in alluding to these two systems is referring to his own collection of words, or Didymus'. As to contents, from looking at Galen's use of Old Comedy elsewhere in his works his preferences can be seen to be very similar to those educated men who either passed judgement on, or sought to emulate or to play with, Atticist usage. In common with some other works of the period, Galen's lost treatise similarly drew on Didymus and a longer scholastic tradition on Attic Old Comedy, so we might speculatively ponder that a set of words similar to those preserved in other ancient works on comedy was also at the core of Galen's work. While this *perhaps* underplays the breadth of Galen's reading, there are nevertheless strong indications that he is engaging closely with lexical collections circulating at Rome and other centres of learning at the period – and even their authors. Correspondences with

---

97   Zecchini (2007) 22–4 outlines Pollux's use of a wide range of non-canonical treatises. More work is certainly needed on the relationships between the works of Galen and Pollux, and as noted in the review of a recent work on Pollux (Rance 2008), also on the setting of Pollux's lexicon in 'the vast output of grammarians and lexicographers of the Antonine period' in general.

Lucian are perhaps most curious: note also that Galen's very rare ἀβυρτάκη is used in Lucian's satirical *Lexiphanes* 6 among a list of foodstuffs (as well as at Pollux 6.56), a work which rejoices in particular in its handling of the vocabulary of Old Comedy – and indeed some have suggested that the doctor character in this work is a mockery of Galen himself.[98] We can thus align Galen very closely with other members of the literary élite of the second century AD who are also looking back to comic exemplars of the fifth century BC, and see the extent to which he was likewise deeply entrenched in Atticising cultures.

While we see Galen using these already seven-hundred-year-old texts to make linguistic points, they are sometimes deployed simply to demonstrate his education. This verges on the use of words as ornaments – the very thing Galen argues should be guarded against. It is not surprising however that Galen, imbued with the *paideia* of the period, should draw on his 'internalisation' of classical literature for its rhetorical power,[99] but the manner in which he does so places him somewhat closer to those he criticises than he has previously been seen to be. In the judgement of history it is a fine – and often subjective – line which separates a positively-viewed Galen, imbued with wide and earnest learning, aptly demonstrated to good purpose, from the schoolish[100] or reductive Galen who slavishly reproduces as fripperies those examples acquired and collected in common with the rest of the educated elite. Galen himself certainly sought to distance himself from elements of the latter and those he would label as 'sophists', composing a strongly militaristic polemic against them at the end of the first book of *On Medical Names*.[101] In this fight over good Greek however, Galen's weapons are remarkably similar to those used by his sophistical foes.

---

98   See the bibliography at Storey (2016) 176, n. 32, who argues for a different identification. Perhaps it is significant that the words put into the fictional Galen's mouth by Athenaeus are on wine (1.26c–27d) and bread, grains and their nutritiousness (3.115c–116a) – was Galen known to his contemporaries to be particularly vociferous on such topics? See Wilkins (2007) 78–9 on these two passages and the 'reality' of Athenaeus' Galen *passim*.

99   Rosen (2013) 188.

100   As Karavas & Vix 2014, 185.

101   Meyerhof-Schacht (1931) 37 = 107v: "Ich habe dieses mein ganzes Buch um jener Sophisten willen verfaßt; es ist ein Buch, das, wenn es in der Welt keine Streitfrage über diese Angelegenheit gäbe, ein nutzloses Gefasel und eine Sinnlosigkeit wäre; so wie der Mensch genötigt ist, die Waffe zu ergreifen und zu seiner Ausrüstung zu machen, nur wegen der schlechten Menschen – nur wenn in der Welt nicht ein einziger von den Menschen schlecht wäre, wäre es überflüssig, sie zu ergreifen und bereitzuhalten –, so ist meine Rede in diesem meinem Buche gleichsam eine Waffe und Ausrüstung zum Kampfe gegen die Sophisten."

Acknowledgements

My thanks are due to the many people who have commented on this paper, both in Warwick and since, in particular to Vivian Nutton for supplying me with a copy of Polemis 2011, Laurence Totelin for kindly sharing with me then forthcoming work, and Nicky Bigwood for help with the German. This paper is an offshoot from a Leverhulme Trust Early Career Fellowship (2013–2016) hosted by the Department of Classics and Ancient History at the University of Manchester; the support of both the Trust and the Department is here gratefully acknowledged.

References

Bakola, E. *Cratinus and the Art of Comedy.* Oxford: OUP, 2010.

Barnes, J. 'Logique et pharmacologie: à propos de quelques remarques d'ordre linguistique dans le *De simplicium medicamentorum temperamentis ac facultatibus* de Galien'. In *Galen on Pharmacology*, ed. A. Debru, 3–33. Leiden: Brill, 1997.

Bowie, E. 'The Ups and Downs of Aristophanic Travel'. In *Aristophanes in Performance 421 BC–AD 2007*, ed. E. Hall & A. Wrigley, 32–51. London: Legenda, 2007.

Coker, A. *Aspects of Grammatical Gender in Ancient Greek.* Manchester: PhD. diss. University of Manchester, 2010.

Cucchiarelli, A. 'La commedia greca antica a Roma'. *Atene e Roma* 51.4, (2006): 157–77.

Daly, L. A. *Contributions to a History of Alphabetization in Antiquity and the Middle Ages. Collection Latomus* Vol. XC. Bruxelles: Latomus, 1967.

Deichgräber, K. (1957) 'Parabasenverse aus Thesmophoriazusae II des Aristophanes bei Galen', *Sitzungsberichte der Akademie der Wissenschaften zu Berlin, Klasse für Sprache, Literatur und Kunst* 1956.2. Berlin: Akademie Verlag, 1957.

De Lacy, P. 'Galen and the Greek Poets'. *GRBS* 7.3 (1966): 259–66.

Dickey, E. *Ancient Greek Scholarship.* Oxford: OUP, 2007.

Erbse, H. *Untersuchungen zu den atticistischen lexica.* Berlin: Akademie Verlag, 1950.

Flemming, R. 'Galen's imperial order of knowledge'. In *Ordering Knowledge in the Roman Empire*, ed. J. König & T. Whitmarsh, 241–277. Cambridge: CUP, 2007.

Hankinson, J. 'Usage and abusage: Galen on language'. In *Language. Companions to Ancient Thought 3*, ed. S. Everson, 166–87. Cambridge: Cambridge University Press, 1994.

Hanson, A. E. 'Galen: Author and Critic'. In *Editing Texts/Texte edieren, Aporemata* Band 2, ed. G. W. Most, 22–53. Göttingen: Vandenhoeck & Ruprecht, 1998.

Hardy, G. & L. Totelin. *Ancient Botany.* London: Routledge, 2016.

Johnson, W. A. *Bookrolls and Scribes in Oxyrhynchus.* Toronto: University of Toronto Press, 2004.

Jones, C. P. 'Greek Drama in the Roman Empire'. In *Theater and Society in the Classical World*, ed. R. Scodel, 39–52. Ann Arbor: The University of Michigan Press, 1993.

Kajava, M. 'Cities and Courtesans'. *Arctos* 41 (2007): 21–29.

Karavas, O. & J.-L. Vix. 'On the Reception of Menander in the Imperial Period'. In *Menander in Contexts*, ed. A. H. Sommerstein, 183–198. London: Routledge, 2014.

Kim, L. 'The Literary Heritage as Language: Atticism and the Second Sophistic'. In *A Companion to the Ancient Greek Language*, ed. E. J. Bakker, 468–82. Oxford: Wiley Blackwell, 2010.

Kollesch, J. 'Galen und die Zweite Sophistik'. In *Galen: Problems and Prospects*, ed. V. Nutton, 1–11. London: The Wellcome Institute for the History of Medicine, 1981.

König, J., K. Oikonomopoulou & G. Woolf. *Ancient Libraries.* Cambridge: CUP, 2013.

Le Guen, B. 'The Diffusion of Comedy from the Age of Alexander to the Beginning of the Roman Empire'. In *The Oxford Handbook of Greek and Roman Comedy*, ed. M. Fontaine & A. C. Scafuro, 359–77. Oxford: OUP, 2014.

Manetti, D. 'Galen and Hippocratic medicine: language and practice'. In *Galen and the World of Knowledge*, ed. C. Gill, T. Whitmarsh & J. Wilkins, 157–74. Cambridge: CUP, 2009.

Manetti, D. & A. Roselli. 'Galeno commentatore di Ippocrate'. *ANRW* II 37.2, (1994): 1529–635.

Marshall, C. W. & T. Hawkins. *Athenian Comedy in the Roman Empire.* London: Bloomsbury, 2016.

Meyerhof, M. & J. Schacht 'Galen, Über die medizinischen Namen, arabisch und deutsch', *Abhandlungen der preussischen Akademie der Wissenschaften.* Berlin: Verlag der Akademie der Wissenschaften, 1931.

Morison, B. 'Language'. In *The Cambridge Companion to Galen*, ed. R. J. Hankinson, 116–156. Cambridge: CUP, 2008.

Nervegna, S. 'Contexts of reception in antiquity'. In *The Cambridge Companion to Greek Comedy*, ed. M. Revermann, 387–403. Cambridge: CUP, 2014.

Nicholls, M. C. 'Galen and Libraries in the *Peri Alupias*'. *JRS* 101 (2011): 123–42.

Nutton, V. 'Galen's Library'. In *Galen and the World of Knowledge*, ed. C. Gill, T. Whitmarsh & J. Wilkins, 19–34. Cambridge: CUP, 2009.

Nutton, V. 'Avoiding Distress'. In *Galen. Psychological Writings*, ed. P. N. Singer, 45–106. Cambridge: CUP, 2013.

Pfeiffer, R. *History of Classical Scholarship.* Vol. 1. Oxford: Clarendon Press, 1968.

Polemis (2011) = Ι. Πολέμης. 'Διορθωτικά στο *Περὶ ἀλυπίας* του Γαληνού'. In *Επιστημονική Επετηρίδα της Φιλοσοφικής Σχολής του Πανεπιστημίου Αθήνων* 43 (2011): 1–8.

Powell, O. *Galen on the Powers of Foodstuffs.* Cambridge: CUP, 2003.

Quadlbauer, F. 'Die Dichter der grieschischen Komoödie im literatischen Urteil der Antike'. *Wiener Studien* 73 (1960): 40–82.

Rance, P. Review of *L'onomasticon Giulio Polluce. Tra lessicografia e antiquaria*, ed. C. Bearzot, F. Landucci & G. Zecchini, 3–16. Milano: Vita e Pensiero, 2007. BMCR 2008.11.28.

Roselli, A. 'Notes on the *doxai* of doctors in Galen's commentaries on Hippocrates'. In *Ancient Histories of Medicine. Essays in Medical Doxography and Historiography in Classical Antiquity, SAM* 20, ed. P. van der Eijk, 359–81. Leiden: Brill, 1999.

Rosen, R. M. 'Galen on Poetic Testimony'. In *Writing Science. Medical and Mathematical Authorship in Ancient Greece*, ed. M. Asper, 177–189. Berlin: De Gruyter, 2013.

Rosen, R. M. 'Philology and the Rhetoric of Catastrophe in Galen's *De indolentia*'. In *Galen's* De Indolentia. *Essays on a Newly Discovered Letter*, ed. C. K. Rothschild & T. W. Thompson, 167–172. Tübingen: Mohr Siebeck, 2014.

Rosen, R. M. 'Lucian's Aristophanes: On Understanding Old Comedy in the Roman Imperial Period.' In *Athenian Comedy in the Roman Empire*, ed. C. W. Marshall & T. Hawkins, 141–162. London: Bloomsbury, 2016.

Ruffell, I. 'Old Comedy at Rome: Rhetorical Model and Satirical Problem.' In *Ancient Comedy and Reception. Essays in Honor of Jeffrey Henderson*, ed. S. D. Olson, 275–308. Berlin: De Gruyter, 2014.

Rusten, J. (ed.) *The Birth of Comedy: texts, documents, and art from Athenian competitions, 486–280.* Baltimore: Johns Hopkins University Press, 2011.

Schmidt, M. *Didymi Chalcenteri grammatici Alexandrini fragmenta quae supersunt omnia.* Leipzig/Amsterdam, 1854/1964.

Schmitz, T. *Bildung und Macht. Zur sozialen und politischen Funktion der Zweiten Sophistik in der griechischen Welt der Kaiserzeit.* Munich, 1997.

Sidwell, K. 'Athenaeus, Lucian and Fifth-Century Comedy.' In *Athenaeus and his World. Reading Greek Culture in the Roman Empire*, ed. D. Braund & J. Wilkins, 136–152. Exeter: University of Exeter Press, 2000.

Skoda, F. 'Galien Lexicologue'. In *Dieux, héros et médecins grecs*, ed. M. Woronoff, S. Follet & J. Jouanna, 177–95. Paris: Presses Universitaires Franc-Comtoises, 2001.

Sluiter, I. 'The embarrassment of imperfection: Galen's assessment of Hippocrates' linguistic merits.' In *Ancient Medicine in its Socio-Cultural Context*, Volume 2, ed. P. van der Eijk, H. F. J. Horstmanshoff & P. H. Schrijvers, 519–535. Amsterdam: Rodopi, 1995.

Sommerstein, A. H. 'The History of the Text of Aristophanes'. In *Brill's Companion to the Study of Greek Comedy*, ed. G. W. Dobrov, 399–422. Leiden: Brill, 2010.

Staden, H. von 'Science as text, science as history: Galen on metaphor'. In *Ancient Medicine in its Socio-Cultural Context*, Volume 2, ed. P. van der Eijk, H. F. J. Horstmanshoff & P. H. Schrijvers, 499–518. Amsterdam: Rodopi, 1995.

Staden, H. von 'Gattungen und Gedächtnis: Galen über Wahrheit und Lehrdichtung'. In *Gattungen wissenschaftlicher Literatur in der Antike*, ed. W. Kullman, J. Althoff & M. Asper, 65–94, *Scripta Oralia* 95. Tübingen: G. Narr, 1998.

Storey, I. C. *Eupolis. Poet of Old Comedy.* Oxford: OUP, 2003.

Storey, I. C. 'Exposing Frauds: Lucian and Comedy'. In *Athenian Comedy in the Roman Empire*, ed. C. W. Marshall & T. Hawkins, 163–180. London: Bloomsbury, 2016.

Strobel, C. 'The Lexica of the Second Sophistic: Safeguarding Atticism.' In *Standard Languages & Language Standards: Greek, Past and Present*, ed. A. Georgakopoulou & M. Silk. Farnham: Ashgate, 2009.

Swain, S. *Hellenism and Empire. Language, Classicism & Power in the Greek World AD 50–250.* Oxford: OUP, 1996.

Tosi, R. 'Polluce: struttura onomastica e tradizione lessicografia'. In *L'onomasticon Giulio Polluce. Tra lessicografia e antiquaria*, ed. C. Bearzot, F. Landucci & G. Zecchini, 3–16. Milano: Vita e Pensiero, 2007.

Tribulato, O. '"Not even Menander would uses this word!" Perceptions of Menander's Language in Greek Lexicography.' In *Menander in Contexts*, ed. A. H. Sommerstein, 199–214. London: Routledge, 2014.

Vegetti, M. 'Tradition and truth. Forms of philosophical-scientific historiography in Galen's *De placitis*'. In *Ancient Histories of Medicine. Essays in Medical Doxography and Historiography in Classical Antiquity, SAM* 20, ed. P. van der Eijk, 333–57. Leiden: Brill, 1999.

West, S. 'Chalcentric Negligence', *Classical Quarterly*, 20.2, (1970): 288–96.

Wilkins, J. 'Galen and Athenaeus in the Hellenistic Library'. In *Ordering Knowledge in the Roman Empire*, ed. J. König & T. Whitmarsh, 69–87 Cambridge: CUP, 2007.

Wilson, N. 'The transmission of comic texts'. In *The Cambridge Companion to Greek Comedy*, ed. M. Revermann, 424–32. Cambridge: CUP, 2014.

Zadorojnyi, A. V. 'Libraries and *paideia* in the Second Sophistic'. In *Ancient Libraries*, ed. J. König, K. Oikonomopoulou & G. Woolf, 377–400. Cambridge: CUP, 2013.

Zecchini, G. 'Polluce e la politica culturale di Commodo'. In *L'onomasticon Giulio Polluce. Tra lessicografia e antiquaria*, ed. C. Bearzot, F. Landucci & G. Zecchini, 17–28. Milano: Vita e Pensiero, 2007.

Texts and Editions

Galen. *The Order of My Own Books* (*Ord. Lib. Prop.*), *On My Own Books* (*Lib. Prop.*). Ed. V. Boudon-Millot. Paris: Les Belles Lettres, 2007. English trans. P. Singer, *Galen: Selected Works.* Oxford: OUP, 1997.

Galen. *On Avoiding Distress* (*Ind.*). Ed. V. Boudon-Millot, J. Jouanna & A. Pietrobelli. Paris, Les Belles Lettres, 2010. (= *BJP*) English trans. V. Nutton, v. 'Avoiding Distress'. In *Galen. Psychological Writings*, ed. P. N. Singer, 45–106. Cambridge: CUP, 2013.

Galen. *On the Natural Faculties* (*Nat. Fac.*). Trans. A. J. Brock. London: Heinemann, 1916.

Galen. *On Medical Names* (*Med. Nom.*) Arabic text and German translation M. Meyerhof & J. Schacht. Berlin: Verlag der Akademie der Wissenschaften, 1931.

Galen. *On the Properties of Foodstuffs.* Trans. O. Powell. Cambridge: CUP, 2003.

Abbreviations

CMG V 4.1.2 = De Lacy, P. *Galeni De placitis Hippocratis et Platonis, CMG* V 4.1.2. Berlin, 1978–1984. (= *PHP*)

CMG V 4.2 = Helmreich, G. *Galeni De alimentorum facultatibus libri III, De bonis mal-isque sucis, CMG* V 4.2. Berlin, 1923. (= *Alim. Fac.*)

CMG V 9.1 = Helmreich, G. *Galeni in Hippocratis De victu acutorum Commentaria IV, CMG* V 9.1. Berlin, 1914. (= *HVA*)

CMG V 10.2.2 = Wenkebach, E. & F. Pfaff *Galeni in Hippocratis Sextum Librum Epidemiarum commentaria I–VI, CMG* V 10.2.2. Berlin, 1956. (= *Hipp. Epid.* on book 6)

PCG = *Poetae comici Graeci*, 8 volumes, ed. R. Kassel & C. Austin. Berlin: Walter de Gruyter, 1983–2001

CHAPTER 4

New Light and Old Texts: Galen on His Own Books

P. N. Singer

My aim in this chapter is to show how the new material from the περὶ ἀλυπίας (*Ind.*) contributes to our understanding of Galen's attitude, practices and intentions in relation to the composition and distribution of his own books. The new text, I suggest, not only provides fresh perspectives but, perhaps more importantly, assists us to evaluate and see more clearly the evidence which was already available in the other most relevant texts in this area, especially *My Own Books* (*Lib. Prop.*) and *The Order of My Own Books* (*Ord. Lib. Prop.*) The 'new light' is thus shed in a process of mutual illumination between περὶ ἀλυπίας and other texts, rather than by the sudden availability of radically new and divergent information.

1   Galen's Losses

A good starting-point for this discussion might be: which of Galen's own writings did he actually lose in the fire which is the subject of περὶ ἀλυπίας? The answer turns out to be surprisingly elusive. Let us consider Galen's account of his losses overall. They are summarized in brief at sections 4–6. Galen lists: items made of precious metals; financial documents; drugs (both simple and compound) medical instruments; books (both copies of classical writings corrected in his own hand his own compositions); antidotes. The list is then elaborated, with, in particular, a lot more detail about the books, between this point and section 30, and with a further category, that of pharmacological recipes, added and discussed in some detail at 31–36.

For simplicity, then, Galen's losses may thus be listed under two main heads: books and other possessions.[1] The books can again be divided: into books by other people and Galen's own compositions. Now, we would probably think

---

[1]   The category of pharmacological recipes, which in a sense could be thought of as books, is interesting here: they seem in fact to be considered by Galen as valuable commodities, rather like the *materia medica* itself, not as texts in any normal sense. This relationship of such unique, collectible, recipes to Galen's own pharmacological writings presents an interesting problem, though it cannot be explored here.

that the loss of his *own* compositions would be what Galen – or any author – would find most agonizing (or, as Galen has it, would create the greatest challenge for his absence of distress). Certainly, as we shall see, there are some specific books of his own composition that do fall into that category. But Galen begins his discussion with a different category of works, and it is the irreplaceability of these, in particular, that he emphasizes: items in his personal library of other authors.[2] At section 5, Galen distinguishes three sub-categories of these:

(i)   rare works in his collection, which are irreplaceable because the only other copies would have been in the Palatine library, destroyed at the same time as his (12–13);

(ii)   copies of works which are not themselves rare, but represent particularly accurate editions of the text in question, because they were prepared by a particular author or scholar (an example is Panaetius' copy of the works of Plato), or because they were, in some sense, autograph copies[3] (14);

(iii)   copies of works which do *not* represent good editions in this way, but where Galen has himself marked corrections to scribal errors – right down to details of punctuation – so as to 'provide almost a new edition' of the work in question; and this includes also some texts of which there is no copy elsewhere. This third category includes works of Aristotle, Theophrastus, Chrysippus and 'all the ancient doctors' (15–17).

The first thing that emerges from all this is the extraordinary level of Galen's scholarly activity: collecting, finding good editions, and correcting and preparing new editions, of a whole range of texts. Texts which include not just those of authors like Plato and Hippocrates, who, as we know, are central to his own intellectual output, but also a whole range of others of much less central philosophical interest, or in some cases just of linguistic interest – Theophrastus, Eudemus, Chrysippus, the orators.[4]

The impression is radically reinforced when we turn (20) to the first explicit mention of a work by Galen himself which was lost: a work on 'words in Attic

---

2   See above, 'Note on MS Vlatadon 14' (henceforth: 'Note'), text (b): if one were to read σεσωρευμένων, rather than συγγεγραμμένων (though I argue against that emendation), then Galen would not be mentioning his own writings until some way down the list of losses.

3   On the differences in interpretation on this point, see 'Note', text (c). On the interpretation of 'Panaetius' Plato', see Gourinat, J.-B. (2008). 'Le Platon de Panétius: à propos d'un témoignage inédit de Galien', *Philosophie Antique* 8, 139–51.

4   As discussed in the 'Note', there is some uncertainty as to which specific texts or manuscripts are being discussed; but the text certainly gives evidence not just for Galen's intense scholarly activity, especially but not only on works in the Aristotelian tradition, but also for the availability to him of a far greater range of works (and or different manuscript traditions) than was previously known.

Greek and everyday language ... in two parts, one drawn from Old Comedy, one from prose-writers'.[5] The work seems to have taken the form of a glossary, explaining to a contemporary audience the usage of the old Attic authors in relation to a whole range of selected words, especially those of significance to medicine and diet (24–27). This, too, then, was a manifestation of his scholarly activity, and a very considerable one, if we are to take seriously the 'forty-eight large books' mentioned, on prose writers alone (28);[6] and indeed, it is perhaps significant that Galen, in making this transition to discuss his own work as opposed to the editions of others just discussed, seems to make no very clear distinction in his syntax: the lost work on Old Comedy appears almost as a continuation of the previous category. And further light on this categorization follows at 29: Galen says that none of the above losses caused him distress ... 'any more than the loss of my own notes (hupomnēmata)'; these latter, he goes on to say (29), were of two sorts: some which had been written up so as to be useful to others, some for a 'reminding' purpose (eis anamnēsin) which was just for his own use.

We shall return to that discussion of hupomnēmata, with its distinction of categories, in due course. At this particular point (29) he gives no further elaboration, but rather proceeds immediately to two other categories: first – again a distinctly scholarly kind of product – that of the 'very many summaries by heading of a very large number of works on medicine and philosophy'; secondly, the recipe collection (which we have already mentioned above). We shall also return in due course to these notes and summaries, as well as to the further remarks on the losses in the fire, especially in Lib. Prop. But only one further work is mentioned by name in the course of Ind. as having been lost in the fire, in addition to that on Old Comedy: his 'treatise on the composition of drugs' (37). But that, surely, is not all. There is, indeed, another characterization of the lost works, though without any titles, in the passage immediately preceding the mention of the work on Old Comedy, at 21–23a: there Galen refers to the loss of copies of 'all his works for distribution' (panta ta pros ekdosin). Before addressing the question of the specific reference of that phrase in its context here, it will be helpful to consider the broader question of Galen's book production and book distribution as evidenced elsewhere in Galen's writings, in particular in Lib. Prop. We might start from what at first blush appears a

---

5   The second part, he goes on to say (20), *does* survive (though it has not come down to us), because a copy was taken and transferred to his country home in Campania.

6   The length indeed seems enormous, although an explanation has been offered in terms of the glossary-style layout: each lexical item would have a fresh line. See del Mastro, G. (2012). 'Μέγα βιβλίον: Galeno e la lunghezza dei libri', in Manetti, D. (ed.) *Studi sul De indolentia di Galeno*, 33–62.

puzzling conundrum: why, given the loss of what Galen describes at one point as 'all my books' (50), do the extant works of Galen occupy a shelf or more in the modern library? How, given the disaster of the fire, is he still the most voluminous author we possess from antiquity?

Of course, the answer, in broad terms, is fairly simple. A work destroyed in the fire was only lost if it had not already been copied and if such a copy – or copies – did not survive elsewhere. This simple answer, though, conceals a rather complex variety of possibilities – possibilities contained or concealed in a number of brief remarks Galen makes in relation to the practice and process of book distribution, or *ekdosis*. Since (a) there has been a considerable volume of recent scholarship on this subject, much of it based on the evidence of Galen, (b) I believe the conclusions of much of this scholarship to be misleading in certain key respects and (c) the new text, περὶ ἀλυπίας, sheds further significant further light in this area, a detailed account of the problem may be of value.

2   Galen and *Ekdosis*

There is a conceptual distinction in ancient discussions of books and their destination audiences, between an apparently private or closed transaction, carried out between friends or within a circle of students or associates, and an apparently wider, more formal kind of distribution or 'publication' of a text; and typically the verb *didonai* and cognates are used for the former, and the verb *ekdidonai* and cognates – especially the noun *ekdosis* – for the latter.[7] In a well-known passage of *My Own Books* (to which we shall return) Galen himself describes a situation whereby works intended to be read only within such an intimate circle, or in some cases only by students at a particular level in their development – works which he typically describes as having been written in response to specific requests from these sources – have been copied and circulated without the author's consent, and thus gained a wider distribution. Such works are explicitly or implicitly characterized as lacking the completeness which one would expect for a work intended for a larger audience. In some cases, a work circulating in this 'bootleg' form, with errors, finds its way back to the author, and is corrected by him before further distribution takes place. An

---

7   Classic studies of the question of *ekdosis* and book circulation in the ancient world are van Groningen, B. A. (1963). ῎Εκδοσις, *Mnemosyne* 4:16, 1–17 and Starr, R. J. (1987). 'The Circulation of Literary Texts in the Ancient World', *CQ* 37, 213–23.

important element of the process of *ekdosis*, as we shall see that the new evidence from περὶ ἀλυπίας makes clear, is the depositing of a copy of one's work in a public library; this – in a process also described by Galen in the new text – enables interested readers not only to consult the work *in situ*, but to have further copies made for their private use. It should also be noted that *ekdosis* is also the term used for an 'edition', or particular version, of a text, especially in the sense of the scholarly edition of a classical author by a particular scholar – e.g. Bacchius' *ekdosis* of Hippocrates – without any reference to a destination audience or process of distribution.

Now, it should always be borne in mind that the process of publication, or distribution, referred to in such discussions has very little in common with those familiar from the modern period. There is no multiple production by the author, or by some 'publisher', of copies for circulation: both the act of 'giving' a work to a friend and that of 'giving-out' a work to a wider public consist, from the author's point of view, of the handing over, or making available, of a single copy, from which further copies may be made. Differences in manner of distribution depend on how many people are given access, and how many further copies are made. This in turn may, of course, depend in some way upon the work's initial manner of composition, its genre and the author's intentions; in this area, however, it is, as we shall see, very difficult to make clear statements or arrive at clear distinctions of type.

But let us look at this process of distribution, and what Galen tells us about it, in a little more detail, beginning with the evidence of *My Own Books* and *The Order of My Own Books*. A clear bipartite distinction has been made by some scholars, following the conceptual distinction given above, between works written for wide circulation or 'publication', on the one hand, and those intended for private use, or circulation within a small circle of friends or colleagues, on the other; and certain passages of Galen's *My Own Books* have provided an important part of the evidence for this supposed *pros ekdosin/ou pros ekdosin* distinction.[8] Let us look at what Galen actually says in this regard. We

---

8   See in particular Dorandi, T. (2000). *Le stylet et la tablette: dans le secret des auteurs antiques* and (2007). *Nell' officina dei classici: come lavorano gli autori antichi* (Dorandi's analysis is not confined to Galen, but uses the Galenic material as an important part of his argument; other relevant composition practices are those mentioned by Iamblichus, *Vit. Pyth.* 23,104, talking of *hupmnēmastismoi kai huposēmeiōseis*; and of Neoplatonist commentators on Aristotle who divide *his* work into *hupomnēmatika* and *suntagmatika*); Gurd, S. (2011). 'Galen on ἔκδοσις', in Schmidt, T. and Fleury, P., *Perceptions of the Second Sophistic and its Times: Regards sur la seconde sophistique et son époque*, 169–84. The bipartite distinction seems to have become widely accepted by scholars working on Galen's literary activity and self-presentation;

shall start with a passage fairly late in *My Own Books*, in which Galen is listing his works on logical demonstration.

ἔγραψα δ' ἄλλα πολλὰ γυμνάζων ἐμαυτόν, ὧν ἔνια μὲν ἀπώλετο κατὰ τὴν γενομένην πυρκαϊάν, ἡνίκα τὸ τῆς Εἰρήνης τέμενος ἐκαύθη, τινὰ δὲ φίλοις δεδομένα διασωθέντα παρὰ πολλοῖς ἐστι νῦν, ὥσπερ καὶ τἆλλα τὰ ἡμέτερα. καὶ μέντοι καὶ τῶν ὑπομνημάτων ὧν ἔγραψα τὰ μὲν ὑπ' ἐμοῦ δοθέντα φίλοις, τὰ δ' ὑπὸ τῶν οἰκετῶν κλεψάντων ἐκδοθέντα παρ' ἄλλων ἔλαβον ὕστερον ... τούτων τῶν ὑπομνημάτων ἁπάντων οὐδὲν πρὸς ἔκδοσιν ἐγράφη ...

I wrote many others as an exercise for myself, some of which perished in the fire in which the Temple of Peace was destroyed, but some had been given to friends and now survive in copies in many people's possession, just like our other works. Even of the *hupomnēmata* that I wrote, some were given by me to friends, while others, which had been stolen and distributed by servants, I later received back from other persons ... None of these *hupomnēmata* were written for distribution (*pros ekdosin*) ...

> *Lib. Prop.* 14 [11] (XIX.41 K. = 166,1–8 Boudon-Millot; XIX.42 K. = 166,18–19 Boudon-Millot)[9]

This text does indeed seem to follow our terminological distinction: Galen himself 'gives' (*dedomena*) works to friends; his household staff steal works and 'give them out' or distribute (*ekdothenta*) them more widely. Two other things, however, are striking in this passage. One is that although Galen identifies a category of works as 'for his own exercise' (*gumnazōn emauton* – we shall consider this description further below), he then adds that he gave such works to his friends. Such a slippage, whereby a type of work which is claimed to be for private use is in fact given to others, gives us an early warning of the difficulty that we shall have in identifying clear categories of works for different destinatees in Galen's accounts.[10] Even more revealing, though, is that though

---

see also Boudon-Millot, V. (2007). *Galien, Tome 1*; Mansfeld, J. (1994). 'Galen's Autobibliographies and Hippocratic Commentaries', in *Prolegomena: Questions to be Settled Before the Study of an Author, or a Text*; Vegetti, M. (2013). *Galeno: nuovi scritti autobiografici*.

9   Translations are my own unless otherwise stated. The chapter numbers of *Lib. Prop.* were altered by the discovery of the Vlatadon MS: in references here the new number is followed by the old in square brackets.

10   Even more strikingly – and even more problematically from the point of view of the literalness with which the terminology can be taken – Galen elsewhere uses exactly the same phrase in a general characterization of his motivation in writing: he always used to write either 'as a favour to friends or *gumnazōn emauton*', *MM* 7.1 (X.456 K.).

these 'private' works were given only to friends, they are now preserved and in the hands of many. Galen here not only sheds light on a process whereby 'giving' a book to friends will lead to its wide (παρὰ πολλοῖς) distribution; he also makes clear implicitly that (in spite of the explicit dismay expressed, as we shall see, elsewhere at such unauthorized distribution) such wider distribution was to be expected and, in the case of an unexpected loss of his own copy, might even be relied upon to fill the gap.

The phrase 'just like our other works' (*hōsper kai talla ta hēmetera*) is tantalizing here, and again we shall see similar phrases elsewhere: it is, by implication, certainly, the term opposed to 'as an exercise for myself', and so seems to suggest a non-private category – the works that Galen *did* intend for distribution. But this is not stated. What, then, of the category of *hupomnēmata*, which is introduced immediately after these other two categories (the sequence is: works of 'self-exercise'; 'our other works'; *hupomnēmata*)? This term, as we shall discuss further below, has a potentially very broad reference in Galen,[11] although it is also true that at some point it became the standard Greek word for 'commentaries'. Whatever the term refers to, Galen asserts that *none* of the works in that category – though some achieved circulation through having been given to friends, and some through theft by his servants – was intended for *ekdosis*. Given the context – Galen goes on to list a number of works on specific classical texts of logic – it seems that the translation 'commentaries' is appropriate here. This would mean that Galen is stating that none of his commentaries on works of logic was intended for *ekdosis*; and this, as we shall see, directly mirrors what he says about his commentaries on Hippocrates in ch. 9 [6]. To sum up: Galen has here identified three categories: about two of them he has made clear that they were not intended for distribution, though distribution in many cases in fact took place; the reference of the third, *talla ta hēmetera*, is quite vague. We should, finally, consider the context of this passage, beginning as it does with a mention of 'many other works': what are the previously-mentioned works with which these 'private' works are contrasted? One might think that the phrase must follow on a list of works which definitely *are* for *ekdosis*. The truth is rather more complicated. In fact, after a lengthy preamble about his own formation in logic and the shortcomings of certain teachers and philosophers, the chapter has so far mentioned one other work by name, before moving to the 'private' categories of the above passage. Certainly,

---

11   On this point see von Staden, H. (1998). 'Gattung und Gedächtnis: Galen über Wahrheit und Lehrdichtung', in Kullmann, W., Althoff, J. and Asper, M. (eds), *Gattungen wissenschaftlicher Literatur in der Antike*, 65–94, pointing to lack of any clear distinction between the different nouns which Galen uses in reference to his works.

it is a work – his *De demonstratione* – which he strongly recommends to the serious student at the beginning of his studies; clearly, then, he must both believe and intend it to have a fairly wide distribution, at least amongst serious students. Yet there is, it should be emphasized, no explicit mention of a *pros ekdosin* category, to contrast with the term *ouden pros ekdosin* which we have noted. Indeed, as we shall see, Galen's own deliberate act of distribution, of *ekdosis*, in this text is extremely elusive.

A converse example to the above one of works not 'given out', but nevertheless extant is provided by the major pharmacological treatise, *De compositione medicamentorum per genera*: here, Galen gives an account of books which *have* been distributed (ἐκδοθέντων, προεκδοθέντων), but are *not* extant. In the proem to the now extant version of this work, Galen claims that he is rewriting the first two books, which were lost in the fire, and that he is doing so *even though they had previously been distributed*:

> Ἤδη μοι καὶ πρόσθεν ἐγέγραπτο πραγματεία, δυοῖν μὲν ἐξ αὐτῆς τῶν πρώτων βιβλίων ἐκδοθέντων, ἐγκαταλειφθέντων δὲ ἐν τῇ κατὰ τὴν ἱερὰν ὁδὸν ἀποθήκῃ μετὰ τῶν ἄλλων, ἡνίκα τὸ τῆς Εἰρήνης τέμενος ὅλον ἐκαύθη, καὶ κατὰ τὸ παλάτιον αἱ μεγάλαι βιβλιοθῆκαι. τηνικαῦτα γὰρ ἑτέρων τε πολλῶν ἀπώλοντο βιβλία καὶ τῶν ἐμῶν ὅσα κατὰ τὴν ἀποθήκην ἐκείνην ἔκειτο, μηδενὸς τῶν ἐν Ῥώμῃ φίλων ἔχειν ὁμολογούντος ἀντίγραφα τῶν πρώτων δυοῖν. ἐγκειμένων οὖν τῶν ἑταίρων αὖθίς με γράψαι τὴν αὐτὴν πραγματείαν, ἀναγκαῖον ἔδοξέ μοι δηλῶσαι περὶ τῶν προεκδοθέντων, ὅπως μή τις προεντυχὼν αὐτοῖς ποτε ζητοίη τὴν αἰτίαν τοῦ δίς με περὶ τῶν αὐτῶν πραγματεύσασθαι.

I had written a treatise previously, too, of which the first two books had been distributed, and also deposited in my storehouse alongside the others, when the whole of the Temple of Peace was destroyed by fire, as well as the great libraries on the Palatine. The books of many others perished at that time, as did all those of mine which were located in that storehouse; and none of my friends in Rome admitted to having copies of the first two books. Since, then, my followers prevailed upon me to write the same treatise again, I thought that I should give this explanation regarding the previously distributed books, in case anyone in the future finds them and wonders why I should have written a treatise twice on the same subject.

Comp. Med. Gen. 1.1 (XIII.362–3 K.)[12]

---

12   Cf. the vaguer reference to the loss in *Ind.* 37, on which more below.

By contrast with the previous case, where informal 'giving' leads to widespread copying and distribution, here books were 'given out' (as well as being deposited in Galen's storehouse) but, after the fire of 192, cannot be found, even amongst friends in Rome. The specific phrase 'in Rome', combined with the implied expectation that the lost books may after all turn up again, suggest that Galen may have grounds to believe that the *ekdosis* has led to the preservation of copies elsewhere, perhaps in a library in Asia.[13] But another point should be made here: elsewhere in this very same work Galen makes clear that its explicitly intended readership is his followers or students: καὶ ταῦθ' ὑμῖν τοῖς ἑταίροις ὑπομνήματα γράφω, 'I write these *hupomnēmata* too for you, my followers'.[14] At least formally, this is a work for a group of intimates; already here, then, we see that the term *ekdosis* may be used in relation to works which are not, formally, intended for a wide audience. (And note that in the above text, again, Galen refers to a process of distribution that has taken place without explicitly admitting any personal role in it.) But let us return to *My Own Books*, and to the preface of that work – a central text on which scholarship identifying the *pros ekdosin / ou pros ekdosin* distinction has based itself.

τοῦ μὲν δὴ πολλοὺς ἀναγιγνώσκειν ὡς ἴδια τὰ ἐμὰ τὴν αἰτίαν αὐτὸς οἶσθα ... φίλοις γὰρ ἢ μαθήταις ἐδίδοτο χωρὶς ἐπιγραφῆς ὡς ἂν οὐδὲν πρὸς ἔκδοσιν ἀλλ' αὐτοῖς ἐκείνοις γεγονότα δεηθεῖσιν ὧν ἤκουσαν ἔχειν ὑπομνήματα.

Well, as for the fact of my works being passed off by many people under their own name you know the reason yourself: ... it is that they were given without inscription to friends or pupils, since they had been written in no way for distribution, but simply at the request of those individuals, who had desired a written record of lectures they had heard.

    Lib. Prop. praef. (XIX.10 K. = 135,11–20 Boudon-Millot)

---

13   On this process see *Ind.* 21 and the discussion of that passage below.

14   *Comp. Med. Gen.* 3.1 (XIII.562 K.). Galen repeatedly uses the term ἑταῖροι in reference to the intended audience of his major medical works. It seems to me, *pace* Mattern, S. P. (2008). *Galen and the Rhetoric of Healing*, 14–16, that ἑταῖροι for Galen has a specific sense, essentially referring to his pupils, or close followers of his medical instruction (a claim which I hope to support in detail in a forthcoming article). But even if this specific interpretation is not accepted, the term ἑταῖροι undoubtedly suggests a fairly small set of associates, not a wider audience. For an important recent discussion of the intellectual community implied by or addressed in Galen's medical works see van der Eijk, P. 'Galen and the Scientific Treatise: A Case Study of *Mixtures*', in Asper, M. (2013). *Writing Science: Medical and Mathematical Authorship in Ancient Greece*, 145–75.

Again, the action which Galen is claiming as his own is *didonai*, not *ekdido-nai*: that is, he himself gives books to his friends or pupils; other people have been responsible for the wider distribution. But note that what Galen is very definitely *not* doing, here, is identifying two categories of books, one for distribution and one not; rather, he is making a general statement about his writings (even if quite *how* general is not perfectly clear[15]), and putting this forward as a reason for people having appropriated his works as their own. The notion of an opposite implied by the negative οὐ(δὲν) πρὸς ἔκδοσιν, that is to say an actual category of books which definitely *were* πρὸς ἔκδοσιν, is something imported into the text – if we choose to import it. Nothing of that sort is stated here, and without support from other contexts this passage would be taken as referring to his books in quite general terms.

What, then, of those other contexts? A few lines later, Galen continues:

γεγραμμένων οὖν, ὡς ἔφην, οὐ πρὸς ἔκδοσιν αὐτῶν ἀλλὰ κατὰ τὴν τῶν δεηθέντων ἕξιν τε καὶ χρείαν εἰκὸς δήπου τὰ μὲν ἐκτετάσθαι, τὰ δὲ συνεστάλθαι καὶ τὴν ἑρμηνείαν αὐτήν τε τῶν θεωρημάτων τὴν διδασκαλίαν ἢ τελείαν ὑπάρχειν ἢ ἐλλιπῆ. τὰ γοῦν τοῖς εἰσαγομένοις γεγραμμένα πρόδηλον δήπου μήτε τὸ τέλειον τῆς διδασκαλίας ἔχειν μήτε τὸ διηκριβωμένον, ὡς ἂν οὔτε δεομένων αὐτῶν οὔτε δυναμένων ἀκριβῶς μανθάνειν πάντα, πρὶν ἕξιν τινὰ σχεῖν ἐν τοῖς ἀναγκαίοις.

Since, then, as I have stated above, they were written not for distribution but to fit the particular level and needs of those who had requested them, it follows naturally that some of them are rather extended, while others are compressed; and that their manner of communication, and indeed the actual exposition of theoretical material, vary in their completeness. Those works which were written for beginners would, quite evidently, be neither complete nor perfectly accurate in their teaching. That was not their requirement – nor would such individuals have been able to learn the whole subject matter accurately, until they had first reached a certain basic level in the fundamentals.

Lib. Prop. praef. (XIX.10–11 K. = 136,4–13 Boudon-Millot)

15   It would, perhaps, be possible to take *ouden* in this sentence not adverbially (as above, cf. the 1997 translator, 'with no thought for', similarly Boudon-Millot: 'aucunement') but pronominally (albeit with a mild anacolouthon, shifting from the plural of *ta ema* and *gegonota* to the singular): '*none* [of them was] written for distribution'; that would make the usage directly parallel to that already observed in the passage from ch. 14 [11].

He then proceeds to explain that certain works intended purely 'for beginners' circulated more widely, because they had not been explicitly so labelled. The subject of the whole paragraph, however, that referred to by *gegrammenōn* at the beginning of this extract, is exactly the same as that of the previous extract: it is the general 'my books'. Galen is still telling a story about his writings in general, not a sub-category of them; indeed, he is analysing a problem which arises precisely from the very wide differences that exist across all his writings (because of their different original destinatees).

Let us turn to the final passage of *My Own Books* which sheds light on Galen's own account of his attitude to *ekdosis* – again a passage which has been central to constructions of a distinction of 'private' and 'public' works in the output of Galen, and indeed of other ancient authors. It comes in the chapter where he makes the transition to discussion of his works of Hippocratic commentary. The passage has been interpreted as stating that Galen wrote such works in two distinct styles, with two distinct sets of recipient in mind, and at two distinct periods. That is, after a period in which he had written commentaries purely for his own use or for that of his close associates, he made an abrupt transition, in response to a particular event, to the writing of works intended for a wider audience and engaging in detail with rival commentators. In the former category, then, are the commentaries on *Aphorisms, Fractures, Joints, Prognosticon, Regimen in Acute Diseases, Wounds to the Head* and *Epidemics I*, in the latter those on *Epidemics II, III* and *VI, Humours, Nutriment, Prorrhetic, Nature of Man, De officina medici* and *Airs, Water, Places*. But this, we shall see, is not what Galen actually says; moreover, even if it could, on a simplistic reading, be taken to be what he says, such an account is substantially undermined by the much fuller, more detailed, chronological account of the same subject which he gives elsewhere in his writing.

Before coming to the precise words in which Galen distinguishes and lists his different Hippocratic commentaries, let us look at the preamble to that. This passage itself contains some problems, both textual and interpretive, which are in need of elucidation; it will therefore be worth our while to consider it in some detail, and with the assistance of an apparatus criticus for the problematic passages.

οὔτ' ἄλλο τι τῶν ὑπ' ἐμοῦ δοθέντων φίλοις ἤλπισα πολλοὺς ἕξειν οὔτε τὰ τῶν Ἱπποκρατείων συγγραμμάτων ἐξηγητικά· τὴν ἀρχὴν γὰρ <οὐδ'> ἐμαυτὸν γυμνάζων ἐγεγράφην εἰς αὐτὰ ποθ' ὑπομνήματα, καθάπερ ἐποίησα τῆς ἰατρικῆς θεωρίας ἁπάσης καθ' ἕκαστον μέρος ἐμαυτῷ παρασκευάσας οἷς ἅπαντα τὰ κατὰ τὴν ἰατρικὴν τέχνην ὑφ' Ἱπποκράτους εἰρημένα περιέχεται διδασκαλίαν ἔχοντα σαφῆ θ' ἅμα καὶ παντοίως ἐξειργασμένην· ἰδίᾳ μὲν γὰρ περὶ κρισίμων ἡμερῶν

ἔγραψα κατὰ τὴν Ἱπποκράτους γνώμην, ἰδίᾳ δὲ περὶ κρίσεων, ἰδίᾳ δὲ περὶ
δυσπνοίας ἑκάστου τε τῶν ἄλλων ὅλην τε τὴν θεραπευτικὴν μέθοδον ὡσαύτως
ἐν τέσσαρσι καὶ δέκα βιβλίοις ἐποιησάμην, ἅπαντα [δὲ] τὰ θεραπευτικὰ καὶ
πρὸς αὐτοῖς [ταύτην], ἃ κατὰ τὴν ἐκείνου γνώμην …

2 αὐτὸν οὐδὲν Α οὐδὲν αὐτὸν Vlat. ἐμαυτὸν Corn. Ar. ΒΜ οὐδὲν πρὸς ἔκδοσιν ἀλλ᾽
ἐμαυτὸν Müller οὐδ᾽ ἐμαυτὸν scripsi 9 δὲ add. Corn. 9–10 ἅπαντα … γνώμην secl.
Müller 10 ἃ κατὰ τὴν ἐκείνου γνώμην om. Ar. ταύτην secl. ΒΜ

Before proceeding we must consider some textual uncertainties. In line 2,
ἐμαυτὸν was Cornarius' emendation: it is supported by the Arabic translation,
whereas both Greek MSS have instead a negative expression (αὐτὸν οὐδὲν Α,
οὐδὲν αὐτὸν Vlat.); Müller also felt it necessary to add a further 'not for distribution' comment to make sense of the passage. But one should consider whether
the negative, supported by all the Greek MSS, may after all be preserved: if we
read οὐδ᾽ ἐμαυτὸν – a minimal emendation of the Vlat. οὐδὲν αὐτὸν – we have
a solution which makes sense of the Greek MS tradition while also preserving
the ἐμαυτὸν suggested by the Latin and Arabic ones; it also fits better syntacti-
cally with ποθ᾽ in the next line. The sense would then be: 'To begin with I *did not
ever* write notes/commentaries on them *even* as an exercise for myself, as I did
in each individual part of the whole art of medicine …'; and this in fact would
be perfectly consistent with the explanation that he goes on to give: he did not
need to write commentaries on Hippocrates because Hippocrates' views were
already contained in Galen's individual medical works. The difference, on this
reading, is that Galen is claiming *not even* to have made 'private' commentaries at an earlier stage, whereas according to both Müller's and Boudon-Millot's
readings he is saying that at that time he wrote *only* private commentaries. My
emendation would of course make the present discussion even less relevant to
the chronological 'private–public' distinction that has been perceived: Galen
is not writing (commentary-style) private notes early on, and moving to works
for publication later, because he was not writing such notes early on at all. Such
a chronological distinction of types of commentary activity is not in play. This
also seems consistent with what is said in *Hipp. Epid. III* (see n. 25 below): at
the earliest stage he is simply not writing commentary on Hippocrates.

    The above emendation will not seem convincing to all; nor is it essential
to my argument in what follows. It should, however, be noted that two quite
substantial interpretive difficulties remain, if we do *not* adopt that negative.
On such a (non-negative) reading, Galen identifies a personal-exercise category (let us call it 'A') of Hippocratic commentaries which he wrote at an
early stage, and sets it alongside another category or writings ('B'), also termed
hupomnēmata, introduced by the phrase καθάπερ ἐποίησα. The first problem,

then, on this reading, is that it is quite difficult to make sense of the opposition between categories A and B. B must now be *hupomnēmata* on the whole of medicine, considered subject by subject as opposed to by Hippocratic treatise. Such an opposition makes sense; but what relationship between category B and the Hippocratic texts is Galen then making in the phrase that follows, οἷς ... ἐξειργασμένην, which must mean something like 'in which are contained all things stated by Hippocrates in relation to the art of medicine, things which have an exposition[16] which is both clear and completely elaborated'? Having made the distinction between categories A (private-exercise notes on Hippocrates) and B (similar notes on each branch of medicine), Galen is immediately insisting on the close relationship of the latter set of notes to Hippocratic texts – a relationship then further insisted upon by the description of these medical works as 'according to the opinion of Hippocrates' κατὰ τὴν Ἱπποκράτους γνώμην ... κατὰ τὴν ἐκείνου γνώμην. If, as this reading requires, Galen is identifying two parallel sets of 'exercise' works, the first on works of Hippocrates, the second on branches of medicine, the distinction between them seems to collapse as he insists on the essentially Hippocratic nature of the latter.

The second, related, problem is that category B includes the works *Critical Days, Crises* and *The Therapeutic Method.* These major medical works – so far from being for 'distribution' in any sense – are, on this reading, claimed by Galen to have been written as a private intellectual exercise: 'I made notes for my own exercise, *as I did* in the individual parts of medicine [and then the reference to those works]'. The adoption of the negative makes the association less close: rather than considering two parallel sets of 'exercise' notes, it is then at least possible to take the καθάπερ ἐποίησα clause, more loosely, as referring simply to the writing of *hupomnēmata*, rather than as picking up the whole phrase including ἐμαυτὸν γυμνάζων. So: 'I did not even make notes on Hippocratic works for my own exercise; I did [by contrast] make notes on the individual parts ...'

---

16   The phrase raises a further interpretive problem: does the participle ἔχοντα refer to the statements of Hippocrates or to those statements as mediated by Galen; in other words, is the 'clear exposition' that of Galen in his explication or that of the master? Either interpretation brings problems. On the one hand, talk of clarity and fulness of Galen's exposition, as opposed to Hippocratic concision, would seem consistent with what Galen says elsewhere about the relationship between his writing and Hippocrates' and about the function of commentary; it might seem odd, indeed, for him to refer to Hippocrates' own writings in such terms. On the other hand, such a reading is grammatically difficult: it is quite hard to take the participle phrase διδασκαλίαν ἔχοντα, appearing without any adversative particle, as suddenly introducing Galen's, not Hippocrates', contribution.

The end of the passage brings more textual and interpretive uncertainties. Müller secluded the whole of the phrase ἅπαντα to γνώμην, thus removing the second statement of the double function of Galen's texts as medical and Hippocratic; yet it seems no more challenging that what has already been said, and is supported by both Greek MSS and (as far as αὐτοῖς), by the Arabic. However, the phrase makes better sense without Cornarius' δὲ, for then it can be taken in apposition to ὅλην τε τὴν θεραπευτικὴν μέθοδον. That is, Galen is *glossing* 'the whole of *The Therapeutic Method*' with the phrase 'all the therapeutics and also what is in accordance with Hippocrates' view'; and this agrees perfectly with the sense of the argument so far. Although the words from καὶ πρὸς αὐτοῖς might seem to suggest a separate work, Boudon-Millot's removal of the ungrammatical ταύτην assists us in seeing that this is not the intention; in any case (see further below), to what additional work could Galen possibly be referring? On balance, this whole last phrase from ἅπαντα must be taken appositionally: again, Galen is presenting his own works of therapeutics as *simultaneously* works on Hippocrates.

To summarize: Galen is about to say that he did not, in an earlier phase, write line-by-line commentaries of Hippocratic works, because he found that unnecessary. The present passage is laying the foundations for this claim by making the point that all Galen's own works on specific medical topics 'contain all things stated by Hippocrates in relation to the art of medicine, things which have a form of exposition which is both clear and completely elaborated'. This is, indeed, a remarkable claim. The interpretive focus on the apparent 'private–public' distinction, and on the classification of the Hippocratic commentaries that follows has, perhaps, taken attention away from how remarkable it is. Galen is saying that his own works on medical topics – central works like *Critical Days, Crises* and *The Therapeutic Method* – in fact perform the function of commentaries on Hippocrates: they are in a sense proto-commentaries, or adequate commentary-substitutes; and he is stating this as his reason for his having carried out no direct commentary work on Hippocrates until a late stage in his career. The only way of resisting this interpretation is by taking the whole phrase περὶ κρισίμων ἡμερῶν ἔγραψα κατὰ τὴν Ἱπποκράτους γνώμην to refer to the composition of a specific work 'On Critical Days According to Hippocrates' – which is indeed what the phrase seems most naturally to mean – and therefore taking this whole passage to refer to works *specifically* on Hippocrates' views. Yet the context, amid the known works *Crises* and *The Therapeutic Method* – especially with the specific reference to *The Therapeutic Method* as having fourteen books, which makes it clear that this is the extant *The Therapeutic Method* – and the absence of any reference elsewhere to these separate 'According to Hippocrates' works, makes this clearly impossible.

And we should note that this very striking claim, in the latter part of the passage quoted, remains *whether or not* we adopt my proposed reading in the first lines. My suggestion, however, is that doing so gives us a progression of thought which is more consistent with this claim: Galen is explaining his *non*-writing of direct commentaries on Hippocrates (even for personal use) by the fact that his other works at this stage were, in a sense, commentaries on Hippocrates. A couple of points of clarification, however, should be made before we proceed. One is that the term *idiai* in this passage must, indeed, be taken to mean 'specifically', not 'privately'.[17] In such contexts Galen uses the term in the former sense quite regularly. The distinction at this point is not between 'for private use' and the (unstated) opposite, 'for publication', but between an organization of his own literary output according to *specific medical subject* (while simultaneously clarifying Hippocrates' views), and the alternative activity of writing line-by-line Hippocratic commentaries. Galen is not here outlining a private–public distinction within his own works. What he is doing is either – on *any* of the previously accepted readings of the above passage – explicitly insisting on the private character of even his most central works of medicine, which he claims to have been written in a process of intellectual self-exercise, or at least – on my reading – associating them quite closely with that intellectual activity.

Let us then offer a translation of this whole introductory passage, before proceeding to that in which Galen does, apparently, mention an *ekdosis* of his own Hippocratic commentaries.

> As with my other works given to friends, so especially with the works of Hippocratic commentary, I had no expectation that they would reach a wider audience. In the first instance, indeed, I did not ever write notes on those works even as an exercise for myself – as I did [on the other hand], preparing them for myself, in each individual area of medical theory – notes by means of which is contained all that Hippocrates had said of relevance to the art of medicine, having a clear and fully elaborated exposition. For I wrote specifically on critical days, in accordance with Hippocrates' views, but also specifically on crises, specifically on difficulty in breathing, and on all the other subjects; and in the same way I produced the whole therapeutic method, in fourteen books: [that is to say,] all of therapeutics, and in addition those things which are in accordance with his views.
>
> *Lib. Prop.* 9 [6] (XIX.33–4 K. = 159,10–160,1 Boudon-Millot)

---

17   As Boudon-Millot *ad loc.*: 'à usage privé'.

That status of *The Therapeutic Method* as – not, to be sure, for personal exercise, but – 'purely for a friend', is, indeed, asserted within the work itself.[18] And this same idea, that Galen 'gave to friends' many of his central medical works – with the further claim that he *would not have done so if he had known that they would be distributed (ekdothēsesthai) to the unworthy* – is asserted also in the autobiographical work, *Prognosis*.[19] In the latter case, the works mentioned include not only *Crises* but also the major treatises in the pulse, all of which, again, feature prominently in the curriculum of study in *My Own Books*.

The fact that a work as central to his own corpus as *The Therapeutic Method* can be referred to in the category 'given to friends' and 'with no expectation that it would reach a wider audience' suggests two rather important things. The first is that the 'giving' in question here can include formal literary dedication to a named addressee (as indeed appears in *The Therapeutic Method*), rather than some private transaction; the second is the disingenuous nature of the 'not-for-distribution' claim itself. The claim that works were never, in the first place, intended for a wider audience, and not written with a view to reputation, is indeed a repeated one throughout Galen's work;[20] it is undoubtedly, at least at some level, a literary trope, whereby the author anticipates or defends himself against criticisms based on a work's apparent incompleteness or other shortcomings.[21] This is not, however, to deny the historical reality behind such claims. There is no reason to doubt, either that the dedicatees of *The*

---

18   See *MM* 7.1 (X.456–7 K.).

19   πάντι τούτῳ τῷ χρόνῳ πολλὰς πραγματείας ἔγραψα φιλοσόφους τε καὶ ἰατρικάς, ἃς
      ὑποστρέψαντος εἰς τὴν Ῥώμην τοῦ βασιλέως αἰτήσασι τοῖς φίλοις ἔδωκα, παρὰ μόνοις ἐκεί-
      νοις ἐλπίσας αὐτὰς ἔσεσθαι· ὡς εἴ γ᾽ἠπιστάμην ἐκδοθήσεσθαι τοῖς ἀναξίοις οὐκ ἂν οὐδ᾽ἐκείνοις
      ἔδωκα, *Praen.* 9 (XIV.650–1 K. = 120,1–4 Nutton): the period referred to is the same one
      mentioned in *Lib. Prop.* as that in which he 'wrote up' his main medical and scientific
      works, on which see pp. 122–3, with n. 45, below.

20   Above we saw the example of *MM*, and below we shall see the same claim with regard to
      the Hippocratic commentaries. Note further that within the preamble to the former work,
      MM 1.1 (X.1–2 K.), Galen laments the current intellectual climate and the likely fate – in
      terms of its reputation – of a work of intellectual value, thus at least implicitly and nega-
      tively acknowledging his ambition for his own works with a broader public.

21   For analysis of Galen's techniques of self-presentation see Boudon, V. (2000). 'Galien par
      lui-même: les traités bio-bibliographiques (*De ordine librorum suorum* et *De libris pro-
      priis*)', in Manetti, D. (ed.) *Studi su Galeno: scienza, filosofia, retorica e filologia. Atti del
      seminario, Firenze, 13 novembre 1998*, 119–33, as well as Boudon-Millot's 'Introduction
      générale' to *Galien, Tome 1*; Gleason, M. W. (1995). *Making Men: Sophists and Self-
      Presentation in Ancient Rome*; von Staden, H. (2009). 'Staging the Past, Staging Oneself:
      Galen on Hellenistic Exegetical Traditions', in Gill, C., Whitmarsh, T. and Wilkins, J. (eds),
      Galen and the World of Knowledge, 132–56; Boudon-Millot, V. 'Galen's *Bios* and *Methodos*:
      From Ways of Life to Path of Knowledge', in ibid., 175–89; more explicitly on such literary
      tropes in Galen, and their relatives elsewhere, König, J. (2009). 'Conventions of Prefatory

Therapeutic Method were Hiero and Eugenianus, in the sense that the text was in some way formally presented to them, or that the Hippocratic commentaries were for the use of – or even in response to the requests of – students and friends, and were given to them in that context. The point is that such a dedication, or such a transaction, is made in the clear expectation that the works will be further circulated and, in at least some cases, with a reliance on this procedure for the dissemination of one's views and the development of one's reputation. The public reception, and criticism, of a work is being anticipated at precisely the same time that its original destination for an inner circle of students is asserted. A good example is the preface to Galen's commentary on the Hippocratic *Epidemics* VI. Here Galen simultaneously anticipates the criticisms of a wider audience who will be impatient with a long exposition which engages in detail with previous commentators, admits that he has compromised with such expectations in the composition of the work, *and* reasserts the fundamental nature and origin or the commentary as a work for his own *hetairoi* (he also seems to imply that the main concession that he is making to the wider public is the very writing of this preface which explains the situation; on this point see further below).[22] Or consider, as a particularly striking example of the non-contradiction of private 'giving' and public dissemination, the magna opera *De usu partium* and *De placitis Hippocratis et Platonis*. These were, at least formally, written in response to the request of a patron, Flavius Boethus, not for *ekdosis*. The first book (at least) of the former, and the first six of the latter, were presented to him, as indeed were early drafts of *Anatomical Procedures*.[23] But no serious student of Galen can doubt that is on precisely these works that Galen in fact built his early reputation in Rome. The

---

Self-Presentation in Galen's *On the Order of My Own Books*', in ibid., 35–58. See also Mattern, *Rhetoric of Healing*.

22   ... εἰ μὲν τῷ μήκει τῶν ὑπομνημάτων οὐδεὶς ἔμελλε <τῶν> ἀναγνωσομένων αὐτὰ δυσχεραίνειν, ἁπάντων μεμνῆσθαι κάλλιον εἶναι, μεμφομένων δὲ πολλῶν οὐ τούτοις μόνον, ἀλλὰ καὶ τοῖς συμμέτρως ἔχουσι καὶ μόνα σπουδαζόντων τὰ χρήσιμα, μέσην τινὰ τούτων ἀμφοτέρων ποιήσασθαι τὴν ἐξήγησιν καὶ τοῦτο εὐθέως ἐν ἀρχῇ προειπεῖν, ὅπως ἀπαλλάττωνται τῶνδε τῶν ὑπομνημάτων οἱ μὴ χαίροντες τούτοις. ἐγὼ μὲν γάρ, ὥσπερ καὶ τἆλλα πάντα πολλοῖς τῶν δεηθέντων ἑταίρων χαριζόμενος ἐποίησα, καὶ τὰς ἐξηγήσεις ταύτας ἐκείνων ἔνεκα συνέθηκα. θεωρῶν δ' εἰς πολλοὺς ἐκπίπτοντα τὰ γραφόμενα προοιμίων τοιούτων ἐδεήθην, *Hipp. Epid. VI* praef. (XVIIA.795–6 K. = 4,19–5,3 Wenkebach).

23   See *Lib. Prop.* 1 (XIX.15–16 K. = 139–40 Boudon-Millot); cf. *AA* 1.1 (II.215–17 K.), which also mentions a number of other anatomical works given to Boethus. Note also that the account in *AA* clearly states that the entire seventeen books of *UP* were sent to Boethus during his lifetime (ἔτι ζῶντι τῷ Βοηθῷ), although he had left Rome (II.217 K.), whereas the *Lib. Prop.* account speaks of one being written before his departure, but then is less clear about the process of the work's subsequent completion (with the above passage cf. *Lib. Prop.* 2, XIX.20 K. = 143,7–12 Boudon-Millot).

further books, and further fortunes, of *De usu partium* are also highly relevant here: Galen speaks very clearly of the text's wide dissemination and influence amongst doctors, and again it was clearly a major work in the formation of his reputation. He does not, however, ever state (*pace* Vegetti) that he wrote or re-wrote it for *ekdosis*.

A further complication should be considered here, which is the relationship of written-up accounts to public lectures or demonstrations. Galen does not deny the competitive and public nature of his activities in this area, especially in the field of anatomy: indeed, he gives us a very clear picture of the social and intellectual climate within which this persuasive and rhetorical activity takes place; he also claims to have ceased such activity at a particular historical moment. In many cases, the texts we have are prefaced as being the written version of such public lecturing. The anatomical works just mentioned are one such example; *The Therapeutic Method* and *De locis affectis* are also so present-ed; so too is the short philosophical work *Affections and Errors of the Soul.* But we note, again, that such prefaces describe this writing-up as being for par-ticular individuals, or for *hetairoi* more generally, even though the original oral context may have been a more public one. There is potentially a complex dy-namic in play here: it may indeed be true, for example, that a work like *De locis affectis*, or even *The Therapeutic Method*, can best be read, not as a stand-alone text but in conjunction with the oral exposition of which it claims to be a re-cord or reminder. Still, the same point already made will apply: the writing-up, though officially defined as being for an individual, is a way of putting the work in the (or at least some) public domain, of ensuring a further dissemination, even if we have no way of being specific about the extent or precise nature of that dissemination.

But we should return to chapter 9 [6] of *My Own Books* and read a little further, because it is here at last that we get, apparently, a positive mention of Galen's own role in *ekdosis* (all the other mentions in *My Own Books* were de-nials). It is in fact the only place in Galen's work – before the discovery of περὶ ἀλυπίας, that is – where we get such a positive admission; it will therefore be important to consider what is actually being stated here.

> ἐξηγήσεις δὲ καθ' ἑκάστην αὐτοῦ λέξιν ἤδη πολλοῖς τῶν πρὸ ἐμοῦ γεγραμμένας
> οὐ φαύλως εἰδώς, εἴ τι μοι μὴ καλῶς ἐδόκουν εἰρηκέναι, περιττὸν ἡγούμην
> ἐλέγχειν· ἐνεδειξάμην δὲ τοῦτο δι' ὧν πρῴην ἔδωκα τοῖς παρακαλέσασι,
> σπανιάκις ἐν αὐτοῖς εἰπών τι πρὸς τοὺς ἐξηγουμένους αὐτάς ... πάντα κατὰ τὴν
> ἐμαυτοῦ γνώμην εἶπον ἄνευ τοῦ μνημονεῦσαι τῶν ἄλλως ἐξηγουμένων ... μετὰ
> ταῦτα δέ τινος ἀκούσας ἐξήγησιν ἀφορισμοῦ μοχθηρὰν ἐπαινοῦντος ὅσα τοῦ

λοιποῦ τισιν ἔδωκα, πρὸς κοινὴν ἔκδοσιν ἀποβλέπων, οὐκ ἰδίαν ἕξιν ἐκείνων μόνων τῶν λαβόντων, οὕτως συνέθηκα ...

Line-by-line commentaries had already been written by many before me, which I knew perfectly well; and I considered it superfluous to refute anything in those which appeared to me incorrect; I had indicated this previously in what I gave to those who made requests to me, where I seldom made reference to other commentators ... I stated everything in accordance with my own opinion, without mention of those who gave other interpretations ... but after this I heard someone praising a bad interpretation of one of the aphorisms, and then whatever I gave to people I composed with an eye to general distribution, not to the level of those people alone who were the recipients ...

Lib. Prop. 9 [6] (XIX.34–5 K. = 160,1–21 Boudon-Millot)

This, then, is the passage that has led to the clear distinction, in modern scholarship, between two actually distinct categories of Galenic commentaries on Hippocrates: the first, intended for limited circulation, and not engaging with the commentaries of others, the second for a wider public and engaging in such argument.[24] But again, let us consider what Galen actually says. The phrase on which this intention to publish, or to engage in wider distribution, has been based, is πρὸς κοινὴν ἔκδοσιν ἀποβλέπων – that is, 'with an eye to' or 'with consideration of' a more general distribution. And it must be taken with the following phrase, οὐκ ἰδίαν ἕξιν ἐκείνων μόνων τῶν λαβόντων. The claim is, still, that there is a specific group of individuals (Galen's own followers; see further below) who are the works' actual *recipients*; it is just that in writing works for them, after a certain point, Galen takes into account that they will, as a matter of fact, reach a wider audience. This is entirely consistent with the picture that emerges throughout this book and elsewhere – the picture, indeed, which Galen wishes to give us – that he is writing for individuals, and that *ekdosis* is something that he is aware will happen, not something which

---

24 The classic work on Galen's Hippocratic commentary activity (and classic statement of this distinction) is Manetti, D. and Roselli, A. (1994). 'Galeno commentatore di Ippocrate', in *ANRW* II.37.2, 1529–1635. But see von Staden, 'Staging the Past', 140–50, who while in broad terms accepting the private–public distinction, also draws attention to a number of specific ways in which such a distinction is not borne out – at least not straightforwardly – by the actual content of the texts. This seems to me extremely significant: the clear division of Galen's commentaries into two categories is frequently stated, while detailed analysis of the commentaries themselves is a much less common enterprise.

he initiates. In this text, he is indeed admitting that in the composition of the later Hippocratic commentaries he 'had an eye' to *ekdosis*. He does not claim to have carried out the *ekdosis*, nor does he give us any information about the broader group that this, as opposed to earlier commentaries, was intended to reach. Certainly, the reason for the reference to *ekdosis* is (at least implicitly) that he believes that his works can be of some public benefit: they can refute errors which are current because of other people's Hippocratic commentaries. But he has stopped short of admitting his own role in self-distribution.

But there is much stronger evidence for Galen's own account of his own distribution – or rather non-distribution – of his works, specifically in the more detailed account of the genesis and progress of his Hippocratic commentaries given in his commentary on *Epidemics* III; let us therefore now turn aside from the rather summary, we might say flitting, account of *My Own Books* – an account which is, as we have seen, not devoid of both interpretive and textual difficulties – to that more detailed and informative one. What is in fact stated, very clearly, in this longer version is that *all* Galen's commentaries were written in response to individual requests, in particular those of his *hetairoi*. If the account of the genesis of the commentaries in *My Own Books* has three stages – those treatises which covered Hippocrates' thought and so were quasi-commentaries; line-by-line commentaries written in response to requests; commentaries responding directly to other commentaries – then that in the commentary to *Epidemics* III has fully seven, each presented as a response to requests, either of *hetairoi* or of a wider group.[25] First (i), we have the stage of writing nothing except at the request of *hetairoi* who want notes of previous oral instruction; then (ii), the writing of works on 'all parts' of medicine, in response to the fact that these previous works have been distributed more widely and found useful by others too. Next comes (iii) the writing of specific works on Hippocrates in response to *hetairoi*, which is followed by (iv) the writing of commentaries on *Regimen in Acute Diseases* and *Humours* in response to specific, urgent requests, (v) the urgings of both *hetairoi* and other friendly doctors to write commentaries on *all* Hippocrates' works and (vi) a begging request to write a commentary on *Prorrhetic*. This was a pressing need because of the problems that arise from failure to understand the status and limitations of that work – an enterprise which in the process leads to the refutation of false exegetes. Related to this last point, there then came (vii) the urgings of *hetairoi* which caused Galen, in moving from the commentary on *Epidemics* II to that on *Epidemics* III, to address false interpretations so precisely that a whole book of the commentary is dedicated to three case-histories.

25   *Hipp. Epid. III* 2, praef. (XVIIA.576–84 K. = 60–66 Wenkebach).

The account seems almost self-parodic in its repetition and elaboration of the theme of the reluctant writer, giving way by stages to the importunings of his followers and of other interested persons. But the essential point is that here, once again – and as typically throughout the Galenic corpus – it is personal requests that have been responsible for every fresh development – and in particular every new prolixity – in Galen's writings. Note in particular that the very last phase of this progress – part of the public distribution project according to the traditional view – is here again a phase carried out at the request of Galen's own *hetairoi*. Now, it is true that Galen is here indeed describing a relationship between the author and his intended audiences; but it is undeniable, also, that any reference to some larger group, as opposed to the close circle of his own *hetairoi*, is extremely limited. Certainly nothing as straightforward as an opposition between works 'for *ekdosis*' and 'not for *ekdosis*' emerges from this text. Most strikingly of all – and crucially for our understanding of what is going on here – it is Galen's response to individual, *private* requests which are, time and again, presented as the occasion for his most prolific literary outputs as well as those which would on other grounds have the strongest claim to be seen as 'for distribution' (*The Therapeutic Method, De placitis Hippocratis et Platonis*,[26] the later Hippocratic commentaries).

We have seen, then, that Galen in *My Own Books* does not identify a category of books 'for *ekdosis*' contrasted with another, 'not for *ekdosis*'; and we have seen, further, that he has a consistent policy of denying or concealing his own role in *ekdosis*. He does not with any clarity identify two audiences, a closer and a wider group;[27] he admits to writing works only (or almost only) at the request of friends, patrons or students; he writes and gives works – including and especially those with the largest public impact – for and to those persons; either as a result of that or through some other clandestine activities they end up in the hands of 'many'; it is also clear that this wider distribution – whatever his protests – is something that he expects to happen.

3   *Ekdosis* and Galen's *Oeuvre*: the New Evidence of περὶ ἀλυπίας

The text of περὶ ἀλυπίας contains some striking new information on Galen's attitude to *ekdosis*. Before turning to that, let us conclude our survey of Galen's

---

26   See *PHP* 7.1 (v.586–7 K. = 428,4–17 De Lacy) for its own internal account of its composition – in a very public, competitive context – in response to the urgings of his own *hetairoi*.

27   But on this point see further below.

attitude to *ekdosis* as evidenced elsewhere in the corpus. Outside περὶ ἀλυπίας, the term is in fact used by Galen between twenty-six and twenty-eight times (depending on textual readings in *Lib. Prop.*). In six of the instances, he is using the term in the specific sense of a particular *edition* of a previous author's work – the author in question being usually Hippocrates.[28] There is then a usage whereby Galen refers to an author's *ekdosis* – or non-*ekdosis* – of his own works. One such case involves a philosopher producing a 'second *ekdosis*' of his book in response to criticism;[29] but by far the most frequent use is to refer to Hippocrates' attitude to his own works, in particular the different books of *Epidemics*.[30] Here Galen is justifying the interpretive approach that he has towards *Epidemics* I and III, on the one hand, and *Epidemics* II and VI, on the other. The backward projection by Galen on to Hippocrates of his own attitudes and compositional practices is in itself interesting. It is noteworthy, here, that although Galen does attribute some kind of *ekdosis* activity to Hippocrates, here too the preponderance of the references is in the negative: the fact that works were *not* for *ekdosis* explains their incomplete or elliptical nature. Finally, we have the four (five if we follow Müller's reading for the ch. 9 [6] text) cases which we have already considered in *My Own Books*, to which we may add one instance in *Anatomical Procedures* – again, a general denial that his works were written *pros ekdosin*.[31] It is also worth noting that in only two of all these cases is the phrase *pros ekdosin* coupled with an article, e.g. *tois*

---

28   The 'Attican' edition of Plato (*In Plat. Tim.* frag. 2); Artemidorus Capito's edition of Hippocrates (*HNH* 1.2, XV.21 K. = 13,19–20 Mewaldt); that of Bacchius (*Hipp. Epid. III* 2.8, XVIIA.619 K. = 87,11 Wenkebach); Dioscorides' edition of Hippocrates (*Hipp. Epid. III* 3.74, XVIIA.732 K. = 158,8–9 Wenkebach; ibid. 1.18, XVIIA.559 K. = 47,2 Wenkebach; cf. *Hipp. Off. Med.* 1 praef. XVIIIB.631 K.).

29   *De marcore* 2 (VII.670 K.).

30   *Epidemics* II and VI were not for *ekdosis*, as were books I and III: *Hipp. Epid. III* 3.1 (XVIIA.648 K. = 109,8–10 Wenkebach); similarly: *Hipp. Epid. VI* 1 praef. (XVIIA.796 K. = 5,4–7 Wenkebach); ibid. 2.15 (XVIIA.922 K. = 75,25 and 76,4–5 Wenkebach); ibid. 2.46 (XVIIA.1001 K. = 118,24–5 Wenkebach); ibid. 3.3 (XVIIB.12–13 K. = 130,12–14 Wenkebach); ibid. 3.17 (XVIIB.52 K. = 151,9 Wenkebach); ibid. 4.11 (XVIIB.153 K. = 208,2 Wenkebach); ibid. 4.20 (XVIIB.183 K. = 227,28 Wenkebach); ibid. 5.3 (XVIIB.241 K. = 264,14 Wenkebach); similarly (only the first and the third were written *hōs pros ekdosin*): *Hipp. Art.*, XVIIIA.530 K.; cf. *Hipp. Off. Med.* 2.26 (XVIIIB.790 K.; ibid. 3,29, XVIIIB.879 K.).

31   *AA* 1.1 (II.217 K.) There is one further possible case in *Lib. Prop.*, though it has been deleted by both modern editors. In ch. 16 [13], in his account of Platonic works, the reference to *Quod animi mores* in both Greek MSS (but not in the Arabic) contains the phrase: β΄· καὶ ἄλλο καθ᾽ἑτέραν ἔκδοσιν (XIX.46 K. = 171,3–4 Boudon-Millot). The suggestion that *QAM* had a two-book version, or indeed that it circulated in two versions, is intriguing, though unsupported by other evidence. It is, however, worth remarking that if this phrase were genuine, it would constitute the only explicit reference by Galen, using this terminology, to two different *ekdoseis* of his own works.

pros ekdosin, thus indicating a distinct category of works so intended; and both these cases refer to Hippocrates, not to Galen himself.[32] That is, in no case – before the discovery of the περὶ ἀλυπίας – does Galen use the phrase *ta pros ekdosin*, 'works for distribution', in relation to any category of his own work.

Which makes the material in περὶ ἀλυπίας all the more interesting. For here Galen does indeed use precisely such an expression. The uniqueness, within the Galenic corpus, of both that formulation and the information contained in it, has not, I think, been properly noticed. It will, then, be of some importance to understand what is actually being stated here.

The crucial passage, which follows on from the mention of his work on Old Comedy, is as follows:

> ... ἀλλὰ κατὰ τύχην γε τῆς ἑτέρας εἰς Καμπανίαν ἐκεκόμιστο τἀντίγραφα. καὶ εἴ γε μετὰ δύο μήνας ἐνεπέπρηστο τὰ κατὰ τὴν Ῥώμην, ἔφθανον ἂν οὖν εἰς Καμπανίαν πασῶν τῶν ἡμετερῶν πραγματειῶν τὰ ἀντίγραφα. διπλᾶ γὰρ ἐγέγραπτο πάντα τὰ πρὸς ἔκδοσιν ἤδη, χωρὶς τῶν ἐν Ῥώμῃ μελλόντων μένειν, ἀξιούντων μὲν καὶ τῶν ἐν τῇ πατρίδι φίλων ἁπάσας αὐτοῖς πεμφθῆναι τὰς ὑπ᾽ἐμοῦ γεγονυίας πραγματείας ὅπως ἐν βιβλιοθήκῃ δημοσίᾳ στῶσι, καθάπερ καὶ ἄλλοι τινὲς ἤδη πολλὰ τῶν ἡμετέρων ἐν ἄλλαις πόλεσιν ἔθηκαν, ἐννοοῦντος δὲ κἀμοῦ πάντων ἔχειν ἀντίγραφα κατὰ τὴν Καμπανίαν. ἦν οὖν διὰ τοῦτο διπλᾶ πάντα τὰ ἡμετερὰ χωρὶς τῶν ἐν Ῥώμῃ μελλόντων μένειν ὡς ἔφην. ἡ μὲν οὖν πυρκαϊὰ τελευτῶντος ἐγένετο τοῦ χειμῶνος, ἐγὼ δὲ ἐνόουν ἐν ἀρχῇ τοῦ θέρους εἰς τὴν Καμπανίαν κομίσαι τά τε αὐτόθι μέλλοντα κεῖσθαι καὶ τὰ πεμφθησόμενα τῶν ἐτησίων πνεόντων εἰς Ἀσίαν. ἐνήδρευσεν δὲ ἡμᾶς ἡ τύχη πολλὰ ... τῶν ἡμετέρων ἀφελομένη βιβλίων ...

> ... but by chance the copies of the second [*sc. part of my work on Attic terms*] had already been transported to Campania. And if the buildings destroyed by fire at Rome had been destroyed two months later, by then there would already have been copies of all our treatises in Campania. For all those for distribution had already been written in two copies, apart from those which were to remain in Rome, since my friends in my homeland, too, asked for all the treatises produced by me to be sent to them so that they might be put in a public library, in the same way that certain others, in other cities, had already deposited many of our works, and I, too, planned to have copies of them all in Campania. This, then,

---

32   At *Hipp. Epid.* VI 2.15 (XVIIA.922 K. = 75,25 Wenkebach) and *Hipp. Off. Med.* 3.29 (XVIIIB.879 K.), though the latter is a reference to *hypothetical* work which might have been distributed to give the fuller account.

is why all our works had been done in two copies, apart from those that were to remain in Rome, as I said. Now, the fire happened towards the end of winter, whereas I planned that at the beginning of the summer I would send to Campania both those works that were to stay there and those that would be sent to Asia once the Etesian winds had started. But chance waylaid me, taking away many ... of our books ...

> *Ind.* 20–23b (8,15–9,13 BJP)[33]

Three phrases here seem to me particularly worthy of note, and of analysis. First, the expression *panta ta pros ekdosin*. In the light of our previous survey, we now see that this is an almost unique case of Galen acknowledging (at least implicitly) his own role in an *ekdosis* process of his own works, and a completely unique case of his use of the phrase *pros ekdosin* with the article, again in relation to his own (rather than Hippocrates') works – thus denoting a specific category of works so intended. To which works is Galen so referring, and what is the nature of the *ekdosis* in question? We must also simultaneously deal with a related problem of interpretation: what is meant by *chōris tōn en Rōmēi mellontōn menein* (8,20–21 BJP)? Thirdly, what is the reference of *panta ta hēmetera* (9,6 BJP)?

To take the last phrase first: we noted above, in the passage from ch. 14 [11] of *My Own Books*, that the similar formulation, *talla ta hēmetera*, seems to refer to a category implicitly separate from the 'private' one for his own exercise (some of which were also informally circulated). The fact that the phrase here clearly functions as the equivalent of *panta ta pros ekdosin* – it substitutes for that earlier phrase in a recapitulation of the identical information a few lines later – strengthens that interpretation. Both phrases, it seems, may be taken to refer to some formal, 'official' group of Galen's own works. Although (as already remarked), Galen's choice of nouns in reference to his own writings is notoriously fluid, this group seems – in the present passage at least – also to be co-extensive with *pragmateiai*, treatises. Thus, it seems, at least on a fairly natural reading of the present passage, that Galen is here – in apparent contradiction of the picture that I have been painting – suggesting a distinct list of those works which constituted his public output: works for *ekdosis*. This set, he further suggests, would be preserved both by his making of a 'backup' copy for his

---

33   My translation. Note that I have used one-to-one correspondences to reflect the distinction between terms used by Galen in each of the references to his own works (even if the distinction of terms may not in fact correspond to a significant conceptual distinction): 'treatise' renders *pragmateia*, 'book' renders *biblion* and 'works' is used where Galen simply has a neuter plural adjective without noun. (See further below on the significance (or not) of the use of the term *hupomnēmata* for certain works.).

house in Campania and by their being deposited in public libraries. This, then, seems also to make natural sense of the phrase *chōris tōn en Rōmēi mellontōn menein*, which in itself might admit of a number of interpretations. The official catalogue of his *oeuvre*, Galen is (on this interpretation) suggesting, exists in a single copy deposited in his storehouse in Rome, to which further copies may be added, to be held elsewhere.[34]

This new picture, then, of the official *oeuvre* which is both deposited in the storehouse and simultaneously *pros ekdosin*, reminds us rather strikingly of the passage which we have already considered from *De compositione medicamentorum per genera*. There, we saw, there is an explicit pairing of precisely these two concepts: 'having been distributed and deposited in the *apothēkē*' (ἐκδοθέντων, ἐγκαταλειφθέντων δὲ ἐν τῇ κατὰ τὴν ἱερὰν ὁδὸν ἀποθήκῃ). But that passage, in conjunction with the present one and other usages which we have seen, suggests another important dimension of *ekdosis* and its cognates, namely that what is referred to in these terms is not, or not only or primarily, a process of distribution, but includes crucially the notions of *editing, writing-up* or *completion* of a pre-existing text.

This, of course, is quite consistent with the process which previous scholars have identified: works previously existing in note or outline form (for private use or informal circulation) are written up for *ekdosis* for a wider audience.[35] But two crucial points need to be made in qualification of such a picture. The first is that – as we have already seen – such a formal list of 'public' works will, in fact, include works which Galen explicitly describes as having been written for his own *hetairoi*; in fact, it seems impossible – at least as far as Galen's main medical output, including the Hippocratic commentaries, is concerned – to identify any works in the 'public' list which are *not* officially so intended. The second, related, point is that what is at stake in the 'private–public' distinction is then a difference in editions of the same work, not a distinction between different works.

---

34   The interpretation is consistent with the translation of BJP ('... tous mes livres qui étaient destinés à la publication ... sans compter les exemplaires qui devaient rester'), i.e. there are three copies in all. A more literal grammatical reading would want *chōris*, etc. to be an exclusion clause, so referring to a *subset* of those for distribution, i.e. 'all those for *ekdosis* had been written in two copies, except for those which were to remain in Rome [which had not been so copied]'; the *chōris* clause would thus introduce a new category. One might in that case further suppose that the *chōris* phrase is applied rather loosely, and what is meant is not 'all works for *ekdosis* had been copied, except for those for Rome ...' but 'all works for *ekdosis* had been copied, except that some [not for *ekdosis*], which were for Rome, had not been copied'. On balance, our first interpretation seems both the most natural and that which will best assist us with the categories of works which then follow.

35   See the literature already cited in n. 8, especially the discussions of Dorandi.

In this context, we should consider also the other two occurrences of the word *ekdosis* in περὶ ἀλυπίας. One clearly falls in the category of scholarly 'edition' or 'version', which, as we already saw, is a common usage, especially in relation to commentators on Hippocrates; the interesting variation here is that it is Galen himself who has produced an *ekdosis* of another author.[36] The other is a mention, in relation to drugs or drug recipes, of τὰς περὶ αὐτῶν ἐκδόσεις γεγονυίας (*Ind.* 50b, 16,13–14 BJP); here Galen is referring to his own compositions; and the context, which is that of a recapitulation of items already mentioned, makes it clear – consistently with what we have just observed – that the term *ekdoseis* here corresponds to what was earlier referred to (at 37, 12,22–3 BJP) as a *pragmateia*. The work in question is, in fact, that on the composition of drugs, already discussed. The term *ekdoseis* here can, indeed, be seen as related to the reference which we saw to that work as *ekdothenta* (a reference which, as we also saw, is for Galen quite consistent with the claim that it was written for *hetairoi*). But this interpretation, or focus on the sense of *ekdosis* as referring to an editorial process or version, raises further problems. In principle, the notion of a later, more formal, writing-up of works which had previously circulated in a smaller circle, seems an eminently plausible one. Yet, as has been pointed out by others,[37] Galen very seldom in fact acknowledges that he has produced more than one version of the same work. If he had done so, one might, indeed, expect that more than one version of the same work would be in circulation. Galen does, indeed, acknowledge the problem of the circulation of faulty, or superseded, versions of his writings; but this seems to be a problem confined to an early phase of his writing, and one which he regards as largely resolved early on in his career.[38] If more than one version – an earlier, informal one and a later, official one – of a range of his mature works were in circulation, one would surely expect some discussion by Galen of the problems that would inevitably ensue. In one case, that of *AA*, where Galen does explicitly state that he wrote a subsequent version of an earlier text (see n. 23 above), the overdetermined nature of his explanation seems revealing. That is, while he claims that the earlier – not-for-*ekdosis* – version is lost, he gives an additional reason for rewriting, namely that he had acquired more accurate anatomical knowledge.

Crucially, indeed, Galen does not describe processes of rewriting or revision of the *same* text, but rather – precisely to the contrary – uses his original

36   *Ind.* 14 (6,11 BJP).
37   See Gurd, 'Galen on ἔκδοσις'.
38   The phenomenon of books of his own composition in need of correction being returned to him, after his first visit to Rome, is discussed in ch. 2 of *Lib. Prop.*

authorial intent as an explanation of the content of the final version of the text which is in the public domain. We have seen, for example, how the changing demands and requests of his own *hetairoi* are used to provide an account of the process of development of his own Hippocratic output: those individual demands and requests, that is, explain the content of the last commentaries – those which were written 'with an eye to wider *ekdosis*' and are 'works for publication' if any are. What, then, can be made of the process of 'editing' which I have suggested gives at least a partial account of what is meant by *pros ekdosin* in this passage from περὶ ἀλυπίας? What, if anything, would be the substantial difference between a *pros ekdosin* version and the original which has circulated informally? As has been noted, the accounts of his own works in *My Own Books* and elsewhere represent a retrospective creation by Galen of an *oeuvre*, the establishment of a curriculum and canon of his own works by an author who claims to have been reluctant to put any of them in the public domain in the first place.[39] But this process or organization and canonization involves not just the listing and categorization of his works in these autobibliographical books. There are also – as very clearly seen above, in the example of *Hipp. Epid. III* – explanatory, apologetic and orientating remarks within the texts themselves, especially in their prefaces. Consider the preface to the first book of the commentary on Hippocrates' *Epidemics* VI.

> ἐγὼ μὲν γάρ, ὥσπερ καὶ τἆλλα πάντα πολλοῖς τῶν δεηθέντων ἑταίρων χαριζόμενος ἐποίησα, καὶ τὰς ἐξηγήσεις ταύτας ἐκείνων ἕνεκα συνέθηκα. θεωρῶν δ' εἰς πολλοὺς ἐκπίπτοντα τὰ γραφόμενα προοιμίων τοιούτων ἐδεήθην.

> Just as I composed all the rest for the benefit of many of my followers, who had asked for them, I put together these commentaries for their sake too. But observing that what was being written fell into the hands of many, I needed such prefaces.
>
> *Hipp. Epid. VI* 1, praef. (XVIIA.795–6 K. = 4,25–5,3 Wenkebach)

The passage incidentally gives yet another affirmation of Galen's claim – which we have now seen many times – to have written all such works for his followers. Our main concern here, however, is with the reference to prefaces. Of course, a preface containing such information on the previous history of the text is, by its very presence, an explicit acknowledgement that this version – the *ekdosis*, if one will – is not identical with that which has previously circulated. By the

---

39   The point is well made by Boudon-Millot, 'Galien par lui-même'; cf. also Vegetti, *Nuovi scritti*.

same token, however, and as we saw very clearly in the example of *Hipp. Epid.*
III, it functions as an apologetic for the extent to which the two forms of the
text *are* the same.

Could it be that to produce the *ekdosis* of a previously circulated work consists in little more than in adding a preface to it? Such framing – such self-
positioning – is, as we have seen, of enormous importance to Galen. There
would, doubtless, be other processes involved: checking and correction,
perhaps the writing *eis katharon edaphos*, the production of a clean copy
which, again in the context of editions of other authors, is mentioned elsewhere in περί ἀλυπίας.[40] But the fact that such apologetics as are found in the
prefaces speak to the substantial identity of the previous, circulated version
with the final, written-up article is highly significant, though easily ignored. A
work may – as indeed Galen essentially claims for his works in general – have
not originally been *intended* for *ekdosis* (and of course how seriously one takes
that claim may be a matter of individual interpretation); but in principle any
work, whatever its origin, could end up in the *pros ekdosin* list; and that destiny,
one might suppose (though we will return to this question in due course), may
correspond also to its ultimate inclusion in the list in *My Own Books*.

We should proceed to enquire what – in the specific context of the passage from περί ἀλυπίας which we are now considering – is the opposed term to
the *panta ta pros ekdosin* category. Before doing so, we should consider a little
more closely what else this particular passage is telling us about *ekdosis*. For in
the immediately preceding paragraphs I have focussed on *ekdosis* as process
of edition; but our passage tells us something about *ekdosis* as process of distribution, too. Here, let us again emphasize the point: this is by far the clearest
account Galen gives us of his own role in the *ekdosis* of his own works; it is a
unique admission in the corpus. His clearest account, however, is still very far
from clear. He does not tell us either which works the *panta ta pros ekdosin*
were, nor what was involved in the process of preparation or editing; and we
have to engage in an intricate, not to say speculative, process of analysis to
arrive at the answer to this. And the context of Galen's admission of his own
ekdosis activity is surely relevant here: he is making as vivid as possible the
account of his own losses, and he can hardly do that without mentioning the
full extent of the texts that were lost. It is only in such a rhetorical context that
Galen has allowed himself to be forced into the admission – still reluctantly,
and of course only in the passive voice – that he had works of his own copied
for distribution. The loss of these copies – so soon before they would have been
safe – makes the events all the more dramatic. Moreover, and still consistently

---

40   *Ind.* 14 (6,9 BJP).

with what we saw above, where Galen only explicitly admits that he intended to *give* books to friends, rather than *giving them out* to a public – the only actual process of *ekdosis* he admits as his own remains that of giving his works to friends back home, at their request. (It happens that they have made this request because they want the works to exist in a public library – but such a provision is, of course, their act and not his.)

One final point on the actual *ekdosis* process. It seems possible, as already suggested, that the term *panta ta pros ekdosin* does indeed correspond to Galen's 'back-catalogue' – to the set of his works which he regards as his canon, and which have been written up at a certain level, so that they may be consulted by others. The peculiar historical accident and atrocious timing to which Galen refers, however, require a little more attention. If Galen indeed had such a central repository of his own writings in his storehouse in Rome, then the destruction of the whole collection in the fire was indeed a monumental loss. It is, as I have already suggested, remarkable in this context that Galen makes so little of it, in terms of the extent of his own works lost, focussing rather on a couple of his own works and devoting more attention to editions of other authors, not to mention drug collections and other valuables. That focus is, as I have also suggested, explicable precisely in terms of the actual networks of distribution that functioned in relation to a successful author's work: put simply, he could be confident that the vast majority of his works were, in fact, extant in other collections.

But there is another detail worth considering here. Granted that Galen may have had such a comprehensive collection of his own writings in their *pros ekdosin* form, is it plausible that he had just now, at this precise historical moment, had two further copies made, of the entire set? If one pauses for a moment to consider the situation, one soon realizes that such a possibility would, indeed, beggar belief, from three points of view. First, the coincidence in that case – the fire came at the precise point when Galen had just decided to make two additional copies of all his works, constituting his lifetime's *oeuvre*, and take them out of Rome, for distribution and safe-keeping – would be truly staggering; secondly, this would imply that Galen had just made a decision, in his mid-sixties, radically to change his longstanding practices in relation to *ekdosis*, both producing a back-up and instigating a particular form of distribution – to libraries via friends in Pergamum – never previously contemplated; thirdly, the copying, twice, of his entire output – even if we take that output by 192 to have run to only about three-quarters of its final extent (a very conservative estimate) – would have entailed the writing of about seven-and-a-half million words by his scribes in a single phase. If the accident of timing had involved such a truly massive loss, Galen would surely have made more of it than the few phrases contained in the passage above; as for the second hypothesis, that Galen has suddenly now revolutionized the distribution practices of a lifetime, that is something that could hardly have been passed over without discussion: indeed, it would mean that the *ekdosis* referred to here was, in a sense, a completely new project. And as for the seven-and-a-half million words – such an undertaking, even by the standards of Galen's undoubtedly hard-worked teams of scribes, would have been more than prodigious.

A far more plausible interpretation of what Galen means, I submit, is that two copies had been made of those works which were intended for *ekdosis* at this particular time. The reference to sending works to Asia once the weather turns is, surely, a reference to a regular, very probably yearly, practice; Galen's friends back home (even if one takes this story at face value) have not, on any plausible account, suddenly requested his whole *oeuvre*; and the notion that a successful author, conscious of his reputation and keen to secure his *Nachleben*, would, on a regular basis, in batches, both make a backup copy and send his works to libraries in Asia, is a wholly reasonable and likely one. Such a process, again, helps explain Galen's – in the circumstances – comparatively relaxed attitude to the losses: previous batches of work, once they reached the *pros ekdosin* state, have already been sent to Asia (and possibly also to the house in Campania); it is only the latest batch which causes concern. And that, indeed, is precisely why the only two mentioned by name are the commentary on Old Comedy – just written – and the work on the composition of drugs – apparently written earlier, but by whatever quirk of fate not extant (or at least not locatable in Rome). We thus have, in conclusion, two distinct, but I suggest complementary, interpretations of the phrase *pros ekdosin* in this particular passage, referring both to a phase of completion or edited form, and to an intention to initiate wider circulation of works which have reached this form.

4   *Pros Ekdosin; Hupomnēmata* and Notes; Non-Surviving Works

I turn, then, finally, to the identity of the 'other' implied by the term *ta pros ekdosin* in this passage, and to the distinctions made between different types or levels of work, amongst those lost in the fire. For we do here get discussion of something like a 'private' category, and an attempt to identify it will be of some value to our enquiry.

> τούτων οὖν οὐδὲν ἠνίασέ με … ὡς οὐδὲ ἡ τῶν ἡμετέρων ὑπομνημάτων ἀπώλεια, διττῶν κατ᾽ εἶδος ὄντων· ἔνια μὲν γὰρ οὕτως ἐγεγόνει σύμμετρα ὡς καὶ τοῖς ἄλλοις εἶναι χρήσιμα, τινὰ δὲ ἐμοὶ μόνῳ καίτοι τὴν αὐτὴν ἔχοντα παρασκευὴν εἰς

ἀνάμνησιν, ἔπειτα αἱ κεφαλαιώδεις πλεῖσται συνόψεις πολλῶν πάνυ βιβλίων
ἰατρικῶν τε καὶ φιλοσόφων⁴¹· ἀλλ᾽οὐδὲ ταῦτα ἐλύπησαν.

None of these things, then, grieved me ... nor did the loss of my notes,
which were of two kinds: some had been produced in such a well-balanced way as to be useful to others, too, while others, although they had
the same form of preparation as those, for reminding, were for myself
alone; then there was the very large number of summaries by main heading, of an extensive list of medical and philosophical books.

    Ind. 29–30 (10,24–11,7 BJP)

The passage comes at the climax of the account of the loss of his books,
just after the discussion of his work on words in Old Comedy. The term
hupomnēmata here seems to introduce a fresh category – although at some
distance in the text – in addition to the *pros ekdosin* works and *pragmateiai* already mentioned.⁴² For that reason, as well as to point up the relationship between this characterization of works and the term 'for reminding', εἰς
ἀνάμνησιν, I have here used the admittedly not unproblematic translation
'notes', rather than the more neutral 'writings' or 'works'. It should be understood that the term *hupomnēmata*, although it has an etymological and indeed
apparently, for Galen, a conceptual relationship with the idea of notes, of an
original oral context or of usefulness for delivering lectures, is used by him
with a very broad and fluid application, and no clear distinction can be made
consistently across his works between his use and application of this term and
that of the terms 'treatises' (*pragmateiai*), 'compositions' (*sungrammata*) or
'books' (*biblia*).⁴³ It seems, however, that in this context we here have a counterpart to *ta pros ekdosin*.

    The *hupomnēmata* themselves are immediately subdivided into two kinds –
produced in such a well-balanced way as to be useful to others, and for himself alone; and then there is added a further, definitely private, category of

---

41   Although the form seems odd here, and BJP emend to φιλοσοφικῶν, I print the phrase
    in this form because of the identical pairing of adjectives at both *Praen.* 9 (XIV.650 K. =
    120,1 Nutton) and *Lib. Prop.* 3 (XIX.19 = 143,2 Boudon-Millot): it seems that Galen may use
    φιλόσοφος as an adjective applied to books, discussions or problems – a usage for which
    there is perfectly good precedent, e.g. Plato, *Phaedrus* 257b.

42   It is also a possible, in view of Galen's fluidity of use of the term *hupomnēmata*, already
    noted, as well as his frequently repetitive manner in this text, that he is here simply giving
    another recapitulation of the works already lost (cf. 20–23b), with slightly different termi-
    nology; but the parallels which we shall see with the similar passage about *hupomnēmata*
    in *Lib. Prop.* speak against this.

43   On this point see n. 11 above.

'summaries by main heading' of works of doctors and philosophers.[44] But what precisely does Galen mean by *hupomnēmata* here? Some were just for his own use, some distributed, but none (implicitly) were intended for *ekdosis*. The primary reference of *hupomnēmata* may be similar to that of a group of lost and unidentified works in ch. 3 of *My Own Books*, namely commentary-style notes on other authors or specific problems. Or, the reference here may be a broader one: *hupomnēmata* are, quite simply, those works of his own composition which have not reached the *pros ekdosin* state. But I note that there are – if we take it that this whole passage is intended as in contradistinction to *ta pros ekdosin* – three categories identified: *ta pros ekdosin; hupomnēmata* which might be shared; purely private *hupomnēmata* (together with which we may group the purely private 'summaries'). It is indeed tempting to map this on to the passage from ch. 3 of *My Own Books*, which we have already considered, where the term was *gumnazōn emauton* rather than *hupomnēmata*, but where a similar three-way division seems to be in play; and we shall return to that passage shortly.

First, it is worth pointing out that some such 'private' categories of notes would, plausibly, have been the main victims of the fire, in terms of irrecoverable losses. Certainly, no such *synopseis* survive (with the apparent exception of a summary of Plato's *Timaeus*, extant in Arabic); on the other hand we would probably not expect them to: some kinds of scholarly writing are too note-like and ephemeral to be expected to survive, even without a fire. But this consideration leads us to our final two questions: (a) can one identify *any* specific extant, or indeed non-extant but listed, works of Galen's as belonging to this 'for himself' category? (b) does belonging to this private category give an explanation, at least in some cases, of the loss of a specific work of which we know the title? Let us return to the passage from *My Own Books* which, we have suggested, quite closely parallels this reference to lost *hupomnēmata* in sections 29 and 30 of *Ind.*

κατὰ τοῦτον οὖν τὸν χρόνον συνελεξάμην τε καὶ εἰς ἕξιν ἤγαγον μόνιμον ἅ τε παρὰ τῶν διδασκάλων ἐμεμαθήκειν ἅ τ' αὐτὸς εὑρήκειν, ἔτι τε ζητῶν ἔνια <ἃ>

---

44   I have preferred the translation 'summaries by main heading', rather than 'chapter summaries', for *kephalaiōdeis synopseis*: certainly, the term *kephalaion* can mean chapter in Galen, but he also specifically mentions the scholarly or intellectual practice of collecting all an author says on a topic, and uses the term *kephalaion* in that context. Such sets of notes accumulating, with quotations and references, all an author says on a particular topic (rather than strictly linear chapter summaries) would then have constituted a valuable database to be drawn upon in the composition of one's own works. Cf. Ammonius, *In Cat.* 4, 3–13 Busse, where there is a description of note composition, including the term *kephalaia*.

περὶ τὴν εὕρεσιν αὐτῶν εἶχον ἔγραψα πολλὰ γυμνάζων ἐμαυτὸν ἐν πολλοῖς
προβλήμασιν ἰατρικοῖς τε καὶ φιλοσόφοις, ὧν τὰ πλεῖστα διεφθάρη κατὰ τὴν
μεγάλην πυρκαϊάν, ἐν ᾗ τὸ τῆς Εἰρήνης τέμενος ἅμα καὶ ἄλλοις πολλοῖς ἐκαύθη.

During this time, then, I collected together and brought into permanent
form both what I had learned from my teachers and what I had discovered myself; I was also still engaged in research on some topics, and wrote
down a lot that I had which was relevant to those enquiries, training myself in many medical and philosophical problems. But most of this material was lost in the great fire in which the Temple of Peace was consumed
along with many other buildings.

> *Lib. Prop.* 3 (XIX.19 K. = 142,25–143,4 Boudon-Millot)

Galen here makes a swift transition, from the first part of the sentence (up to
εὑρήκειν), in which he seems to be talking of the final writing-up (*eis hexin ...
monimon*), at a critical time in his career, of a core body of his works, to a category related to ongoing research and self-training (*eti ... zētōn ... gumnazōn
emauton*).[45] Though the speed of the transition – from a clause summing up
most of his core works to one referring to a whole different category of now
lost ones – is confusing, it does seem clear that it is indeed the latter, 'ongoing
research and private exercise' writings that are referred to as having been lost
in the fire. There is another place where Galen mentions the losses in the fire –
a passage which we have already considered in a different context.

I also wrote a large number of other works as an exercise for myself; of
these some were lost in the fire which consumed the Temple of Peace,

---

45   The period in question is 169–76, to which, it seems, a majority of Galen's extant scientific
      and medical works may be dated (not including the bulk of the pharmacological works
      or most of the Hippocratic commentaries). Great caution must be exercised in assign-
      ing clear dates to Galenic works: there were clearly drafts and – as indeed the present
      text makes clear – subsequent writings-up, and in some cases later revised versions; it is
      also clear, simply from a consideration of the totality of cross-references between works,
      and the inconsistent chronological picture that emerges from them, that material can be
      added to texts at different phases. A useful overview of relative dates is nonetheless still
      that of Bardong, K. (1942). 'Beiträge zur Hippokrates- und Galenforschung', *Nachrichten
      von der Akademie der Wissenschaften in Göttingen, Philologisch-Historische Klasse*, Nr.
      7, 577–640 (who is not insensitive to these complexities). He assigns 23 treatises to this
      period. See also Peterson, D. W. (1977). 'Observations on the Chronology of the Galenic
      Corpus', *Bulletin of the History of Medicine* 51, 484–95; and Boudon-Millot, *Galien, Tome I*,
      'Introduction' and ad loc.

others had been given to friends and are now extant in many private collections, as is the case with my other works.

Lib. Prop. 14 [11] (XIX.41 K. = 166,1–5 Boudon-Millot)

It is true that we have seen considerable fluidity, even unreliability, in Galen's
use of the phrase *gumnazōn emauton*. But the context here may be informative. As we saw earlier, the discussion of 'personal-exercise' works here leads
into a discussion of *hupomnēmata*, and a long list of commentaries and works
on individual philosophical problems. Broadly speaking, again, it seems that
a similar category of note-like, private-use writings on individual philosophical texts or questions, is being referred to here and in *Ind.* 29–30, as discussed
above. But we are left with the following puzzle. In the later course of ch. 14
[11] of *My Own Books* Galen goes on to list literally dozens of such works on individual texts and questions in the area of logic and demonstration.[46] If these
correspond to the large group of *gumnazōn emauton* and *hupomnēmata* works
which, Galen says, were lost in the fire, that would give us an at least partial
answer to our initial question, and a neat account of why so many works on
these particular issues are lost to us. But are we to imagine that Galen is, in fact,
listing works which he knows to be lost? The earlier passage, in ch. 3, seems at
least to imply that he is refraining from listing works in that category (and this
would be consistent, too, with the suggestion that he has omitted mention of
Prognosis in *My Own Books* because he believed that work to be lost). If, on
the other hand, he has made a decision to list his lost works too, it is odd, to
say the least, that he lists them without mentioning whether they are extant
or not.

If, on the other, most or all of these works are extant at the time of the writing of *My Own Books*, then we have to accept that a fairly vast number of works
of Galen have been lost to us, but in a way which has nothing to do with the
fire at the Temple of Peace. Of course, many works by ancient authors are lost,
and one does not perhaps need any explanation for the partial nature of the
transmission other than the central authority role that Galen came to have, in
later antiquity and the middle ages, in medical curricula, as against his much
less exalted role in logic or philosophy.

---

46   To these we may add some of those mentioned also in chs 16 [13], 17 [14] and 18 [15], with
      which, however, there is some overlap: those latter chapters list works under the head-
      ings Plato, Aristotle, the Stoics and thus (especially in the case of Plato) include works of
      broader philosophical interest; this chapter concentrates on works of a highly technical,
      logical bent.

Still, returning to the former hypothesis, there are, I suppose, two possible explanations for the presence in *My Own Books* of a number of works which had already been lost at the date of that work's composition. One is that – as we have seen in other contexts – Galen may hope that someone else has a copy of a work, even if he does not. That possibility would, admittedly, be in literal contradiction with the characterization of the works as for his own use alone; on the other hand, we have already seen Galen committing this contradiction. Another explanation, however, may lie in a closer consideration of this very concept: the date of composition of *My Own Books*.

This text, it seems to me, is likely to have been composed provisionally as a list and added to over years. Even if works composed after the early 190s are, in general, absent from it, and in that sense such a date is to be seen as that of its completion, it could still have undergone revision and updating at later times. It may be that the sentences mentioning the fire of 192 belong to such a later updating – an updating which nonetheless did not extend to the deletion of all references to works lost in the fire. Such non-deletion may seem odd; but the matter could be explained by some uncertainty – of a kind, I suppose, familiar to most scholars in relation to the organization of their most informal or private sets of notes – in Galen's own mind as to precisely what he still had, and where. At any rate, I think we may say that – if my account of *My Own Books* as a work which was composed over a period of time is correct – it is also possible that its revision was partial and incomplete. Or it may be that the vast body of works mentioned in ch. 14 [11] were indeed more 'note-like', sketchy and private in their use than others, and that this smaller circulation, or non-circulation, accounts for their loss – even though they were extant after the fire. On this interpretation, we are given no further information about the *gumnazōn emauton* category in which Galen claims to have lost so many books, and can in no way map it on to any existing list. We would also, on this view, have solved the problem of identifying a genuinely 'not for publication' category, within Galen's explicit list of his own works; but would still be left with the puzzle as to the precise identity of the *gumnazōn emauton* works which were lost (and it might also seem strange that this vast set of listed works, if they genuinely were for private use and not copied, *did* survive the fire). Some puzzles, certainly, remain; but I hope that the above has shown with greater clarity what we learn from περὶ ἀλυπίας, taken in conjunction with Galen's 'autobibliographical' remarks elsewhere, about book composition and distribution in the Graeco-Roman world, about Galen's own practices in particular, and about what can and cannot be deduced from what he himself says – or fails to say – about *ekdosis*.

5   Different Audiences?

We should add, finally, that the above analysis should not be taken as denying that Galen does, indeed, intend certain of his works for different audiences, or that some such distinctions can be discovered.[47] Rather, my claim is that such a distinction, within the extant works, cannot be mapped on to a theoretical one between works for *ekdosis* and works not for *ekdosis* – a distinction which Galen does not in fact make in this form – and further that those works which we do possess are, typically, both not for *ekdosis* (in the sense that this is Galen's claim about his intention when writing them) and for *ekdosis* (in the sense that these same works are subsequently made available in an edition for distribution, with minimal if any differences between that *ekdosis* and the previous version, indeed with so complete an overlap between the original and the *ekdosis* that the author feels obliged to explain features of the final version on the basis of their original composition).

There are, however, other kinds of distinction in audience and intent, though these are seldom clear-cut. There is, to be sure, the distinct category of works for beginners. There are also works which can be understood, on the basis of what Galen himself says, as intended for a broader audience than the usual medical one consisting of his *hetairoi*. For example, Galen uses the phrase 'for all' to characterize his intention in writing *De sanitate tuenda* – a work which on other grounds too can be identified as aimed at a non-medical, or broader, readership.[48] It is interesting to place this 'for all' alongside a similar formulation in *My Own Doctrines*, in relation to his shorter ethical writings: ethical philosophy, he says there, is something both useful and possible *for all* to train themselves in, and he in this context mentions his composition of two books on the subject (presumably *Affections* and *Errors*).[49] These are available for *all*

---

47   In relation to this discussion see also the bibliography cited at n. 14 above.

48   'The function [I so translate here *dunamis*] of them [*sc.* the short works *De optima corporis nostri constitutione, De bono habitu* and *De inaequali intemperie*] is contained also in the work on *Matters of Health*, in which the different types of constitution of our body are stated *for all* (πᾶσιν)', *Ord. Lib. Prop.* 2 (94,12–14 Boudon-Millot; n.b. not in the pre-Vlatadon text); within the work itself he makes the distinction that it is for *philiatroi*, people interested in or friendly to medicine, as opposed to *The Therapeutic Method* which is 'only for doctors' (ἐν ἐκείνῃ... μόνοις διαλέγομαι τοῖς ἰατροῖς, ἐνταυθοῖ δὲ καὶ τοῖς ἄλλοις ἅπασιν, οὓς ὀνόματι κοινῷ προσαγορεύουσιν ἔνιοι φιλιάτρους, *San. Tu.* 4.5, VI.269 K. = 118,31–3 Koch).

49   *Prop. Plac.* 14 (188,17–19 Boudon-Millot and Pietrobelli): τὴν ἠθικὴν φιλοσοφίαν... χρησίμην τε ἅμα καὶ δυνατήν... πᾶσι τοῖς βουλομένοις ἀσκῆσαι. The same text, incidentally, has a reference (if we trust the Greek MS rather than the Arabo-Latin tradition) to *De naturalibus facultatibus* as having been written 'for all' - an interesting notion in relation to the following point about *De placitis Hippocratis et Platonis* and *De usu partium* and their

to train towards virtue. And this may apply also to a range of other 'occasional' works on ethical and more popular themes (without their being extant, it is difficult to judge); indeed, the listing of such works in a series of separate chapters towards the end of *My Own Books* seems to highlight their separate status; certainly they stand outside the main curriculum of scientific, anatomical and medical works recommended for his students. And, as we have seen, there is a range of commentary-style works on specific philosophical texts and themes, mainly lost, which it seems that Galen does not intend for the majority of his readers, or even for the majority of his medical students, and which (although, as we have seen, certainty in these areas is impossible) probably never achieved a wide circulation.

There are also, of course, considerable variations, within the central list of Galen's work presented to us with an order for reading in *My Own Books* and *The Order of My Own Books*, as to how directly relevant they are to medical training or practice. Indeed, the latter work explicitly states two different possible starting-points, or courses, for readers, within that central list. The only substantial difference made explicit is whether one starts with the great work (also lost), *De demonstratione*, or omits this – that is to say, whether one's medical training or knowledge will be based on the understanding of what constitutes a logically secure demonstration, and on the ability to produce such. But apart from that explicit distinction, there are others. Galen does not himself present the sliding scale of the course, from more theoretical areas – element theory, physiology – to the more practical, clinical ones, as a difference based on audience; that is, he does not explicitly suggest that a more practically, less theoretically, inclined student should cut to a later point in the curriculum. On the other hand, there are certain works which clearly belong both to an early phase in Galen's clear and to the project of establishing his intellectual reputation, in anatomy and related theoretical areas, in a highly competitive and public context, amongst the intellectuals of Rome. We have seen that on both internal grounds and the basis of what Galen tells us about the circumstances leading to their composition, both *De usu partium* and *De placitis Hippocratis et Platonis* – or, to be more precise, these works in a certain phase of their composition – belong to that phase. These works are in that sense more 'public', and it is also true that their content, theoretical and scientific in nature – indeed, laying out the most central of Galen's views on the functioning and structure of the body – is less closely tied to medical usefulness.

---

broader, theoretical content: ἅπασι τοῖς ἰατροῖς τε καὶ τοῖς ἄλλοις ἅπασιν ἀνθρώποις, *Prop. Plac.* 3 (174,22–3 Boudon-Millot and Pietrobelli).

On the other hand, such differences of original intent are occluded by Galen by the very fact of his listing, all together, of a central body of works in terms of suggested order of reading. This is, we have seen, a retrospective construction, which to a considerable extent tends to obscure those questions of original audience and argumentative context. And, as we have also seen, Galen repeatedly claims that his central body of works – including also the Hippocratic commentaries – is aimed at, and written at the request of, his *hetairoi*, students, people with serious medical interests. Dual intent runs throughout this corpus. The claim that works were written for this specific group – or even for one member of it – is, for Galen, in no way in contradiction with the ambition to gain for them a wide distribution which will both enhance his reputation and disseminate his views throughout the intellectual world.

Acknowledgements

The author gratefully acknowledges the financial support of the Wellcome Trust and the Alexander von Humboldt-Stiftung during the research and writing of this paper. Heartfelt thanks go also to the editor, Caroline Petit, for her invitation to participate in the conference from which this chapter arose, and especially for her very helpful advice and encouragement during its subsequent development. The faults which it retains are, of course, my own.

References

Bardong, K. 'Beiträge zur Hippokrates- und Galenforschung', *Nachrichten von der Akademie der Wissenschaften in Göttingen, Philologisch-Historische Klasse*, Nr. 7 (1942), 577–640.

Boudon, V. 'Galien par lui-même: les traités bio-bibliographiques (*De ordine librorum suorum* et *De libris propriis*)'. In *Studi su Galeno: scienza, filosofia, retorica e filologia. Atti del seminario, Firenze, 13 novembre 1998*, ed. D. Manetti, 119–33. Florence, 2000.

Boudon-Millot, V. 'Un traité perdu de Galien miraculeusement retrouvé, le *Sur l'inutilité de se chargriner*: texte grec et traduction française'. In *La science médicale antique: nouveaux regards (Études réunies en l'honneur de Jacques Jouanna)*, ed. V. Boudon-Millot, A. Guardasole and C. Magdelaine, 73–123. Paris, 2007.

Boudon-Millot, V. 'Galen's *Bios* and *Methodos*: From Ways of Life to Path of Knowledge'. In *Galen and the World of Knowledge*, ed. C. Gill, T. Whitmarsh and J. Wilkins, 175–89. Cambridge: CUP, 2009.

Boudon-Millot, V. (ed., trans. and notes) *Galien, Tome I*, Paris: Les Belles Lettres, 2007.

Boudon-Millot, V. and Pietrobelli, A. 'Galien ressucité: édition princeps du texts grec du *De propriis placitis*', *Revue des Études Grecques* 118 (2005), 168–213.

Boudon-Millot, V. and Jouanna, J. (ed. and trans.), with A. Pietrobelli, *Galien, Oeuvres, 4: Ne pas se chagriner.* Paris: Les Belles Lettres, 2010.

Dorandi, T. *Le stylet et la tablette: dans le secret des auteurs antiques.* Paris: Les Belles Lettres, 2000.

Dorandi, T. *Le Nell' officina dei classici: come lavorano gli autori antichi.* Rome: Carocci, 2007.

van der Eijk, P. 'Galen and the Scientific Treatise: A Case Study of *Mixtures*'. In *Writing Science: Medical and Mathematical Authorship in Ancient Greece*, ed. M. Asper, in collaboration with A.-M. Kanthak, 145–75, *Science, Technology and Medicine in Ancient Cultures* 1. Berlin: de Gruyter, 2013.

Gill, C., Whitmarsh, T. and Wilkins, J. (eds) *Galen and the World of Knowledge.* Cambridge: CUP, 2009.

Gleason, M. W. *Making Men: Sophists and Self-Presentation in Ancient Rome.* Princeton, New Jersey: Princeton University Press, 1995.

Gourinat, J.-B. 'Le Platon de Panétius: à propos d'un témoignage inédit de Galien', *Philosophie Antique* 8 (2008), 139–51.

van Groningen, B. A. ' "Εκδοσις', *Mnemosyne* 4:16 1963, 1–17.

Gurd, S. 'Galen on ἔκδοσις'. In *Perceptions of the Second Sophistic and its Times: Regards sur la seconde sophistique et son époque*, ed. T. Schmidt and P. Fleury, 169–84. Toronto University of Toronto Press, 2011.

König, J. 'Conventions of Prefatory Self-Presentation in Galen's *On the Order of My Own Books*'. In *Galen and the World of Knowledge*, ed. C. Gill, T. Whitmarsh and J. Wilkins, 35–58. Cambridge: CUP, 2009.

Manetti, D. (ed.) *Studi sul De indolentia di Galeno*, Pisa and Rome: Fabrizio Serra Editore, 2012

Manetti, D. and Roselli, A. 'Galeno commentatore di Ippocrate'. In *ANRW* II.37.2 (1994), 1529–1635.

Mansfeld, J. 'Galen's Autobibliographies and Hippocratic Commentaries'. In *Prolegomena: Questions to be Settled Before the Study of an Author, or a Text.* Leiden, New York and Cologne: Brill, 1994.

Manuli, P. and Vegetti, M. (eds). *Le opere psicologiche di Galeno: atti del terzo Colloquio Galenico Internazionale, Pavia, 1986.* Naples: Bibliopolis, 1988.

del Mastro, G. (2012). 'Μέγα βιβλίον: Galeno e la lunghezza dei libri'. In *Studi sul De indolentia di Galeno*, ed. D. Manetti, 33–62. Pisa and Rome: Fabrizio Serra Editore, 2012.

Mattern, S. P. *Galen and the Rhetoric of Healing.* Baltimore: The Johns Hopkins University Press, 2008.

Peterson, D. W. 'Observations on the Chronology of the Galenic Corpus', *Bulletin of the History of Medicine* 51 (1977), 484–95.

Singer, P. N. *Galen: Selected Works*. Translation with introduction and notes. Oxford: OUP, 1997.

Singer, P. N. (ed.) *Galen: Psychological Writings: Avoiding Distress, The Diagnosis and Treatment of Affections and Errors Peculiar to Each Person's Soul, Character Traits and The Capacities of the Soul Depend on the Mixtures of the Body*, translated with introduction and notes by V. Nutton, D. Davies and P. N. Singer, with the collaboration of Piero Tassinari. Cambridge: CUP, 2013.

Starr, R. J. 'The Circulation of Literary Texts in the Ancient World', *CQ* 37 (1987), 213–23.

von Staden, H. 'Gattung und Gedächtnis: Galen über Wahrheit und Lehrdichtung'. In *Gattungen wissenschaftlicher Literatur in der Antike*, ed. W. Kullmann, J. Althoff, M. Asper (eds), 65–94. Tübingen, 1998.

von Staden, H. 'Staging the Past, Staging Oneself: Galen on Hellenistic Exegetical Traditions'. In *Galen and the World of Knowledge*, ed. C. Gill, T. Whitmarsh and J. Wilkins, 132–56. Cambridge: CUP, 2009.

Vegetti, M. *Galeno: nuovi scritti autobiografici*. Rome: Carocci editore, 2013.

Texts: Editions, Translations and Abbreviations

Ammonius

In Cat. = *In Aristotelis Categorias*. Ed. A. Busse: Berlin, CAG IV.4, 1895.

Galen

Texts of Galen are cited by volume and page number in Kühn's edition (where available), followed by page and line number in the most recent critical edition, if different.

K. = C. G. Kühn, *Claudii Galeni Opera Omnia*, 22 vols. Leipzig, 1821–1833.

CMG = Corpus Medicorum Graecorum, Leipzig and Berlin, 1908–.

AA = *De anatomicis administrationibus* (*Anatomical Procedures*). [K. II].

Aff. Pecc. Dig. 1 and 2 = *De propriorum animi cuiuslibet affectuum dignotione et curatione* and *De animi cuiuslibet peccatorum dignotione et curatione* (*Affections and Errors of the Soul*). [K. V]. Ed. W. de Boer. Berlin and Leipzig: Teubner, CMG V 4,1,1, 1937; trans. in Singer, *Galen: Psychological Writings*.

Comp. Med. Gen. = *De compositione medicamentorum per genera*. [K. XIII].

De crisibus (*Crises*). [K. IX].

De diebus decretoriis (*Critical Days*). [K. IX].

Hipp. Art. = *In Hippocratis De Articulis*, [K. XVIIIA].

Hipp. Epid. III = *In Hipporatis Epidemiarum librum III* (*Commentary on Hippocrates 'Epidemics III'*). [K. XVIIA]. Ed. E. Wenkebach. Leipzig and Berlin: Teubner, CMG V 10,2,1, 1936.

Hipp. Epid. VI = In Hippocratis Epidemiarum librum VI (*Commentary on Hippocrates 'Epidemics VI'*). [K. XVIIA–B (partial)]. Ed./German trans. E. Wenkebach and E. Pfaff. Berlin: Akademie Verlag, CMG V 10,2,2, 1956.

Hipp. Off. Med = In Hippocratis De officina Medica. [K. XVIIIB]. Ed. (Arabic) M. Lyons. Berlin: Akademie Verlag (CMG Suppl. Or. 1), 1963.

HNH = In Hippocratis De natura hominis. [K.XV]. Ed. J. Mewaldt. Leipzig and Berlin: Teubner, CMG V 9,1, 1914.

Ind. = De indolentia (*Peri alupias*). [Not in K.]. Ed. V. Boudon-Millot and J. Jouanna, with the collaboration of A. Pietrobelli: *Ne pas se chagriner.* Paris: Les Belles Lettres, 2010 (BJP); trans. by V. Nutton in Singer, *Galen: Psychological Writings.*

Lib. Prop. = De libris propriis (*My Own Books*). [K. XIX]. Ed. V. Boudon-Millot. Paris: Les Belles Lettres, 2007; trans. in Singer, *Galen: Selected Works.*

Loc. Aff. = De locis affectis (*Affected Places*). [K. VIII]. Books 1 and 2 ed. F. Gärtner. Berlin: De Gruyter, CMG V 6,1,1, 2015.

MM = De methodo medendi (*The Therapeutic Method*). [K. X]. Trans. I. Johnston and G. H. R. Horsley. Cambridge, Mass.: Harvard University Press (Loeb), 2011.

Ord. Lib. Prop. = De ordine librorum propriorum (*The Order of My Own Books*). [K. XIX]. Ed. V. Boudon-Millot. Paris: Les Belles Lettres, 2007; trans. in Singer, *Galen: Selected Works.*

PHP = De placitis Hippocratis et Platonis (*The Doctrines of Hippocrates and Plato*). [K. V]. Ed. and trans. P. De Lacy, 3 vols. Berlin: Akademie Verlag, CMG V 4,1,2, 1978–84.

In Plat. Tim. = In Platonis Timaeum Commentarii Fragmenta. [Not in K.] Ed. H. O. Schröder. Berlin and Leipzig: Teubner, CMG Suppl. 1, 1934.

Praen. = De praenotione ad Epigenem (*Prognosis*). [K. XIV]. Ed. and trans. V. Nutton. Berlin: Akademie Verlag, CMG V 8,1, 1979.

Prop. Plac. = De propriis placitis (*My Own Doctrines*). [Not in K.] Ed. and trans. V. Nutton. Berlin: Akademie Verlag (CMG V 3,2), 1999. Ed. and French trans. of fuller text by V. Boudon-Millot and A. Pietrobelli, A., 'Galien ressucité: édition princeps du texte grec du *De propriis placitis*', *Revue des Études Grecques* 118 (2005), 168–213. Ed. with Italian trans. by I. Garofalo and A. Lami, *Galeno: L' anima e il dolore.* Milan: Rizzoli, 2012. Italian trans. by M. Vegetti, *Galeno: nuovi scritti autobiografici.* Rome: Carocci, 2013.

QAM = Quod animi mores corporis temperamenta sequantur. (*The Soul's Dependence on the Body*). [K. IV]. Ed. I. Müller, in *C. Galeni Scripta Minora*, 2. Leipzig: Teubner, 1891; trans. in Singer, *Galen: Psychological Writings.*

San. Tu. = De sanitate tuenda. (*Matters of Health*). [K. VI]. Ed. K. Koch. Berlin and Leipzig: Teubner, CMG V 4,2, 1923.

UP = De usu partium. [K. III-IV]. Ed. G. Helmreich, 2 vols. Leipzig: Teubner, 1907–9.

Iamblichus

Vit. Pyth. = De vita pythagorica

PART 2

Galen's Distress: Περὶ Ἀλυπίας *and the Philosophical Tradition*

∴

CHAPTER 5

Galen's Περὶ Ἀλυπίας as Philosophical Therapy: How Coherent is It?

Christopher Gill

In this discussion, I consider Galen's περὶ ἀλυπίας as an exercise in philosophical therapy of the emotions. I focus on the question how far it is a coherent work, when taken in this context. Overall, I conclude that it is largely coherent; but it also raises some significant questions in this respect, and consideration of these questions helps us to define the distinctive character of the work and its contribution to the genre.[1]

1 Galen's Two Therapeutic Works: The Question of Coherence

By Galen's time, Hellenistic-Roman writing on the therapy of the emotions formed a well-established genre. Although there are some earlier precursors (especially Plato),[2] the genre was decisively shaped by Stoic and Epicurean thinkers.[3] It was also adopted by Academic or Platonic thinkers, notably Cicero and Plutarch. Galen contributed to the genre in two surviving works, *Avoiding Distress* (περὶ ἀλυπίας = *De Indolentia*, or *Ind.*) and the first book of *The*

---

1   See also, on περὶ ἀλυπίας, as philosophical therapy, Gill, C. (2010), *Naturalistic Psychology in Galen and Stoicism*, 262–68; *Galien tome IV: Ne pas se chagriner*, eds. V. Boudon-Millot et al. (2010) (=BJP), xxxix–lviii; Nutton, in Galen, *Psychological Writings*, ed. Singer (2013), 61–68; Kaufman, D. H., 'Galen on the Therapy of Distress and the Limits of Emotional Therapy', *Oxford Studies in Ancient Philosophy* 47, 2014, 275–96; Xenophontos, S., 'Psychotherapy and Moralising Rhetoric in Galen's Newly Discovered *Peri Alypias*', *Medical History* 58.4, 2014, 585–603. The present discussion focuses on the question of coherence more than these other treatments, with the exception of Kaufman, 'Therapy', who discusses this question in 276–89. On interpretation of *Ind.*, see also the essays in Rothschild, C. K. Thompson, T. W. (eds.), *Galen's De Indolentia*, 2014.
2   On the earlier history of the genre, see Laín Entralgo, P., *The Therapy of the Word in Classical Antiquity*, 1970; Gill, C., 'Ancient psychotherapy', *Journal of the History of Ideas* 46.3, 1985, 307–25, esp. 320–25.
3   See Gill, *Naturalistic Psychology*, 246–300, on Galen's two works in the context of the genre; also, on Hellenistic-Roman philosophical therapy, Hadot, I. (1994) *Seneca und die griechische-römische Tradition der Seelenleitung*; Nussbaum, M. C. (1994). *The Therapy of Desire*; Sorabji, R. (2000). *Emotion and Peace of Mind*, esp. chs. 11–17.

Diagnosis and Treatment of the Affections and Errors Peculiar to Each Person's Soul (*Aff. Pecc. Dig.*; first book is *Aff. Dig.*).[4] Galen was the only ancient medical writer to do so, as far as we know; and this reflects his exceptional ambition to combine medicine and philosophy. His two writings in this genre are not, in any obvious way, influenced by his work as doctor, and reflect, to a large extent, the characteristic themes of philosophical therapy.[5] Among earlier works of this kind, Galen certainly knew what was probably the key founding text in the genre, Chrysippus' (lost) 'therapeutic' book (Book 4 of *On Passions = peri pathōn*), and criticised it extensively in *The Doctrines of Hippocrates and Plato* (*PHP*).[6] However, he seems to have been more directly influenced by works such as Plutarch's *On Contentment* (*peri euthumias*) and *On Avoidance of Anger* (*peri aorgēsias*). These are shorter and more practically oriented writings; they are also philosophically eclectic, or at least less uniformly shaped by a single intellectual approach than Chrysippus' 'therapeutic' book or subsequent Stoic or Epicurean works in the genre.[7] Even so, all these writings, including Galen's two works, express certain broad conceptual patterns which go back, at least, to the Stoic-Epicurean roots of the genre. They do not only discuss the management or control of emotions (either emotions in generally or a specific emotion), especially negative, disturbing or distressing emotions, and recommend methods for promoting this process. They also reflect the claim, accepted in varying degrees by all the philosophical schools, that the roots of our happiness or well-being (including our emotional state) are 'up to us' or fall within our power as psychological agents. The overall project of philosophical therapy is to find ways of 'curing' painful or 'diseased' emotional states by exercising this agency. This depends, typically, on activating our capacity to develop the virtues, or to do so more fully; this process of development not only rids us

---

4 English titles as in Galen, *Psychological Writings*. Abbreviations of Latin titles of Galen's works as in Hankinson, R. J. (2008). *The Cambridge Companion to Galen*, 399–403.

5 On Galen as author of both medical and ethical writings (though not combining the two approaches), see Singer, general introduction in Galen, *Psychological Writings*, 10–15, 26–30; also Gill, *Naturalistic Psychology*, 300–29. See also Gill, C. 'Philosophical psychological therapy – did it have any impact on medical practice?' in Thumiger, C. and Singer, P. N. (eds) (2018), *Mental Illness in Ancient Medicine*, 365–80.

6 For a reconstruction of Chrysippus' *therapeutikon*, see Tieleman, T. (2003). *Chrysippus' On Affections: Reconstruction and Interpretation*, 140–97, 326; also Gill, *Naturalistic Psychology*, 280–95.

7 On links between Plutarch's *peri euthumias* and Gal. *Ind.*, see BJP, x–xi, xl–xli. On the philosophical approach of Plutarch's essays, see Gill, C. 'Peace of Mind and Being Yourself: Panaetius to Plutarch', in Haase, W. and Temporini, H. (1994). *Aufstieg und Niedergang der römischen Welt* II.36.7, 4599–4640, esp. 4624–31, *Naturalistic Psychology*, 250–1; Van Hoof, L. (2010). *Plutarch's Practical Ethics*, ch. 4.

of vices of character but also of negative or misguided emotions linked with those vices.[8]

Why is the question of coherence an important one to raise in connection with Galen's works in this genre? Both of them offer some grounds for concern in this respect, regarding the choice and organisation of themes and also the conceptual framework applied. *Aff. Dig.*, the longer work, can be seen as breaking down into two halves. The first half (*Aff. Dig.* v.1–27 K. = 3–19 DB), on emotions in general, is rather generic in its approach, and employs themes and methods of emotional management characteristic of a wide range of writings in this genre. The second half (v.27–57 K. = 19–37 DB), increasingly, focuses on a single vice, 'insatiability' (*aplēstia*), presented as underlying a wide range of emotional disturbances (v.45–52 K. = 31–35 DB). This theme is also handled in a more individual way, including a section on Galen's upbringing and his father's influence and the lessons learnt in that way, a section which is similar in content to the latter part of *Ind* (v.40–45 K = 27–30 DB).[9] This contrast between the two parts of *Aff. Dig.* corresponds to the use of two distinct addressees, characterised in significantly different ways.[10] The question of coherence also arises as regards the philosophical framework informing the approach to therapy. As I have argued elsewhere, *Aff. Dig.* displays an uneasy combination of Stoic-Epicurean and Platonic-Aristotelian approaches, marked by two main points of contrast. Stoicism and Epicureanism assume a unified conception of human psychology, in which emotions and desires are shaped by beliefs and reasoning, whereas the Platonic-Aristotelian framework, as understood in this period, assumes a substantive division between rational and non-rational parts of the psyche. Second, Stoicism and Epicureanism presuppose that human beings are all naturally capable of developing towards virtue and happiness. By contrast, the Platonic-Aristotelian view is that ethical development depends on a combination of the appropriate kind of inborn nature, family or communal upbringing, and intellectual education. Elsewhere in his writings (notably in *PHP* and *QAM.*, ch. 11), Galen underlines these points of contrast and argues strongly for a Platonic-Aristotelian approach on both topics.[11] However, in *Aff. Dig.*, Galen's discussion reflects both approaches, without acknowledging the rather different implications they have for the management of emotions, the scope for change at different points in one's life and for methods of therapy.

---

8   See Gill, C. 'Philosophical Therapy as Preventive Psychological Medicine', in Harris, W. (ed) (2013). *Mental Disorders in the Classical World*, 339–60, and refs. in n. 3.

9   See text to nn. 18–21.

10   Gal. *Aff. Dig.* v.1, 13–14; 37, 48–51 K. = 3, 11; 25, 32–34 DB. See also Singer, introduction to *Aff. Dig.*, in Galen, *Psychological Works*, 218–19.

11   See Gill, *Naturalistic Psychology*, 214–29.

Although, in the first part, the Stoic-Epicurean influence is more marked, and in the second part, the Platonic-Aristotelian approach is more evident,[12] the distinction is not systematically maintained. For instance, the therapeutic method consistently recommended is rational self-monitoring and conscious self-correction, a method that matches the Stoic-Epicurean approach rather than the Platonic-Aristotelian.[13] So, when examined closely, *Aff. Dig.* exhibits problems of cohesion both in structure and philosophical consistency, despite presenting itself as a unified study of the management of emotions.

On the face of it, *Ind.* also exhibits problems of structure or organisation of themes, and raises questions about its philosophical coherence. As regards structure, there is an obvious division between the first half, cataloguing Galen's many losses in the great fire in Rome of AD 162 (1–37) and the second half, which presents themes characteristic of the therapy of emotions (38–84).[14] Of course, the two halves are explicitly linked: the overall aim, signalled in the initial address and underlined subsequently, is to explain why Galen was not distressed by losses, detailed in the first half, which would be expected to cause distress, and which caused distress to others.[15] Even so, the scale and detailed elaboration of the catalogue of Galen's losses is quite exceptional, within the genre of philosophical therapy, and it is not obvious why this degree and kind of detail is needed for this purpose. Also, the second half seems to break down, into a number of distinct sections or phases, and the rationale for the ordering of these sections is not immediately clear. The first and last sections (39–48 and 79–84) are centred on a critique of insatiability (*aplēstia*), the first of which is rather generic (typical of the genre of philosophical therapy of emotions). Another element, rather puzzlingly repeated, is a quotation from Euripides, which was often cited in connection with a well-known method of therapeutic training, the 'preparation for future evils', alluded to in *Ind.* 52–57,

---

12   See e.g. v. 4–5, 7, 16–17, 24 K. = 5, 7, 12–13, 17 DB) (Stoic-Epicurean view: all or most emotions/passions, *pathē*, are psychological sicknesses or forms of 'madness' to be cured or extirpated, and ethical progress can be correlated with this process); v. 27–34 K. = 19–23 DB (Platonic-Aristotelian view: distinction between 'education', *paideusis*, and 'disciplining', *kolasis*, and stress on 'habituation', coupled with distinction between rational and non-rational parts of psyche).

13   Methods recommended are sustained self-scrutiny, using a critical adviser, adjusting your ideas about what you really need: see e.g. v.6–7, 8–14, 20–21, 51–3, 55–6 K. = 6, 7–11, 15, 34–35, 36–37 DB. See Gill, *Naturalistic Psychology*, 252–62; also Singer, introduction to *Aff. Dig.*, in Galen, *Psychological Writings*, 220–28. However, Hankinson, R. 'Actions and passions', in Brunschwig, J. and Nussbaum, M. C. (eds), *Passions and Perceptions*, 1993, 198–204, sees Galen's approach in *Aff. Dig.* as more coherent.

14   Numbers of sections in *Ind.* as in BJP (2010) and Galen, *Psychological Writings*, 2013.

15   See text to n. 25.

76–7.[16] Along with these more standard features of philosophical therapy, we also have, as well as the recollection of the horrors of Commodus' rule (54–5), the more personal reminiscence of the psychological and ethical influence of Galen's father (54–68). This incorporates a series of philosophical or quasi-philosophical reflections, presented as underlying Galen's equanimity in the face of losses (61–68). Another section seems to offer a more pragmatic or qualified version of the philosophical principles just outlined, setting out the minimum standards needed, in Galen's view, for an endurable form of human life (69–78). Although I think there is an underlying rationale for this set of topics and for their linkage with the opening catalogue of losses, it is easy to form the impression of a rather miscellaneous, even ramshackle, structure.[17]

One can also question whether there is a coherent philosophical, or at least conceptual, framework. The most densely philosophical section is the resumé of ideas in 61–68, which hovers, rather awkwardly, between reportage of Galen's father's advice and Galen's own, philosophically informed, conclusions. Although this section seems to evoke the ethical positions of various philosophical schools, it is less clear which theories are being evoked and whether the section as a whole hangs together and adds up to an overall framework for maintaining equanimity. The dominant note has sometimes been seen as Aristotelian; but there is a strong case for seeing it as Stoic. However, exactly, we interpret this resumé, we need also to correlate it with the following section in which Galen explicitly distances himself from Stoic and Epicurean ideals of emotional invulnerability from disaster, 69–75. Further, though less obviously, there is the question how the two middle sections in the second half (61–8, 69–78) relate to Galen's advice on avoiding insatiability, which comes earlier and later (39–48, 79–84).

The difficulty of gauging the structure and conceptual framework just high-lighted emerges more strongly if we compare the second part of *Ind.* with the closely analogous section of *Aff. Dig.* (v.37 K.–52 K. =25–34 D B). In *Aff. Dig.*, we find similar motifs to those just noted in the second half of *Ind.*: (1) explanation why Galen shows exceptional equanimity (v.37–38 K. = 25–26 D B); (2) clarification of the respective roles of inborn nature (v.38–40 K. = 26–27 D B), family upbringing (v.41 K. =28 D B), and intellectual education, combined with his father's advice (v.41–43 K. =28–29 D B); (3) the personal impact of these factors

---

16   Euripides fr. 814 Mette = fr. 94 Nauck; also cited in Gal. *PHP* v.418 K. = De Lacy 282.17–23,
      [Plu.] *Consol. Ad Apoll.* (*Moralia*) 112 D, and (in Latin), Cic. *Tusc.* 3.29. It was regularly cited
      in connection with the therapeutic strategy of 'preparation for future evils', recommend-
      ed by both Cyrenaics and Stoics; see Cic. *Tusc.* 3.28–31, 52; also Tieleman, *Chrysippus*,
      311–14, Gill, *Naturalistic Psychology*, 290, BJP, 139–42.

17   On this whole sequence of topics, see BJP, xxix–lviii.

on Galen and his view of the minimum conditions for an endurable human life (v.43–5 K =29–30 DB); (4) a sustained critique of insatiability and correlated commendation of self-sufficiency (*autarkeia*) (v.46–52 K. =31–34 DB).[18] Although the themes themselves are highly comparable in both works, the ampler scale and fuller explication in *Aff. Dig.* make it easier to discern the overall line of thought. Galen's main point is that a proper realisation of the misguided character of the emotional force of insatiability, and its corrosive effect on human happiness, is crucial for achieving both self-sufficiency and equanimity in the face or prospect of material losses (v.51–52 K. = 34 DB). However, a crucial prerequisite for grasping this point properly and making it genuinely part of one's character is the kind of nature, upbringing and education that Galen had. This, presumably, explains the difference emphasised between Galen and his addressee. Although they are both wealthy members of their society, Galen is more ready to spend his income and to do so in a way that benefits others, and is also not worried about money. The addressee is much richer, but also less willing to spend on himself or others, and is also much more anxious, because he is gripped by the insatiable desire to have more money than others, without any need to do so (v.47–51 K. = 32–34 DB). This may also explain the points made subsequently that Galen's advice to others has been generally ineffective and that in people more advanced in years this vice is too ingrained to be removed (v.53–54 K. =35–36 DB).

Another feature that is clearer in *Aff. Dig.* is the precise content of the advice offered by Galen's father (which is cited as direct quotation in v.42–43 K. = 29 DB). In *Ind.*, by contrast, it is less evident what is and is not being ascribed to Galen's father. The quotation of his father's view in *Aff. Dig.* also makes it plain that the paternal advice is neutral between philosophical theories, and is presented as a kind of 'consensus-position', shared also by non-philosophers. It is also more apparent in *Aff. Dig.* that the intellectual eclecticism or independence which is also implied, I think, in *Ind.* 61–8 (and which is Galen's typical stance) is the product of his father's advice.[19] Also, Galen here ascribes to his father the account of the minimum level of possessions needed for a life free from distress, namely what is enough to keep one from hunger, thirst or cold, which is presented in *Ind.* as Galen's own opinion.[20]

---

18   On these similarities, see also BJP xlv–xlix, lv–lviii; Nutton, introduction to *Ind.* in Galen, *Psychological Writings*, 65–66; Xenophontos, 'Psychotherapy', 2014, 598–600.

19   See para. including n. 46. See also Hankinson, R.J. 'Galen's Philosophical Eclecticism', in Haase, W, and Temporini, H. eds, *Aufstieg und Niedergang der römischen Welt*, II.36.5, 1992, 3502–22. On Galen's philosophical eclecticism in *Ind.*, see also Kaufman, 'Therapy', 286–7, and the appeal to his father's authority, 'Therapy', 291.

20   *Aff. Dig.* v.44 K. = 30 DB: *Ind.* 78.

In the light of the fuller articulation of themes and the clearer specification of the father's influence, I am inclined to see *Aff. Dig.* as the later work, and as a reworking (at least in the sections discussed) of similar themes. This dating matches some of the other evidence bearing on this question. The main obstacle to this view of their relative dates is the curious omission of any reference in *Aff. Dig.* v.44 K. = 30 DB, where more minor losses are noted, to the substantial losses so fully emphasised in *Ind* (1–37). However, the losses in the fire of 192, even if they had been mentioned, were not enough to cause Galen any real material discomfort or loss of social standing, let alone leaving him hungry or cold (the levels of loss he specifies as really significant in *Aff. Dig.* v.44 K. =30 DB). Also, although Galen presents himself as exemplary in both works, it is on rather different grounds. In *Ind.* Galen's equanimity in the face of his losses is central for the whole work and the therapeutic strategy. In *Aff. Dig.*, shortly after this passage, Galen sets up a contrast between himself and the addressee, in which both are presented as wealthy people, but Galen is willing to use his resources for himself and others, whereas the other man hoards his resources because of the insatiable desire to accumulate property for its own sake (v.48–49 K = 32–33 DB). It may be that Galen de-emphasises his earlier losses in *Aff. Dig.* because they are not relevant for this specific contrast.[21]

2   Galen's De Indolentia: Underlying Cohesion

In the light of this analysis of the latter part of *Aff. Dig.*, I return to *Ind.*, taking up the question whether there is more underlying cohesion than is initially obvious. In fact, I think that the pattern of thought just outlined in *Aff. Dig.* also forms the organising framework for *Ind.*, both for the second half and also, though less obviously, for the work as a whole. The aim of the quasi-philosophical reflections in 61–68 remains rather puzzling; but the opening catalogue of losses makes good sense in this framework. The core theme emerges most clearly towards the end of the work. The key prerequisite for gaining freedom from distress (*alupia*) is freeing yourself from 'insatiability' (*aplēstia*), the restless desire for more (especially more material possessions) that afflicts many

---

21   On the dating question, see Nutton, introduction to *Ind.* in Galen, *Psychological Writings*, 2013, 45–48, which I follow, by contrast with BJP, lviii–lxi, which places *Aff. Dig.* before *Ind.* The fact that Galen presents himself in *Therapeutic Method*, probably written in the late 190s (i.e. later than *Ind.* or *Aff. Dig.*) as intensely distressed for long periods (MM x.456–457 K.) (cf. Nutton, ibid. 67) suggests that Galen's self-presentation is often shaped for the needs of the context of writing. On Galen's self-presentation and authority, see Xenophontos, 'Psychotherapy', 2014, 590–93.

people, but especially the rich (79–84). A correlative of this advice is recognising what is really needed to make a human life that is free from distress – more precisely, recognising how *little* is needed to achieve this. Galen spells out several times what is required: namely, an adequate level of bodily and psychological health, combined with enough material possessions to avoid physical discomfort (71–6, 78). However, this minimum level needs to be accompanied by the right mental attitude, which enables one to regard this standard of living as acceptable. Achieving this attitude depends on psychological training, formulated here (77, cf. 52) in terms of a Euripidean passage frequently cited in support of the philosophical therapeutic method of 'preparation for future evils'.[22] As brought out earlier in the work, the effectiveness of this training depends, in turn, on nature, upbringing and education.[23] Although this overall line of thought is spelled out most clearly here (in what seems to be signalled earlier as Galen's 'second' explanation for equanimity),[24] it also makes sense of the previous part of the second half and also, in a different way, of the catalogue of losses in the first half of the work.

To some extent, the function of the catalogue of losses is made apparent from the start. The work is presented as a letter in response to an invitation 'to show you what kind of training, what arguments or what considerations had prepared me never to be distressed' (1).[25] Galen's equanimity in the face of the very extensive losses experienced in the great fire at Rome in AD 162 represents the most striking expression of a fortitude shown by him in earlier losses (1–2). The losses are outlined in 4–6, together with a pointed contrast between Galen's equanimity and the terminal or funereal despair of others in the same situation (7). This prepares the ground for the promised explanation for Galen's absence of distress (1) in the latter half of the work (38–84). However, this rationale is not quite sufficient, at least, if we are interpreting the work as a contribution to the philosophical therapy of emotions. The main relevant features of the situation are set out in 1–7. Why then do we need, for this purpose, another 30 chapters cataloguing Galen's losses in such detail? Admittedly, Galen does not only list losses. He also underlines features that made the losses particularly severe, notably the impossibility of replacing Galen's, often

---

22   See n. 16.

23   See *Ind.* 79, also 51, 57, 65. In these passages, by contrast with *Aff. Dig.* v.48–52 = 32–4 DB, Galen stresses the similarity of character between himself and the addressee. See also on this point Kaufman, *Therapy*, 2014, 292–3.

24   I take it that *Ind.* 70–83 amplifies the explanation said to be complete in 69, and thus provides the 'second' explanation signalled in 39.

25   Translations taken from Galen, *Psychological Writings*, 2013. For an alternative English translation, see Rothschild, C. K., Thompson, T. W. (eds.), *Galen's De Indolentia*, 2014.

personally annotated, books (12b–19), losses intensified by the timing, just before Galen sent a substantial number of copied works to Campania (20–29). Galen also concludes the catalogue (30–37) by enumerating a unique collection of drug recipes, of immense value for his medical work, along with many other medical items lost in the fire. While accentuating these very substantial losses, which were items hugely valuable as support for Galen's intellectual life and his mission as a medical writer and practitioner, Galen stresses, repeatedly, that he was not distressed by their loss (11–12a, 29–30, 37). So it might seem that, even for therapeutic purposes (setting aside any purely autobiographical objectives), the catalogue of losses is fully explained.

However, I think we can see one further salient objective, if we bear in mind the aim of counteracting 'insatiability' (aplēstia), apparent at the close of the work (78–84, esp. 80–81). Galen, here and in *Aff. Dig.*, does not simply identify this vice in general terms. He also spells out, often in precise numerical terms, the scale of the desires and ambitions of those afflicted by this vice. He specifies in the same numerical terms the attitudes of those, such as Aristippus, who endured significant losses without distress.[26] By the end of the work, we are also in a position to recognise the sharp contrast between these extravagant desires and the minimum level that human beings actually need for a life free from distress (78–84). Galen's particularised catalogue of his losses (1–37), like the much briefer sketch of Aristippus' response to his losses (40–42), thus serves as a powerful contrast to those extravagant desires. Whereas insatiability yearns for an ever-increasing amount and plurality of possessions, Galen's catalogue spells out in graphic detail all that one can live without – while still remaining un-distressed. The catalogue of losses can thus be seen as a complement to the later specification of the minimal conditions needed for a human life free from distress: Galen is saying, 'look at how much one can live without', as well as 'look at how little one can manage with'. From this standpoint, the scale and particularity of Galen's catalogue serves a therapeutic function (whatever autobiographical function it may also have). The fact that Galen's list of losses focuses on the destruction of resources for intellectual activity and medical practice, rather than more standard examples of precious objects, is not, perhaps, directly relevant for this broad, moralising point. However, it does illustrate that 'insatiability' can take many different forms, not all of which are obviously moral defects. Also, of course, it takes us to the heart of the significance of these losses *for Galen*. Although this is, on the face of it, a

---

26   *Ind.* 41–48, esp. 42–43, 45, 47, also 83; *Aff. Dig.* v.46–47, 49 K. (=31–32, 33 DB); see also BJP lv–lviii.

purely personal point, it has significant implications for his therapeutic message explored in the final section of this discussion.

How far does the linkage between *aplēstia* and *alupia*, made at the end of the work, together with the parallel with the relevant section of *Aff. Dig.*, help us to make sense of the earlier sections in the second part (38–68) and the overall sequence of thought? The relevance for the opening section of Galen's explanation for not being distressed (39–48) is clear. Galen's use of stock anecdotes and exemplars from the therapeutic tradition (especially Aristippus) illustrates the contrast between insatiability and taking a realistic view of what one has, and thus not being distressed by loss, which is articulated more fully later.[27] However, Galen also underlines the limitations of this initial, and rather generic, set of exemplars for his purposes. He acknowledges, first of all, the difference between his financial situation and that of some of the philosophical exemplars he refers to (notably, the Cynics Crates and Diogenes and the Stoic Zeno, 45, 48). What was left for Galen was 'much more than sufficient' (46). Also, what Galen accentuates was not just his lack of distress at the loss of money or standardly valuable items, but rather the drugs and writings central for his mission in life (50). It was his lack of distress at this loss which constituted 'a prime display of nobility and nigh on magnanimity' (50) that needs to be explained. So the opening illustration of the difference between insatiability and realism is marked as only a preliminary move in Galen's explanation, and his therapeutic strategy.

How is the explanation developed? First, Galen has recourse to another rather standard feature of the philosophical genre, the strategy of preparing for misfortune by anticipating it in your mind, illustrated by the Euripides passage also cited later (52–3, 76).[28] He gives this stock item a more personal force – and one which would have resonated strongly with his contemporary readers – by presenting it as his way of coping with the horrors and unpredictability of the rule of Commodus, only just ended (54–6). However, more significant is his next move, a qualification of the usefulness of this method, or, by implication, of the earlier recommendation to avoid insatiability, taken on its own. 'This prescription cannot be given to those with no natural aptitude for courage or without an excellent education, which a generous fate vouchsafed to me' (57). This point is developed by reference to Galen's father, who was naturally exceptional for his 'justice and self-control' (58) and who had in turn

---

27   *Ind.* 43, 45, cf. 80–2 (also 71–5, 78). The Aristippus anecdotes appear also in Diog. Laert. 2.77, Plut. *peri euthumias* (*Mor.*) 469 C–D.

28   See n. 16. Kaufman, 'Therapy', 2014, 281–4, stresses the importance of this theme in Galen's therapeutic strategy in *Ind.*

been 'trained from childhood in virtue' (59). Galen spells out the inference: 'So you may suppose that I am naturally like my forebears because I was born like this and, moreover, because I had an identical upbringing, I have a similar disposition of soul to them' (60). At this point, as in the comparable section of *Aff Dig.*, Galen signals his adherence to the Platonic-Aristotelian, rather than Stoic or Epicurean, pattern of thinking about ethical development.[29] Philosophical strategies, such as 'preparation for future evils', and indeed philosophical advice generally, are not enough by themselves to shape character and reactions. They are only effective if grounded on the right kind of inborn nature and childhood habituation, a point underlined by reference to the addressee, who is presented as someone who shares these advantages (51, 57, 79).

However, Galen goes on to outline a number of philosophical principles, and to say that these were (presumably, in conjunction with his nature and upbringing) influential on his state of mind: 'Brought up in this way of thinking, I always consider these things of little value, so how could I suppose leisure, instruments, drugs, books, reputation and riches to be precious?' (65) This outline of philosophical ideas and their effect (61–8) is the most problematic part of the work, generating interpretative problems of various kinds. It is difficult, first, to determine whether Galen is reporting his father's ethical principles or offering his own account of them (or of his own ideas). He begins by reporting them (61–2) and implies in 65 that these were the parental ideals that shaped his upbringing. But in 63–4 he seems to be thinking the ideas out for himself. In 64, he refers to his own views or at least his reflections on certain received views, and in 67 he cites his own opinions and, indeed, 'logical proof' of the claims made (67, also 68). A further complication is that, although the passage evokes specific themes in philosophical ethics, Galen says that his father 'did not consort with philosophers in his youth' and that his father's principles were based on his being 'trained from childhood in virtue' (59). Hence, the philosophical connotations of the passage, whether presented as reportage of his father's views or not, must be Galen's addition. As noted earlier, the comparable *Aff. Dig.* passage is much clearer in this respect, explicitly quoting Galen's father's advice, as well as reporting his commendation of a kind of 'consensus-position', shared by many philosophers and ordinary people.[30] Although we may think that a similar view is implied here, emerging out of the various

---

29 See text to nn. 11, 18. Kaufman, 'Therapy, 292–3, also underlines this point.
30 See text to nn. 19–20. As noted there, in *Aff. Dig.*, the specification of a minimum level of life is presented as part of Galen's father's advice (v.44 K. = 30 DB), whereas in *Ind.*, this appears as a subsequent qualification by Galen of the philosophical ideas, which are linked (though loosely) with his father (71–5, 78).

allusions to philosophical positions in 61–8, this is not actually explicit, leaving the overall significance rather unclear.

A second problem lies in establishing which philosophical theories are being evoked in the passage, as well as how far these evocations add up to a single line of thought. The most unequivocal allusion is the rejection, first, of vulgar hedonism, and then of the subtler Epicurean view of pleasure (that of 'being merely free from pain and distress') as a plausible candidate for being the goal of human life (or the good) in 62. This is reinforced by the subsequent dismissal of the idea 'that remaining undisturbed' (*aochlēsia*) is the good, along with Galen's reference to his own *Against* (or *On*) Epicurus (68).[31] The review of principles begins with the striking claim that 'my father despised human affairs as of little worth, and this is exactly the same for me in my old age' (61). The rather lofty, 'god's-eye', stance of this passage, may evoke two striking Platonic passages in the *Republic* (a work Galen knew well), bearing in mind that the whole passage is designed to explain the 'magnanimity' (*megalopsuchia*) with which Galen bore his losses.[32] A later passage, referring to Galen as writing, not 'with zealous enthusiasm or as something tremendous, but simply as a kind of hobby' (67) seems also to allude to a well-marked Platonic comment on the relatively low value of writing in the *Phaedrus*.[33] In 63–4, Galen gives a prominent place to the idea that the good (or goal of human life) is 'knowledge of matters human and divine'. Although some commentators have seen this phrase as Aristotelian in provenance,[34] Teun Tieleman, writing in this volume, argues strongly that the allusion is to Stoic ideas, since this phrase was a standard

---

31   For the Epicurean ideal, see Long, A. A. and Sedley, D. N., *The Hellenistic Philosophers* 1987 (= LS) (refs. to sections and passages), 21 A–B. The ideal of 'remaining undisturbed' is also associated with other thinkers, including the Peripatetic Hieronymus of Rhodes (BJP, 162), but Epicurus seems to be meant here.

32   See *Republic* 486a: the world-view of the 'philosophical nature' is characterised as including the kind of 'magnificence' (*megaloprepeia*) that makes one regard human life as nothing great (*mega*); 604b–c: the rational response to misfortune includes seeing human life as not 'worth great seriousness' (*axion … megalēs spoudēs*).

33   *Phaedrus* 276c–e, philosophical writing (as opposed to oral dialectic) should not be done as something worthy of seriousness (*spoudē*) but as a 'hobby' (*paidia*), 276c7, d3, e1, 5. Galen refers to both Platonic works (esp. *Republic*) a good deal, esp. in *PHP*: see Galen, *PHP*, ed. P. De Lacy, vol. 3, 831 (index locorum). The comment is sometimes taken (BJP, 161) as referring to Galen's writing specifically about ethics ('each of these things', 67), as opposed to medicine; but, bearing in mind his previous dismissal of the importance of 'instruments, drugs, books' in 65, his comments, like Plato's, may apply to writing in general.

34   Nutton, in Galen, *Psychological Writings*, 94, n. 104, cites Arist. *Met.* VI.1, 1026a18–32, XI.7, 1064b1–4; BJP, 156–7, also see Aristotelian influence but offers no refs.

formulation for wisdom (the ideal human state) in Stoicism.[35] Tieleman links this phrase with the 'magnanimity' accentuated in 50–51, pointing out that the relevant sense of this term, namely facing adversities in a courageous spirit, has clear Stoic, rather than Aristotelian, connotations.[36] However, Aristotle's stress on the idea that the goal of life must be an activity not a state may be alluded to in the final comment in the passage, criticising the Epicurean ideal of 'remaining undisturbed' (68).[37]

Even if we are confident about charting these allusions, there remains the problem of making sense of the overall line of thought in the passage, taken in the context of the work as a whole. One approach worth considering is a broadly Stoic reading, building on Tieleman's interpretation of the connotations of the terms. The underlying line of thought would be some version of the Stoic claim that happiness depends wholly on virtue, and that 'external things' such as material goods and reputation are, relatively, 'matters of indifference'.[38] The Stoic conception of magnanimity as fortitude in the face of disaster reflects this general view, as does their belief that possession of virtue brings with it inner peace of mind, regardless of external circumstances (ideas that figure prominently in Stoic or Stoic-influenced therapeutic writings).[39] On this reading, Galen interprets his father's adherence to virtue ('justice and self-control', 58) primarily in Stoic terms. This would explain Galen's conclusion that 'external things' such as 'leisure, instruments, drugs, books, reputation and riches' are 'of little value', that is, in more technical Stoic terms, they are only, at most, 'preferred indifferents' (65).[40] In support of this view is the prominent role played elsewhere by the Euripidean passage linked with the strategy of 'preparation for future evils', which was recognised as a Stoic, rather than Epicurean, method, though it was not peculiar to them.[41] As so interpreted, Galen's exceptional equanimity concerning his great losses in the fire would be explained, primarily, in Stoic terms.

Although this interpretation is coherent, and matches some points in the text, I do not think it is, in the end, tenable. A rather obvious problem is that

---

35   See e.g. SVF 2.35, 36, also 3.362. See also Brouwer, R. (2014), *The Stoic Sage*, 8–41.

36   See e.g. Cic. *Off.* 1.15, also SVF 3.264, 265; contrast Arist. *Eth. Nic.* 4.3.

37   Arist. *Eth. Nic.* 1098a5–18, 1098b30–1099a7. On this theme in later Peripatetic thought, see Inwood, B., *Ethics after Aristotle*, 2014, 69–70, 109–10; see e.g. Cic. *Fin.* 5.55–57 (based on Antiochus, an Academic influenced by Peripatetic ideas).

38   LS 58 and 63.

39   See e.g. Cic. *Off.* 1.66–69, Cic. *Tusc.* 5.40–1, 81–2, Sen. *Tranq.* 11, 14, 16; see Gill, 'Peace of mind', 4609–10, 4615–16, 4621–2.

40   See LS 58; also Xenophontos, 'Psychotherapy', 2014, 596.

41   See n. 16. According to Cic. *Tusc.* 3.32–3, Epicureans favoured, rather, averting the mind from bad things.

in 63–64, Galen adopts a very guarded or cautious attitude towards this ideal, or at least towards putting it into practice. Galen's wording and line of thought is particularly murky here.[42] But the main point seems to be that it is very difficult to gain 'knowledge of human and divine affairs' (the Stoic account of the human good) with sufficient understanding to put it into practice. In fact, the Stoics do believe that wisdom, the human ideal state, is very hard, even virtually impossible, to achieve fully, though they also maintain it is the appropriate target for everyone; and this combination of ideas was often cited by critics of Stoicism as self-contradictory or at least problematic.[43] Galen perhaps has that criticism in view here. He connects this point with a guarded attitude towards engaging in politics, because of its inherent difficulty and the fact that most people are not in fact helped even by genuine efforts in their behalf (64). The link between the two ideas in 63–4 is not obvious. But it may be significant that the Stoics were well-known for maintaining that the wise man (the paradigm for all of us) should, in principle, engage in political life, by contrast with the negative Epicurean attitude towards political involvement.[44] So Galen may be dissenting at this point from two standard features of the Stoic ethical ideal. A further problem for taking 61–8 as marking Galen's adoption of a Stoic approach is that this would run counter to the explicit repudiation of the Stoic (or Epicurean) ideal of invulnerability in 71–75, and the earlier presentation of Zeno's response to misfortune as 'amazing' and well beyond Galen's own (48, cf. 46).[45]

How, then, does 61–68 contribute to Galen's therapeutic strategy in *Ind.* as a whole? Overall in *Ind.*, Galen explains his exceptional equanimity in the face of his losses (his *alupia*) by his having counteracted any tendency towards insatiability (*aplēstia*). Crucial in this respect is forming a realistic picture of the minimum needed to maintain a human life free from distress, namely an adequate level of physical and psychological health supported by enough material possessions to avoid pain and discomfort. Galen has also prepared himself for any such eventuality by dwelling on this prospect in advance, especially

---

42   See BJP, 156–7.

43   See Brouwer, *Stoic Sage*, ch. 3.

44   See e.g. Cic. *Fin.* 3.66, 68, LS 67 W(3); for the Epicurean view, see LS 22 D(1), S.

45   See Gill, *Naturalistic Psychology*, 264–65. This rejection of an extreme standard of invulnerability may also have philosophical echoes: there is a strong vein in Platonic-Aristotelian thought underlining the importance of bodily health and (some) external goods for happiness, often linked with dissent from the Stoic position; see Sharples, R. *Peripatetic Philosophy 200 BC to 200 AD*, ch. 18. BJP, liv–lv, links *Ind.* 73 with Crantor (4th/3rd BC Academic), referred to in Cic. *Tusc.* 3.12, whose position was often cited as part of this strand of thought. However, Galen presents this as his own view.

during the reign of Commodus, when exile and loss of all one's possessions were daily prospects (54–55) – that is, situations much worse than he actually experienced. There remains the question how Galen mustered the inner, psychological or ethical, resources (the 'magnanimity', 50–51) to embrace this tough-minded approach to life. This is explained primarily in terms of his inborn nature and upbringing, and the adoption of the (un-theorised) ethical principles of his father and forefathers (59). Although these principles are expressed (or 'glossed') in terms that evoke specific philosophical ideals, Galen does not identify the principles adopted in terms of any one philosophical framework. Indeed, he explicitly rejects some philosophical ideals (Epicurean ones, 62, 68) and is guarded regarding the achievability of others (Stoic ones, 63–4). The positive element, which is not qualified, is a kind of high-minded indifference to circumstances (or indeed 'human life', 61) that Galen sees as enabling him to regard the things lost as 'of little value' (65) and hence to be free from distress at their loss. What emerges, overall, is not the conception of virtue or the good life (happiness or *eudaimonia*) espoused by any specific theory but, rather, a broadly, 'philosophical' view of life that can support the quality of character, the virtue ('magnanimity') that enables Galen to maintain a realistic view of the scale and importance of his losses. On this view, the resumé of philosophical ideas in 61–68 makes a relatively modest contribution to the overall line of thought, compared with the contribution made by the theoretical framework in more doctrinally focused works of ancient (especially Stoic and Epicurean) therapy of the emotions.[46] But the contribution is one that is consistent with the overall shaping and line of thought of the work: and this helps us to recognise that *Ind.*, taken as a whole and closely examined, has its own coherence and distinctiveness, exceptional though it is in the genre in which it figures.

3   Was This the Whole Truth?

I end this discussion by raising a different, though related, question. Was Galen's explanation for his equanimity actually true – or at least, was it the whole truth? Assuming that he did indeed show exceptional equanimity in

---

46   For a broadly similar interpretation of Galen's line of thought in *Ind.*, see also Kaufman, 'Therapy', 276–89. Contrast Chrysippus' 'therapeutic' book, on which see Tieleman, *Chrysippus*, ch. 4. But works such as Plut. *peri euthumias* are more comparable; see also Gill, *Naturalistic Psychology*, 250–1.

this situation (of course, we only have his word for this),[47] does this explanation ring true in the light of what we know about him from other sources?

Let us briefly call to mind what most of our evidence suggests about Galen's character. He was an utterly driven, obsessive, hugely ambitious, medical practitioner, thinker and writer whose core project in life was to become, and remain, *the* world-leader in his field.[48] In the first half of *Ind.*, his account vividly underlines the threat to this aim from the losses of medical handbooks, recipes, collections and so on in the great fire (5–6, 12a, 29–37). I strongly suspect that what enabled his equanimity in the face of these losses was the confidence that he still had the resources, energy and determination (despite his age, about sixty-three) to maintain and take further this core project. If this was what he felt, he was right, as it turned out; he did rewrite lost works, gather missing resources, and produce more medical writings, though not perhaps on the same scale as before, until his death about seventeen years later.[49] Of course, in 193, when he seems to have written the work,[50] he could not have known that he would be able to continue his career in this way. But he had reasonable grounds for thinking he could do so; and this was, I guess, a key factor, and perhaps *the* key factor, underlying his absence of distress.

However, if I am right in suggesting this, the obvious further question is this: why did he not say so in *Ind.*, which claims to offer the explanation for his equanimity? It is also perhaps surprising, from this standpoint, that, in the section of *Aff. Dig.* (V.44 K = 30 DB) dealing with his response to losses (though not his losses in the fire of 192), he also does not cite this factor explicitly.[51] However, here he comes closer to bringing out this side of his motivation. He makes it clear that at all stages of his life so far he has had ample financial resources and that he feels committed to using these to benefit others, following his father's advice and example. This can plausibly be taken as an allusion to his exceptional social contribution as a medical practitioner and writer, which depended on using his considerable personal wealth for this purpose.

47   See n. 21.

48   This comes out clearly in Mattern, S., *The Prince of Medicine*, 2013, esp. chs. 2, 5, 7. See also Hankinson, R. J. 'The man and his work', in Hankinson, R. J. (ed), *The Cambridge Companion to Galen*, 2008, 23–4; Boudon-Millot, V. 'Galen's *Bios* and *Methodos*', in Gill, C. et al. (eds) *Galen and the World of Knowledge*, 2009, 175–89, on Galen's view of his medical mission in life.

49   On his medical writings after the fire, see Hankinson, 'Man and work', 22–3; Mattern, *Prince*, 274–7.

50   See Galen, *Psychological Writings*: Singer, general introduction, 39–41; Nutton, introduction to *Ind.*, 45–8.

51   Also, of course, since Galen does not cite his losses in the fire in *Aff. Dig.*, it would be inappropriate to refer to this explanation for not being distressed by the losses.

As suggested earlier, Galen's self-presentation in this passage forms part of his therapeutic guidance, showing how his characteristic freedom from distress is linked with his freedom from insatiability.[52] However, if this passage at least allows the possibility of the kind of explanation I am suggesting, this raises still more acutely the question why this explanation is entirely missing in *Ind.*

In considering this question, it is worth noting that this explanation is not only absent from *Ind.*, but is actually ruled out by the line of thought presented there. The catalogue of losses, as noted earlier, gives special attention to the loss of medical books and resources, as factors which *might have* made Galen especially distressed – but which did not in fact do so.[53] Also, the philosophical section in 61–8 excludes this option in two ways. In 64 Galen discounts the idea that aiming to help many people by one's earnest endeavours can, on a realistic view, provide the basis of a human life free from distress (because most people cannot reliably be helped in this way). In 65, he stresses that his upbringing made it inconceivable that he could regard 'drugs, books, and reputation' as precious, although these are things that we might well suppose *were* precious to Galen in his role as world-famous doctor. Also, while acknowledging in 46 that even after the losses, 'what was left was more than sufficient', and thus, by inference that this allowed the renewal of his medical role, his account of the minimal conditions for a life free from distress falls far short of this level. Indeed, Galen there presents himself as happy 'to talk with a friend and to follow what is being read by someone to me' (78). He presents himself as an amiable, if slightly doddery, old man: a picture very different from that of the still active and forceful individual we might reasonably reconstruct from Galen's medical and other writings in the later part of his life.[54] This is also a self-presentation which runs counter to the view I am proposing, that Galen was heartened in his losses by the prospect of engaging fully again in his medical objectives.

To put the point more generally, the therapeutic strategy Galen adopts in *Ind*, rules out reference to the explanation which I am suggesting may have underpinned his equanimity. In focusing on the idea that the key to *alupia* lies in counteracting *aplēstia*, especially by recognising the minimum needed

---

52   See text to nn. 18, 21.

53   *Ind.* 5–6, 10–12a, 31–8.

54   On his writings after the fire, see n. 49. Kaufman, 'Therapy', 284–6, reads this passage (78) as having more positive content, and evoking Epicurus' famous death-bed letter (D. L. 10.22) and the Epicurean therapeutic strategy of avoiding pain by redirecting one's attention to more pleasant things (Cic. *Tusc.* 3.32–3); but I am not persuaded that this short and unemphatic passage carries these larger connotations.

for a pain-free life,[55] Galen set up a framework in which the retention of a specific life-mission had little room. Indeed, it would have run counter to this therapeutic approach, since it would have placed weight on factors (material resources, medical supplies and books, intellectual energy and stamina) that Galen here insists are *not* prerequisites for a life free from distress. So I think this explanation does not appear for this reason – which is not to say it was not, in reality, part of his response at this time. A further question, then, is why he adopted a therapeutic strategy which ruled this possibility out. Galen could have found, for instance, in Stoic thought, support for the idea that one can be sustained in one's losses, which can include loss of loved ones as well as possessions or even your own life, by renewing or continuing one's commitment to a life-project. This set of ideas figures as part of a therapeutic strategy in Seneca's *On Peace of Mind*, for instance, and appears also in Epictetus' *Discourses* and Marcus Aurelius' *Meditations*.[56] Of course, Galen might not have been aware of this line of thought, though he seems to have a good knowledge of the philosophical therapeutic tradition. He might also have had reservations about adopting a strategy that was so closely linked with Stoicism, although *Aff. Dig.* shows a good deal of influence from Stoic therapeutic writings.[57] In any case, this was not the strategy he chose to adopt, in *Ind.* or in the comparable part of *Aff. Dig.*; and the explanation for his equanimity that I am proposing did not fit the strategy he did adopt. However, this does not mean it was not part of his actual experience – though we may never be able to prove this.[58]

References

Boudon-Millot, V. 'Galen's *Bios* and *Methodos*: from Ways of Life to Paths of Knowledge', in *Galen and the World of Knowledge*, eds. C. Gill, T. Whitmarsh, and J. Wilkins, 175–89. Cambridge: Cambridge University Press, 2009.

---

55   See paras including nn. 22, 46.

56   See Gill, 'Peace of Mind', 4609–10, 4614–24, 4627–31; Epict. *Diss.* 1.1–2; on Marcus (whose approach reflects earlier Stoic ideas), see C. Gill. *Marcus Aurelius*, Meditations Books 1–6, xlix–lii.

57   See Gill, *Naturalistic Psychology*, 253–5.

58   This paper has gained from the stimulating discussion at the Warwick conference. It has also benefited from helpful comments made after two papers I gave on Galen's therapeutic writings given in Berlin, at the Topoi Exzellenzcluster and Humboldt University; special thanks to Philip van der Eijk and Roland Wittwer for organising these sessions.

Brouwer, R. *The Stoic Sage: The Early Stoics on Wisdom, Sagehood and Socrates.* Cambridge: Cambridge University Press, 2014.

Gill, C. 'Ancient Psychotherapy', *Journal of the History of Ideas* 46.3 (1985): 307–25.

Gill, C. 'Peace of Mind and Being Yourself: Panaetius to Plutarch', in *Aufstieg und Niedergang der römischen Welt* 11.36.7, eds. W. Haase and H. Temporini, 4599–4640. Berlin/New York: De Gruyter, 1994.

Gill, C. *Naturalistic Psychology in Galen and Stoicism.* Oxford: Oxford University Press, 2010.

Gill, C. *Marcus Aurelius, Meditations Books 1–6.* Translated with introduction and commentary, Clarendon Later Ancient Philosophers. Oxford: Oxford University Press, 2013.

Gill, C. 'Philosophical Therapy as Preventive Psychological Medicine', in *Mental Disorders in the Classical World*, ed. W. Harris, 339–60, Columbia Studies in the Classical Tradition 38. Leiden: Brill, 2013.

Gill, C. 'Philosophical Psychological therapy – Did it Have Any Impact on Medical Practice?' in *Mental Illness in Ancient Medicine: From Celsus to Paul of Aegina*, eds. C. Thumiger and P. N. Singer, 365–80. Studies in Ancient Medicine. Leiden: Brill, 2018.

Hadot, I. *Seneca und die griechische-römische Tradition der Seelenleitung.* Berlin: De Gruyter, 1994.

Hankinson, R.J. 'Galen's Philosophical Eclecticism', in *Aufstieg und Niedergang der römischen Welt*, 11.36.5, eds. W. Haase and H. Temporini, 3502–22. Berlin/New York: De Gruyter, 1992.

Hankinson, R.J. 'Actions and Passions: Affection, Emotion and Moral Self-management in Galen's Philosophical Psychology', in *Passions and Perceptions*, eds. J. Brunschwig and M. C. Nussbaum, 184–222. Cambridge: Cambridge University Press, 1993.

Hankinson, R.J. *The Cambridge Companion to Galen* (ed.). Cambridge: Cambridge University Press, 2008.

Hankinson, R.J. 'The Man and his Work,' in *The Cambridge Companion to Galen*, ed. R. J. Hankinson, 1–33. Cambridge: Cambridge University Press, 2008.

Inwood, B. *Ethics after Aristotle.* Cambridge, MA: Harvard University Press, 2014.

Kaufman, D. H., 'Galen on the Therapy of Distress and the Limits of Emotional Therapy', *Oxford Studies in Ancient Philosophy* 47 (2014): 275–96.

Laín Entralgo, P. *The Therapy of the Word in Classical Antiquity*, New Haven: Yale University Press, 1970.

Mattern, S. M. *The Prince of Medicine: Galen in the Roman Empire.* Oxford: Oxford University Press, 2013.

Nussbaum, M. C. *The Therapy of Desire; Theory and Practice in Hellenistic Ethics.* Princeton; Princeton University Press, 1994.

Rothschild, C. K. Thompson, T. W. (eds.), *Galen's De Indolentia: Essays on a Newly Discovered Letter*. Tübingen: Mohr Siebeck, 2014.

Sorabji, R. *Emotion and Peace of Mind: From Stoic Agitation to Christian Temptation*. Oxford: Oxford University Press, 2000.

Tieleman, T. *Chrysippus' On Affections: Reconstruction and Interpretation*. Leiden: Brill, 2003.

Van Hoof, L. *Plutarch's Practical Ethics*. Oxford: Oxford University Press, 2010.

Xenophontos, S. 'Psychotherapy and Moralising Rhetoric in Galen's Newly Discovered *Peri Alypias*', *Medical History* 58.4 (2014): 585–603.

Texts and Translations Used

De placitis Hippocratis et Platonis. Ed. with translation and commentary P. De Lacy. Corpus Medicorum Graecorum v.4,1,2. Berlin: Akademie, 1978–84, rev. edn. 2005.

Galen. *Oeuvres*, tome IV: *Ne pas se chagriner*. Eds. with translation, introduction, and commentary, V. Boudon-Millot and J. Jouanna, with the collaboration of A. Pietrobelli. Paris: Les Belles Lettres, 2010 (= BJP).

Galen. *De propriorum animi cuiuslibet affectuum dignotione et curatione; De animi cuiuslibet peccatorum dignotione et curatione*. Ed. W. De Boer. Corpus Medicorum Graecorum v.4,1,1. Leipzig/Berlin: Akademie, 1994 (= DB).

Galen. *Psychological Writings*. Ed. P. N. Singer, translated with introductions and notes by V. Nutton, D. Davies and P. N. Singer, with the collaboration of P. Tassinari. Cambridge: Cambridge University Press, 2013.

Long, A. A. and Sedley, D. N. *The Hellenistic Philosophers*. Cambridge: Cambridge University Press, 1987 (= LS).

Sharples, R. W. *Peripatetic Philosophy 200 BC to AD 200: An Introduction and Collection to Sources in Translation*. Cambridge: Cambridge University Press, 2010.

CHAPTER 6

Galen and the Sceptics (and the Epicureans) on the Unavoidability of Distress

R. J. Hankinson

I will be flesh and blood;
For there was never yet philosopher
That could endure the toothache patiently.

> *MUCH ADO ABOUT NOTHING*, V I

•••

For he was not sprung from some ancient oak, nor from a rock
<But from the race of men>.[1]

> *ODYSSEY* 19.163+, QUOTED BY SEXTUS, *AGAINST THE PROFESSORS* [M] 11.161

•••

For this reason, we say that while in the case of matters of opinion, the end for the sceptic is tranquillity, in the case of what is forced upon us it is moderation in affection.

> SEXTUS, *OUTLINES OF PYRRHONISM* [PH] 1.30

∴

One of the most extraordinary scholarly events of recent years was Antoine Pietrobelli's discovery in 2005 of a hitherto unknown manuscript containing, among other things, a previously lost work of Galen, περὶ ἀλυπίας: *Avoiding Distress* (*Ind.*). Since then, it has been edited and translated several times,[2] and

---

1 This half-line is not in our MSS. of Homer, but it is metrical and may well derive from a lost alternative tradition known to Sextus: see Bett, 1997, 166.
2 Notably in Boudon-Millot et al., 2010, to which edition subsequent references will be keyed. An English translation, by Vivian Nutton, appears in Singer, 2013. The text is sometimes also

provoked a flurry of articles. It contains invaluable biographical information, in particular concerning the disastrous fire of 192, in which Galen lost many unique exemplars of his own writings, as well as a vast store of *materia medica* (some of it decades old and very valuable), and a large number of surgical instruments, several of his own devising. His experience of the loss, and his observation of that of others, prompted him to write this short treatise on the subject of how to deal with distress, motivated, or so he says, by his colleagues' astonishment at the equanimity with which he dealt with the catastrophe. The treatise falls recognizably into the category of consolation literature, as well as into that of the ancient anticipations of Cognitive Behavioral Therapy (CBT). It thus bears comparison with Cicero and Seneca's *Consolations*, and also with Galen's own surviving treatise on the *Diagnosis and Cure of the Passions of the Soul*.[3] This latter is aimed against a particular Epicurean, and also retails some anecdotes from Galen's life illustrating his own stoicism (with a lower-case 's') in the face of adversity, as well as his attempts to help people deal with their anger issues, which again connects with both ancient and modern concerns (cf. Seneca's and Plutarch's treatises *On Anger*).

The fire, which began at the Temple of Peace and spread rapidly to neighbouring parts of central Rome, destroying a variety of buildings, including a depository in which Galen stored much of his important professional equipment and library,[4] was a shattering event for many people. Galen himself mentions it, and his loss, in a number of places; and he contrasts his own attitude of quiet resignation with the more extreme reactions of others, such as the grammarian Callistus, who died of a fever caused by insomnia brought on by grief at his losses (*Hipp.Epid.* VI, 486,19–24 Pfaff; see Hankinson, 'The man and his

---

referred to as *Freedom from Distress*, which is perhaps a more accurate rendering of the title, although arguably less appropriate to the actual content of the treatise.

3   *Aff.Dig.* V 1–57; its companion piece, *Diagnosis and Cure of the Errors of the Soul* (*Pecc.Dig.*: V 58–103), is also relevant and important, not least because it *is* a separate treatise – errors, failures of the rational part, are to be rigorously distinguished from the irrational passions, or affections (*pathê*). Both are edited in Marquardt,1884, and De Boer, 1937, and translated in Singer, 1997 (revised in Singer, 2014). In general, on a first reference to a text of Galen, I give a full English title, followed by an abbreviation if it is referred to again, followed by a reference to the Kühn edition, followed by references to later, better editions (if any).

4   Among the works he took to be irretrievably lost (wrongly, as it turned out) was his own *On Prognosis*: "I wrote about these prognoses in one book of the same title. But shortly after its publication this book was consumed in the great fire that burnt down the so-called Temple of Peace, along with many other books which were also burnt" (*On Hippocrates' 'Epidemics'* (*Hipp.Epid.*) VI, CMG V 10,2,2, 495,2–12, Pfaff, 1956. Galen also refers to his losses in the fire at *My Own Books* (*Lib.Prop.*) XIX 19, 41, = 143,2–4, 166,1–5 Boudon-Millot, 2007 (*Lib.Prop.* is also edited in Müller, 1891); see Boudon-Millot, 2007, 198 n 2.

work', in Hankinson ed., *The Cambridge Companion to Galen*, 2008, pp. 21–2). This was not the right sort of response at all, and Galen wrote *Ind.* to underscore this fact, and to explain how it was that he managed to avoid such self-destructive excesses, or even lesser versions of them, such as a decline into melancholic apathy.[5]

My main concern here, however, is not with Galen's response to this, or with the advice he gives to those in danger of being so afflicted. Rather I want to explore a possible, and at first sight surprising, connection between Galen's self-expressed attitude in *Peri Alupias* and that of a group of philosophers to whom he is invariably implacably (indeed frequently offensively) hostile: the sceptics, especially Pyrrhonian sceptics; and, to a lesser extent, with another philosophic persuasion with which he has almost as little sympathy: atomism.[6] But let's start by sketching the relevant parts of Galen's text.

1 Avoiding Distress: the Philosophical Examples and Galen's Own Story

Galen begins by drawing attention to some relevant philosophical examples, starting with the story of the founding Cyrenaic Aristippus's indifference to wealth, exemplified by has calm acceptance of the loss of one of his four fields (*Ind.* 41–2, 13,21–14,7 BJP).[7] He draws the following morals:

(i)   Those unsatisfied with moderate means will be insatiably greedy, and as a result always poor (42–3, 14,7–18)

---

5   A curious inconsistency is worth pointing out here: at the beginning of the second part of *Therapeutic Method* (MM X 456–7), which Galen took up again after a lengthy interruption in the 190s, he writes of his own tendency (well known, apparently, to his addressee) to fall into despondency about such matters. On this, and other Galenic inconsistencies, see Vivian Nutton's Introduction to his translation of *Ind.*, in Singer, 2014, 66–8.

6   Attacks on atomism figure at *Nat.Fac.* II 44–51, = 133,16–138,14 Helmreich, 1893 (on magnetism); *Elements according to Hippocrates* I 416–26, = 58,16–68,24 De Lacy, 1996 (on the inadequacy of a physics that denies genuine alteration to account for such obvious phenomena as pain). He is also relentlessly hostile to the atomist denial of teleology; see *Functionality of the Parts, passim* (Helmreich, 1907–9; May, 1968). On Galen's willingness to countenance some Epicurean approaches to psychotherapy, see now, in the context of *Ind.*, Kaufman, D. H., 'Galen on the therapy of distress and the limits of emotional therapy', *Oxford Studies in Ancient Philosophy* 47, 2014, 275–96 (p. 287–9).

7   Elsewhere Galen recounts another well-known story concerning Aristippus; when asked by people on their way to his hometown of Cyrene if he had any message for his relatives, he replied "tell them to acquire only those goods which can survive a shipwreck", i.e. intellectual ones: *Protrepticus* I 8–9, = Boudon, 2002, 90,4–18.

(ii)   Someone who isn't envious of others' wealth will bear any loss, as long as they still have enough left to live (44, 14,18–15,2)

(iii) But if someone loses everything, they will "be justifiably distressed" (45, 15,2–4)

This is a perfect anticipation of Galen's own view. The self-defeating nature of avarice is an ancient commonplace, one often linked with a contempt for the love of monetary gain for its own sake, and the advocacy of true wealth as consisting in satisfaction with a modest provision of necessary and advantageous possessions. Aristotle expresses the idea trenchantly at *Politics* 1.8–9, 1256b26–58a18; pursuit of wealth for its own sake is both pointless, and, since wealth has no natural limit, intrinsically unsatisfiable. Similar views are expressed by Epicureans (Lucretius 3.59 ff.), and others. But the position outlined in (i)–(iii) is not without its problems, primarily in the interpretation of "enough still left to live"; how much is enough? And to live how? Presumably not as a pauper, a beggar, or a day-labourer, a fact suggested by his attitude to the Cynic Crates: it is indeed remarkable that he was satisfied with no possessions, and even more so Diogenes, who didn't even have a proper house[8] (45, 15,4–10). So Galen's own *alupia* is nothing special, since he was left with more than sufficient, presumably for a decently comfortable life (46, 15,10–13).

Still, it is people's greed and insatiability that are responsible for thinking, wrongly, that fortitude in the face of bearable losses remarkable. What really is remarkable is the indifference to complete loss, as supposedly exemplified by Zeno after losing all his possessions in a shipwreck, when he praised fate for reducing his worldly goods to a coat and a Porch (48, 15,18–16,2).[9]

Galen then turns to his own case, saying that it was no harder for him to shrug off his own losses than it was to adopt the same attitude towards his (mis)treatment by the Imperial court, which, or so he says, he had never

---

8   Galen doesn't really think that the Cynics are praiseworthy exemplars of superhuman moral fortitude; rather the succeeding paragraphs suggest that their indifference is extreme, amounting to an unreasonable, undesirable, and unattainable, *apatheia*, of which more below. Elsewhere, he is acerbically hostile, at least to contemporary adherents of the school: *Pecc.Dig.* V 71–2, = 49,1–22 De Boer (1937) – Cynicism "is a quick route, by way of ignorance, to self-regard". However, he does commend Diogenes for his no-nonsense, Johnsonian refutation of philosophical arguments against motion (*Antecedent Causes* ix 116–17), and for relieving his lust by masturbating, rather than seeking out a prostitute (*Affected Parts* VIII 419). On these passages in *Ind.*, see Boudon-Millot et al., 2010, 124–30.

9   Cf. Plutarch, *Tranquillity of the Soul* 467d; the Porch is a reference to the Stoa itself (hence my capitalization of it); it is probably also intended to recall Cynicism, the porch standing in for Diogenes' kennel (the 'cloak' too may be metaphorical). Zeno was supposedly a pupil of Crates (DL 7.1–5); Diogenes retails several different versions of the shipwreck story (DL 7.5), one of which seems to make it merely metaphorical: see Boudon-Millot et al., 2010, 131.

aspired to be part of in any case (49–50a, 16,3–10).[10] His experience of living in constant apprehension of being unjustly exiled to a desert island (or worse) as a result of slander and the capricious and tyrannical, not to say sociopathic, temperament of the emperor helped inure him against possible loss (54–6, 18,1–13). It was also responsible for his 'magnanimity' when loss, the extent of which he emphasizes in 50b (16,10–18), finally came. He attributes his fortitude not only to this experience of living in unsettled and unpredictable times (he recommends visualizing and preparing for the worst that might happen to you as a way of minimizing the impact of the blows of fate: 56, 18,13–16),[11] but also, characteristically, to his own character and upbringing, particularly to the influence and example of his revered father (57–62, 18,17–20,2).[12]

Here, as elsewhere, the legacy of Galen's father is multifaceted. He is an exemplar not just of moral excellence, but also of the *engagé* life: "he never praised those who despise such [sc. disreputable] pleasures, and who are simply satisfied that their soul is never pained or distressed, proclaiming that the good was in its nature something bigger and better than this" (62, 19,19–20,2). Here too Galen parts company with some of his philosophical contemporaries, notably the Epicureans, but to some extent also the Stoics (not to mention the Cynics). An untroubled life, *ataraxia*, the common goal of a variety of Hellenistic schools, including (but only up to a point, as we shall see) the Pyrrhonists, is sometimes equated with a sort of quietistic withdrawal from the world. This is not something Galen, as a busy and committed professional, has any time for, any more than he has for the unrealizable (indeed inhumane) goal of *apatheia*, lack of affection (or feeling) of any kind.

---

10   The reference seems to be to some slight or slights he underwent during the reign of Commodus, about whom he is generally tight-lipped (although he opens up a little in what follows: 54–7, 18,1–20); elsewhere he emphasizes his reluctance to enter imperial service even under the benign Marcus: *Lib.Prop.* XIX 17–19, = 141,17–142,25 Boudon-Millot, as well as the dangers of being too publicly successful (*Praen.* XIV 599–605, = *CMG* V 8,1, 68,3–74,13 Nutton); Quintus, "the best doctor of his time", was forced into exile from Rome on trumped-up charges by jealous inferior practitioners. See Boudon-Millot et al., 2010, 132–3. The title of a lost text he describes as containing autobiographical material is relevant: *On Slander: Lib.Prop.* XIX 46, = 170,8 Boudon-Millot.

11   On visualization of unpleasant possibilities as a means of drawing their sting, see *The Doctrines of Hippocrates and Plato* (*PHP*) V 417–8, = 282,7–16 De Lacy, 1978, on Posidonius; Kaufman, D. H., 'Galen on the therapy of distress and the limits of emotional therapy', 2014, pp. 281–3, offers a good discussion of this aspect of Galen's account, in the course of stressing the eclecticism of Galen's general approach. He makes no mention of the sceptics, however.

12   Cf. *Aff.Dig.* V 40–3; for more on human insatiability and its malign effects, see ib. 45–8.

2   Ataraxia and Its Antecedents: the Atomists

Let us turn, then, to consider the ideal of *ataraxia*, freedom from disturbance, or tranquillity.[13] As David Sedley ('The motivation of Greek skepticism', in Burnyeat, 1983, 9–29) notes, it is common property to the major Hellenistic schools, Stoic, Epicurean and Sceptic, even if rejected by Peripatetics and Platonists. As such it is supposed to be the appropriate way of understanding *eudaimonia*, happiness or human flourishing, which everybody (at least verbally: see Sextus, *PH* 3.175; *M* 11.35–6), following Aristotle, agrees to be the fundamental human goal, even if they differ as to what it consists in. It amounts, crudely, to the claim that we do best when we are undisturbed by anything, or at least anything which we are capable of controlling, including our emotional, affective reactions to things. The last two riders indicate just how differently the notion may be construed.

The ideal of the undisturbed life had a long philosophical history, stretching back at least to Democritus, who advocated *athambia*, freedom from wonderment: Fr. 68 B 4 DK;[14] as well as the presumably equivalent *euthumia* (B 191).[15] The term *ataraxia* itself was attributed to him, and while that is probably an anachronism,[16] what matters is not the terminology but the attitude and ideal it indicates. In Democritus's case, this seems to amount to an avoidance of excessive states of emotion, indeed of sensations in general. His attitude to sex was at best equivocal, indeed tending towards the disapprovingly prudish, if not without a certain wit: male orgasm "is a mild form of madness – for a man rushes out of a man" (B 32), while the pleasure of sex is not really different from that derived from scratching oneself (B 127). Of the large number of fragments and testimonia attributed to Democritus concerning the good life, pleasure, duty, and so on, many are of disputed authenticity; but the overall picture is clear enough. For Democritus, excessive preoccupation with physical pleasure is self-defeating:

---

13   The literature on the issue is large; see classically, on Timon Fr. 842 (68 Diels, 1901), Burnyeat, M. F., 'Tranquillity without a stop: Timon Frag. 68' *The Classical Quarterly*, 30.1., 1980, 86–93; Striker, G., 'Ataraxia: happiness as tranquillity', *The Monist* 73.1, Hellenistic Ethics, 1990, 97–110; and in general Hankinson, R. J., *The Sceptics*, 1995, chs. 17–18.
14   Presocratic Fragments are referred to, standardly, by way of Diels/Kranz, 1952.
15   Cf. Cicero, *Fin.* 5.87: "he calls the highest good *euthumia* and also frequently *athambia*, that is, a mind free from terror. But though what he says is all very fine, it is still not very polished, for he has little to say, and that not very articulately, about virtue".
16   On the terminological issues, see Striker, G., 'Ataraxia: happiness as tranquillity', *The Monist* 73.1, Hellenistic Ethics, 1990, 97–110 (p. 97–8).

> All those who get pleasure from their bellies, exceeding the measure in food, drink and sex, find the pleasures slight and short-lived ... But the pains are many. For they always desire the same things, and when they obtain what they desire, the pleasure swiftly goes, and they find nothing but a brief joy, and the desire for such pleasures again. (B 235)

Unrestrained desire brings misery, and also injustice, as men are driven to seek to acquire the goods of others, as well as ruining their own health (B 219–24); justice is something that should be welcomed for its own sake (B 62), and its "glory is confidence of judgement and imperturbability" (B 215).

None the less, properly construed as moderate contentment, pleasure is indeed the end: "Joy and the absence of joy are the boundaries of advantage and disadvantage" (B 4, 188); where people go wrong is in their understanding of what pleasure really is. Anticipating Epicurus' distinction between static and kinetic pleasure, "He calls happiness contentment, well-being, harmony, orderliness and tranquillity. It is constituted by distinguishing and discriminating among pleasures" (Stobaeus, 2.7.31). A proper education should involve instilling, by habituation and persuasion, a desire for healthy moderation and avoidance of excess (B 178–83). The desired way of living "with as much contentment and as little distress as possible ... will come about if he does not take his pleasure in mortal things" (B 189), which is another way of exalting the claims of the soul over those of the body (cf. e.g. B 36–7). A recurring theme is satisfaction with what one has. "The man of sound judgement is not distressed by what he does not possess, but rejoices in what he does" (B 231). On the other hand 'fools' who always want more are never satisfied, and terrified of death: "Fools get no pleasure in the whole of their lives" (B 204; cf. 197–206); yet "with self-sufficiency in upbringing, the night is never long" (B 209).

I have outlined Democritus's position at some length because, initial impressions aside, it is not one of unalloyed asceticism. Just as Epicurus was to think that pleasure was the end, and that pleasure was primarily physical (Cicero, *Tusc.* 3.41, = 21L Long and Sedley, 1987 ['LS']; below, 163), and that no pleasure was wrong *per se*, but only unchoiceworthy if it entailed countervailing pains (*Men.* 127–32, = 21 B LS), Democritus, for all his apparent distaste for the pursuit (the excessive pursuit) of some pleasures, does not simply advocate trying to get rid of all desire. Desire is a necessary part of human existence, but it requires careful moderation if it is not to be allowed to take over and ruin a life. Balance is everything, as the perennial truism has it; but properly interpreted it does not entail asceticism and the avoidance of all indulgence.[17]

---

17   Compare B 229: "thrift and hunger are good – but so too on occasion is extravagance; it
      is the mark of a good man to recognize the occasion"; and B 230: "A life without a feast

The key is self-mastery: "Men pray to the gods for health, not knowing that they how the power to attain it within themselves; lacking self-control, they act contrary to it, and sacrifice health to their desires" (B 234; cf. B 69–74). This is underlined by fragment 191:

> Men gain contentment from moderation in joy and a measured life ... Thus you must set your judgement on the possible and be satisfied with what you have, giving little thought to those who are envied or admired ... Consider those who are badly off, so that what you have ... may seem great and enviable and so that you may no longer suffer in your soul by desiring more ... If you hold fast to this judgement, you will live in greater contentment and drive away those not inconsiderable plagues of life, jealousy, envy and malice.
>
>   STOBAEUS, 3.1.210; cf. B 219–24 on the destructiveness of avarice; B 88 on the pains of envy

Money itself is not itself evil, although acquiring it unjustly is "the worst of all things" (B 78); in fact, "when used with thought promotes generosity and charity" (B 282). Indeed, "If you do not desire a great deal, a little will seem a great deal to you; for a small appetite makes poverty as powerful as wealth" (B 284). Properly considered, "Poverty and wealth are names for want and satisfaction, so that one who is in want is not wealthy, while one who is not in want is not poor" (B 283). Resting content with "moderate goods", and being aware of and prepared for life's inevitable disappointments, is critical (B 285–6; cf. 3, 42, 46, 58, 287–92), as is the lack of distress, envy, at what one does not own (B 231, above). Finally, two remarks about courage: "A courageous man not only conquers his enemies, but also ... his pleasures" (B 214); and perhaps most significantly for our purposes: "Courage makes disasters small" (B 213). Many of these attitudes will find their echoes in Galen's own approach to distress.

Epicurus adopts a very similar position, albeit one given a greater theoretical density by his explicit distinction between static and kinetic pleasures, and his elevation of the former at the expense of the latter: all real and enduring pleasure is the static enjoyment of the absence of pain (*Sovereign Maxims* [*KD*] 3, = 21C LS). Equally important is his distinction between desires which are natural and necessary (sc. for the preservation of one's life), natural but unnecessary (fine dining, and certain kinds of sex, perhaps all sex),[18] and 'empty' pleasures,

---

is a long road without an inn" (cf. B 232–3); note also B 271: "if a woman is loved, then no blame attaches to lust".

18   "You say that the movement of your flesh is too inclined to sex; but as long as you do not break the laws or disturb proper and established conventions or distress any of your

which are neither (such as the desire for crowns or honorific statues: sch. to *KD* 29, = 21I LS). The latter are empty because they rest on the mistaken opinion that not satisfying them will cause pain (*KD* 30, = 21E LS). His hedonism, then, is very much in the restrained, Democritean mould: "When we say that pleasure is the end, we do not mean the pleasures of the dissipated[19] ... but freedom from pain in the body and disturbance in the soul" (*Letter to Menoeceus* 132, = 21B(5) LS). Even so, he says, "I cannot conceive of anything as good if I remove the pleasures perceived by taste, and sex, and listening to music, and the pleasant motions felt by the eyes through beautiful sights"; but this is because mental delight consists in remembering and anticipating them, rather than necessarily experiencing them (Cicero, *Tusculan Disputations* 3.41, = 21L(1) LS).

Still, mental pleasures outweigh physical ones, even though they are dependent upon them. The wise man will be comforted in painful circumstances, and his pain thereby alleviated, by reflecting on past pleasures and anticipating future ones; and this what it is to be untroubled. Epicurus himself allegedly exemplified this attitude on his death-bed: "Strangury and dysentery had set in, with all the extreme intensity of which they are capable; but the joy in my soul at the memory of our past discussions was enough to outweigh all of this" (DL 10.22, = 24D LS). Perhaps most importantly from our point of view, "*ataraxia* and *alupia* are static pleasures": DL 10.136, = 21R LS.

So Epicurus's hedonism is, paradoxically, ascetic – indeed, the central claim of his death-bed letter (which is of extremely doubtful authenticity) may seem as extravagantly implausible as the notorious contention that the wise man can remain untroubled even on the rack (DL 10.118). Even so, a weaker and hence more plausible version of the thought is readily constructible, consistently with another unimpeachably genuine feature of Epicureanism, namely the idea that error (typically regarding perceptual judgements, but the idea is readily extendible) involves *prosdoxazomena*, unfounded additional beliefs (this term will become important later on: §5). Physical pain may well in certain cases, such as Epicurus's death, be unavoidable; but it can be mitigated by cultivating certain mental attitudes, and made worse by other suppositions, paradigmatically the idea that death is in itself something to be feared.[20] How

---

neighbours or ravage your body or squander the necessities of life, act in any way you like. But it is impossible not to be constricted by any of these. For sex is never advantageous, and one should be pleased if it does no harm". *Vatican Sayings* [VS] 51, = 21 G LS.

19   Among which Epicurus singles out 'the enjoyment of women, small boys, and fish'.

20   Fear of death is, for Epicureans, the most pernicious and destructive of all irrational fears; the centrality of the attempt to eradicate it is exemplified by the famous slogan "Death is nothing to us": *Letter to Menoeceus* [*Men.*] 124, = 24A(1)–(4) LS; cf. Lucretius 3.830 ff. (= 24E LS).

plausible that might be is another (still much-controverted)[21] issue; but however that may be, the Epicurean prescription does not amount to recommending complete freedom from affective states, or *apatheia*. Painful and damaging mental conditions can be mitigated, but not eradicated. Even so, freedom from distress, *alupia*, is at least something to be aimed at, and secured insofar as that is possible; and is clearly related, as DL 10.136 shows, to the fundamental goal of tranquillity itself.

3   Ataraxia and Its Antecedents: Pyrrho and the Sceptics

There are important points of contact between atomism and scepticism, both genetic and (to some extent) doctrinal[22] (insofar as it makes sense to speak of sceptical 'doctrine': *PH* 1.13–17; cf. 21–4).[23] Anaxarchus, a pupil of the atomist Metrodorus, is a transitional figure, who anticipates some standard sceptical contentions regarding the veridicality of perception.[24] More important from our point of view is the following: "Anaxarchus was called *ho eudaimonikos* (the happy one) because of the *apatheia* and contentment of his life; he was able to induce moderation in the easiest possible way" (DL 9.60, = 1E LS). His *apatheia*, however, was apparently of a superhuman nature; while being beaten to death in a large mortar at the behest of an enraged tyrant, he is said to have remarked: "You may pound the envelope containing Anaxarchus, but not Anaxarchus himself" (DL 9.58). Such heroic *apatheia* anticipates rather the attitude later attributed to the Stoics, and implicitly characterized by Galen as being beyond the capacity of mere humankind. Another, no doubt equally apocryphal, story links him directly with Pyrrho, the eponymous founder of the sceptical way (who was said to have been his pupil: DL 9.61, = 1A(1) LS). One day, as philosophers will, Pyrrho stumbled abstractedly into a dungheap, and Anaxarchus passed by without helping him out; while others present

21   For an influential modern discussion, see Nagel, T., 'Death', *Nous* 4.1, 1970, 73–80; repr. in Nagel, 1979, *Mortal Questions*, Cambridge, CUP, 1979, 1–10.

22   The collection of individual sceptical essays against the practitioners of the various liberal arts (*M* 1–6) contains some arguments explicitly attributed to the Epicureans, against the arts' utility; see Hankinson, R. J., *The Sceptics*, 1995, ch 15; Barnes, J. 'Scepticism and the arts', in R.J.Hankinson (ed.), *Method, Medicine and Metaphysics: Apeiron* 21.2, Supp. Vol. 19 (Edmonton, Alberta: Academic Printing and Publishing), 1988, 53–77.

23   On this issue, see Hankinson, R. J., *The Sceptics*, 1995, ch 17.

24   On Anaxarchus's epistemology, see now Burnyeat, '"All the world's a stage-painting": scenery, optics, and Greek epistemology', *Oxford Studies in Ancient Philosophy* 52, 2017, 33–7.

condemned him for failing to render assistance, Pyrrho himself praised him for his indifference, *adiaphoria* (DL 9.63).

As for Pyrrho himself, Timon, his satirical amanuensis, made him into a paradigm of *ataraxia* (2B–D LS): "This, Pyrrho, my heart yearns to hear: how can you, human though you are, act most easily and calmly, never taking thought and consistently undisturbed (*atarachos*)?" (DL 9.65, = Fr 841, = 2D LD). He is said to have demonstrated his *adiaphoria* by washing pigs (however that was supposed to work: see below, §7), and to have endured surgery "without so much as a frown" (DL 9.66). In the most important testimonium to his philosophical 'position', albeit one that survives only at fourth hand and is multiply controversial, Timon (according to Aristocles, *ap* Eusebius 18,18,1–5, = 1F LS) says that Pyrrho held that being 'unopinionated', 'uncommitted', and 'unswayed' (*adoxastoi, aklineis, akradantoi*) leads first to *aphasia*,[25] and thence to *ataraxia*. Even so, Pyrrho's version of *ataraxia* strays close to a more severe *apatheia*; and Cicero, pairing Pyrrho with the extreme Stoic Aristo, as he often does (cf. 2G–H LS), explicitly describes it as such (*Academica*, 2.130, = 2F LS; cf. *Fin.* 3.11–12), in contrast with Aristo's mere *adiaphoria*.[26]

It is worth emphasizing at this point that *apatheia* comes in different forms, partly corresponding to the varying semantic range of the root-term *pathos*. Galen himself takes care to distinguish the latter's various senses in order to guard against potential fallacies of ambiguity, and to clarify its relation with the various meanings of *energeia* (PHP V 506–13, = 360,15–366,30 De Lacy). Thus a *pathos* may simply be something that happens to something (as opposed to something it does); but it may also be an abnormal affection of something, something in some sense contrary to its nature. In fact:

> In this way both anger and desire will be called both *pathê* and *energeiai*; for since they are certain immoderate and unnatural motions of the soul's intrinsic powers, they are *energeiai* of those powers, because the powers have their motions from themselves; but because they are *immoderate* motions, they are *pathê*. And these motions of the whole soul of the two powers that are themselves set in motion are contrary to nature. This is

---

25   Not literally speechlessness, but the refusal to make dogmatic assertions, positive or negative; the whole fragment is the subject of much dispute, not least as to the appropriate reading of the Greek; see Hankinson, R. J., *The Sceptics*, 1995, 59–64.

26   Here not in the sense of being indifferent to one's circumstances, but rather in supposing that all the things that Stoics considered neither actually good (virtue) nor actually bad (vice), such as health, were not merely technically 'indifferent', but not even the object of rational preference (or dispreference), as the orthodox view, rather paradoxically, held: see 58 A–J LS, esp. (for Aristo) F, G and I.

> so for the irrational powers because of their lack of measure, and for the
> whole soul because we say that it is in accordance with nature for our life
> to be governed by the rational part, not by the motions of the affective
> (*pathêtikos*) part.
>
>   *PHP* V 511–12, = 364,31–366,4 De Lacy

All of this is, obviously enough, Platonic in inspiration (it immediately follows a discussion of the charioteer image of the *Phaedrus*), and as such is
part and parcel of Galen's anti-Chrysippean project of a large part of *PHP*
(effectively the bulk of Books II–VI). This need concern us only insofar as it
is relevant to Galen's understanding of the proper roles of emotion and desire in the well-ordered human soul (and consequently the well-managed
human life). Emotions and desires can get out of hand, and usurp the prop-
erly-governing role of reason; and they are intrinsically non-rational. But for
all that, if properly constrained by reason, they need not render the animal
itself irrational (for Galen's detailed, if polemical, examination of the senses
of *alogos*, see *PHP* V 370–2, 383–5, = 242,12–244,9, 252,20–254,12 De Lacy).
Indeed, so constrained, they are essential components of the overall performance of the complex economy of parts and functions that is the human
soul.

   Here Galen's account leans towards the Peripatetic; it is central to the
Aristotelian tradition that anger (for example), provided that it meets the appropriate criteria of appropriateness, is not only unavoidable: it is actually a
good thing (*NE* 4.5, 1125b27–26b10, esp. 1125b31–26a2). It is not clear whether
Galen would actually endorse this position – certainly he wants to restrict the
terms for anger (*orgê*, etc.) to the excessive, blameworthy (indeed from his
perspective pathological: *Aff.Dig.* V 7–8) conditions. Still, he praises moderation, while admitting that "No-one is free from the *pathê* or errors, not even
the person with best natural endowments, brought up to the best of practices.
Always there will be some failures, especially when one is young" (*Aff.Dig.* V
14). Becoming as good as humanly possible, which in this context means ridding oneself as far as is possible of the tendency of being swayed by irrational
emotions, is a lifelong project (14–16). After much practice, "one may eventually reach the goal of getting only slightly angry even over the greatest matters"
(17), which implies that the goal is that of eliminating all angry impulses, but
only as far as is humanly possible. This is backed up in what follows (17–27):
one must be constantly aware of the ugliness and bestiality of anger indulged,
and keep one's eyes constantly on the prize of freedom from enslavement to
unreason: "If you act in this manner, you may succeed in taming and soften-
ing the irrational power of the spirited part of your soul" (26–7). The Platonic
language is deliberate and unmistakable:

Is not anger a sickness of the soul? Or do you deny the wisdom of the ancients who gave the name of "affections of the soul" to the following five:
distress, rage, anger, desire and fear? The following seems to me to be the
best course of action for one who wants to rid himself as far as possible
of these affections.

   Aff.Dig. V 24, = 17,7–12 De Boer

Desire figures here simply among the irrational affections. Galen thus elides
the Platonic distinction between the spirited and the desiderative (although
later he re-introduces it: 27–34); he is operating, at least provisionally, with a
straightforward distinction between the rational and the non-rational, which
again might be owed to Aristotle (*Nicomachean Ethics* [*NE*]1.13, 1102a16–
1103a10), although Aristotle too subdivides the irrational part of the soul.

   So where does this leave Galen's confrontation with Stoicism? That is an extremely complex question, and one whose details lie beyond the remit of this
study; but ultimately, perhaps, there may be less to the dispute than initially
meets the eye. Galen does indeed think that the outright elimination of the
pathê, even the destructive ones, is not something which is humanly possible;
but then Stoic total *apatheia* is something only achievable by the sage, and
notoriously they were in extremely short supply. Quite a lot also turns on the
precise nature of the Stoics' *eupatheiai*, the desirable counterparts of (at least
some) of the normal human affections (DL 7.115, = 65F LS): joy (*chara*), corresponding to pleasure, in being "a well-reasoned swelling", caution (*eulabeia*:
"a well-reasoned contraction") to fear, and wish (*boulêsis*) to desire. There is no
eupathetic counterpart to *lupê*, perhaps because it is (or is at least consequent
upon) a false judgement concerning a present evil, and there can be no corresponding true judgement for the sage, since for the Stoics true happiness is always within one's grasp. So while the Stoic Sage may be no more than an ideal,
this is exactly the sort of high-minded fantasy which Galen has no time for.

4   Galen and Scepticism

So let us turn at last to Scepticism. In a well-known passage, Galen tells us that,
as a young student of logic, he was so disheartened with the apparently undecidable and interminable (as well as practically useless) disputes among the
representatives of the schools, that he might have succumbed to a Pyrrhonian
despair concerning the attainability of truth, had he not reflected on the un-
assailable certainty of mathematical demonstration (*Lib.Prop.* XIX 39–40,
= 164,2–165,2 Boudon-Millot). He often makes little distinction between the
Pyrrhonian and Academic forms of skepticism in the course of his polemics,

lumping them both together as equally hopeless. Both schools, for example, reject the possibility of distinguishing between veridical perception and delusion:

> There are some things which we think we see, hear, or in general perceive, such as in dreams or delusions, while there are other things which we not only think we see, or in general perceive, but actually do so. In the case of the second class everybody, other than the Academics and Pyrrhonists, thinks that they have arrived at secure knowledge, while they consider everything of which the soul produces images while asleep or delirious to be false.
>
> *The Best Method of Teach.* (*Opt.Doct.*) I 42, = 94,14–18 Barigazzi, 1991

And, in the case of ethical argument,

> Academics and Pyrrhonists, who do not accept that we have scientific demonstration of the matters at issue, believe that any assent is hasty, and may also be false.
>
> *Pecc.Dig.* V 60, = 42,16–18 De Boer

Of course, it is not just in these matters where they (perhaps reasonably) reject the possibility of *apodeixis epistêmonikê*; they do so quite generally. But elsewhere Galen distinguishes between the sceptical schools, and while frequently hostile to what he takes to be Academic excesses (such as Carneades' alleged rejection of the Euclidian equality axiom (cn 1): *Opt.Doct.* I 45, = 96,20–98,9 Barigazzi),[27] none the less he believes that the dispute between Academics and others regarding epistemological justification is largely verbal:

---

27   Galen is sarcastically dismissive of this; reports of this Carneadean 'refutation' as well as "of many others which are evidently and persuasively valid" are attributed to 'his own pupils', pre-eminent among whom was his amanuensis Clitomachus (Carneades, in good Socratic – and subsequently sceptic – tradition left nothing in writing himself). This was almost certainly discussed in Galen's lost *Clitomachus and his Refutations of Demonstration* (*Lib.Prop.* XIX 44, = 168,8–9 Boudon-Millot). This seems the most likely translation of the title; Boudon-Millot renders it 'Sur Clitomaque et ses solutions de la démonstration', which hints at a general 'proof against proof', and could be right; Morison (2008, 67) translates 'On Clitomachus and his solutions to demonstrations', which would require a (very minor) emendation, and suggests a more piecemeal approach. Certainly the denial of the axiomatic status of cn. 1 hints at a general argument against the possibility of discovering unimpeachable axioms, freestanding, certain and necessarily-true fundamental premises; and if there are no such things (or we can't recognize them) then there are no demonstrations (at least none that we can recognize).

Discrimination between these things[28] is reduced to an impression (*phantasia*) which, as the philosophers from the New Academy say, is not only 'persuasive' (*pithanê*), but 'tested' (*periôdeumenê*) and 'unshaken' (*aperispastos*); or which as Chrysippus and his followers put it is apprehensive (*kataleptikê*); or as all men believe in common, it is reduced to evident (*enargês*) perception (*aisthêsis*) and intellection (*noêsis*). These expressions are thought to differ in meaning from one another, but if one examines them more carefully they have the same import; just as, indeed, when someone says that they begin from common notions (*koinai ennoiai*), and sets them up as the primary criterion of all things which is trustworthy in itself (*ex heautou piston*). That the first criterion must be trustworthy without proof is admitted by everyone, although not everyone supposes that it must be natural and common to all men.

> *PHP* V 778, = 586,16–25 De Lacy

I have assessed the plausibility of this claim elsewhere.[29] I think there is something to it; but that need not detain us. What matters is that Galen never shows any such respect, grudging as it might be, to Pyrrhonists, at least when they are considered on their own. Mostly they simply serve as suitable targets for insult. The following is typical:

If you are looking for logical demonstrations in the area of perceptible fact, perhaps you would like to embark on an investigation of snow. Should we think it white (following the way it appears to all men), or not white (following the 'proof' of Anaxagoras)?[30] We could make similar inquiries on the subject of pitch, ravens, or indeed anything else ... Swans should not said to be white without first being subjected to logical investigation ... At this point, we may realize we are faced with a Pyrrhonian *aporia*; or rather with a complete load of bollocks.

> *Mixtures* I 589, = 50,25–51,10 Helmreich, 1904; trans. after – quite a long way after – Singer, 1997

Aporia is indeed a Pyrrhonian technical term (drawn ultimately of course from Plato's Socrates); an *impasse* from which there is no exit, the result of

---

28   I.e. between the plausible but false and the true, and cases where plausible and implausible are very similar and hard to distinguish: *PHP* V 777–8, = 586,9–16 De Lacy.

29   Hankinson, R. J., 'A purely verbal dispute? Galen on Stoic and Academic epistemology', in A.-J.Voelke (ed.) *Le Stoïcisme: Revue internationale de philosophie* 45.3, 1992, 267–300.

30   Reported at *PH* 1.33 (= 59 A 97): "snow is frozen water and water is black; so snow is black" (or perhaps rather 'dark'); cf. Cicero, *Acad.* 2.100.

endemic, undecidable dispute: *PH* 1.26, 165. For Galen, while there are such hopeless cases (in the useless parts of logical theory, but also in 'speculative philosophy': issues such as the eternity of the world, the essence of the divine or of the soul, the existence of an extra-mundane void),[31] resolution of them is of no practical importance. In the practical cases, we have 'natural criteria' (senses and reason),[32] by the practice and refinement of which we can come to legitimate and grounded understanding of the world and its functioning. It is simply a gross, indeed jejune, error to look for demonstration in matters of perceptual clarity (and intellectual clarity as well, such as in the case of the axioms of equality).

Galen's animus against what he takes to be pointless Pyrrhonian resistance to the obvious is particularly apparent in his dismissive language; on numerous occasions he refers to *agroikoi Purrhôneioi*, peasant Pyrrhonists, for instance at *Differences of Pulses* VIII 711; *Blood in the Arteries* IV 727; and *Distinctions of Pulses (Dig.Puls.)* VIII 780–3. In the latter passage, Galen allows that you can, if you are so inclined, adopt an extreme phenomenalist language. Instead of saying things like "excessive rain caused the river to rise in flood and wash away the bridge", you may talk of 'the apparent rain', 'the seeming river', 'the ostensible flood'. and so on; but this doesn't (or shouldn't) make any practical difference whatsoever to the way you behave. Any individual of any degree of sanity will still take rapid and unsceptical evasive action.[33] This is pointedly directed towards Pyrrhonists like Sextus, who insists that the Pyrrhonian is perfectly capable of living (indeed of practising an art), by following the 'criterion' of the appearances (*PH* 1.21–4) It is simply idle and disingenuous, Galen thinks, not to take evident perceptual facts as being true.[34] When he asks the Peripatetic Alexander of Damascus to adjudicate his demonstration of the nerves responsible for vocalization by vivisectional experiments on pigs and goats, and

---

31 See e.g. *PHP* V 766, 779–82, = 576,27–578,2, 588,7–590,11 de Lacy; *Prop.Plac* 2, 56,12–24; 3, 58,22–60,6 Nutton; *Pecc.Dig.* V 67, = 52,13–18 Marquardt; see Hankinson, 'Epistemology', in Hankinson ed., *The Cambridge Companion to Galen*, 2008, 178–80; *eiusd.* 'Philosophy of nature', in Hankinson ed., *The Cambridge Companion to Galen*, 2008, 233–6.

32 On the natural criteria, see *Opt.Doct.* I 48–9, = 102,10–104,2 Barigazzi. 1991.

33 On this passage, see Hankinson, R. J., 'A purely verbal dispute? Galen on Stoic and Academic epistemology', in A.-J.Voelke (ed.) *Le Stoïcisme: Revue internationale de philosophie* 45.3, 1992, 267–300. Relevant here are the ancient characterizations of Pyrrho as being so indifferent to possible physical suffering that his associates had to prevent him from walking over cliffs and in front of oncoming traffic, as we'll as into dungheaps; but they are canards, as Aenesidemus said (DL 9.62, = 1A LS).

34 He is following a tradition here: see Hankinson, 1997; on his refutation of scepticism, Hankinson, 'Epistemology', in Hankinson ed., *The Cambridge Companion to Galen*, 2008, 162–5; see also *SMT* XI 462.

Alexander inquires whether we are supposed to rely on the evidence of our senses, Galen takes characteristic umbrage and walks out, saying that there is no point continuing the discussion if we are to be reduced to such a peasant Pyrrhonism as to fail to credit the clear evidence of the senses (*Prognosis* XIV 626–8, = 96,4–98,8 Nutton, 1979).

So Galen is unequivocally hostile to Pyrrhonian scepticism, and not much friendlier to the Academic variety. At first sight, then, it might seem absurdly quixotic to suggest any serious point of contact between them.

5   Tranquillity and Moderation in Affection

Sceptics – like many other Hellenistic philosophers – aimed (in a sense) at *ataraxia*. Pyrrho, allegedly, managed it in a pretty heroic fashion. However, his later eponymous followers moderated (in a very real sense) this position:

> We do not think that the sceptic is in every respect untroubled (*aochlê-tos*); rather he is distressed by what is forced upon him, for we concede that he is sometimes cold and thirsty, and is affected by things of this sort. But whereas in these cases ordinary people are afflicted by two conditions, namely by the affections themselves and by the belief that these conditions are by nature evil, the sceptic, by doing away with the additional belief (*prosdoxazomenon*) that each of these things is evil in its actual nature, gets off more moderately in these cases as well. For this reason, then, we say that tranquillity (*ataraxia*) is the end in matters of opinion, and moderation in affection (*metriopatheia*) in the case of things forced upon us.
>
> SEXTUS, *PH* I 29–30

The "things forced upon us" are the unavoidable sources of distress that any human life entails, the thousand natural shocks that flesh is heir to. This represents an obvious, and self-conscious, retreat from the pretence of heroic detachment from the travails of the physical which we have seen characterizing a variety of otherwise quite distinct earlier philosophies. Towards the end of *Outlines*, Sextus sums up his sceptical attitude to ethics. The sceptic

> Suspends judgement as to the existence of anything good or bad by nature, or generally which should or should not be done, and in this way distances himself from dogmatic precipitancy and follows the dictates of ordinary life (*hê biôtikê têrêsis*). Because of this he remains unaffected

(*apathês*) in matters of opinion, while in the case of things forced upon him his affections are moderate (*metriopathei*). Being human, he is affected perceptibly (*aisthêtikôs paschei*); but since he does not also believe in addition (*prosdoxazôn*) that what he is affected by is bad by nature, his affections are moderate. For the additional belief that something is actually bad is worse than the suffering itself, just as sometimes those undergoing surgery or something similar put up with it, while those observing it faint away because of their belief that what is happening is appalling.

PH 3.235–6

That latter claim has not commanded universal assent, at least in the stark form in which it is put here; but there is surely something to it. My extreme cowardice makes the anticipation of a visit to the dentist deeply distressing (perhaps not actually as distressing as the visit itself, but at the very least a supplementary source of pain); to the extent I could rid myself of that, no doubt my life would be more tranquil, and as such preferable. But more important is the nature of the "things forced upon" us. There are certain things we can't avoid experiencing, and some of those experiences are unpleasant, some of them extremely so. Philosophy, as Shakespeare's Leonato so rightly said in my epigraph, can't do anything about that. In other words, in Sextus's mature scepticism, the pretence of heroic philosophical indifference has been explicitly abandoned. The example of the surgical operation is pointed, given that Pyrrho supposedly underwent surgery with total equanimity (DL 9.66). But as Sextus says at the end of his programmatic prologue, "We do not think that the sceptic is in every way untroubled; we do say he is troubled by what is forced upon him; for we allow that he is sometimes cold and thirsty and is affected by things of that sort" (*PH* 1.29).

Sextus expands on what he has in mind in his longer treatment of ethics in *M* 11. He again makes the distinction between affections induced by belief, and those forced by necessity. The general injunction to total suspension of judgement only applies to matters of judgement: "In the case of sensory and non-rational judgements, one yields" (148); you can't reason your way out of being troubled by hunger and thirst (149). But for all that, the sceptic is better able to bear distress in presence of the inevitable (150). The unavoidable pains are "not excessively disturbing"; serious pain is not long-lasting (153–5); the *tarachê* which disturbs the sceptic is moderate and not so fearful (155). We are not responsible for unavoidable pains: nature is (156–7). But the additional belief that this is bad by nature, or in itself, is up to us and is the cause of further suffering. Someone who suspends judgement about all things dependent on belief reaps the fullest well-being, and when disturbed by involuntary and non-rational movements, he is affected only moderately (*metriopathôs*); we are not sprung from oak and rock, after all (158–61).[35]

The invocation – and recommendation – of *metriopatheia* has something of a history. It is attributed to the early Platonist Crantor, where the context seems to be that of putting up with physical ailments. According to Chrysippus, the *theôrêtikos* will be *apathês*, while the *spoudaios* will be *metriopathês*. Philo of Alexandria uses the term in the context of Moses and Aaron. There are five occurrences in Plutarch, two of them in the *Consolation to Apollonius* 102cd, where Plutarch stresses that it is normal to feel distress at the death of a son; in fact not to do so would be harsh and callous, a case of fundamentally inhuman *apatheia*: for "*metriopatheia* of grief is not to be censured".[36] Congruently, Alcinous (*Handbook* 30.5) contends that it is not *metriopathês* to feel no grief at all at the death of, or at violence done towards, one's parents, but rather *apathês*, which is clearly here an unreasonable response.[37] *Metriopatheia* is also contrasted with *apatheia* in Clement; while Diogenes says that for Aristotle the wise man not *apathês* but *metriopathês* (DL 5.31); and this is surely right (for Aristotle). Finally Iamblichus, in his *Life of Pythagoras* 27.131, says that his hero cultivated *metriopatheia*. The general tendency among such sources is unmistakable. Not all experience of *pathê*, and specifically of distress, should be avoided, even if such avoidance were humanly possible, which it isn't.

6   Galen and Metriopatheia

Galen himself never deploys the actually terminology of *metriopatheia*; but he is, for all that, clearly in the camp of the moderately affected:

---

35   The Epicurean echoes in all of this are unmistakable: cf. *KD* 4, 33, 59 (= 21C, G LS), *Men.* 133 (= 20A LS).

36   See also *adv Col.* 1119c, where Plutarch attacks Stilpo, a man known among other things and in other contexts for *metriopatheia*. In *Restraining Anger* 458c, he recalls the advice given to Philip of Macedon when attacking Olynthus not to exact too harsh a retribution from the city, since restraint is the way of mildness, pity and *metriopatheia*. These latter cases are not of course technical; indeed they recall several similar usages in Appian concerning Philip's more famous son. But they are significant in the general context of the disapproval of actions performed in the grip of rage, and the corresponding exaltation of the contrasting mildness of disposition.

37   See Dillon, J. M., *Alcinous. The Handbook of Platonism*, 1993, 188; *eiusd.*, 'Metriopatheia and apatheia: some reflections on a controversy in later Greek ethics', in J. Anton ad A. Preus (eds.) *Essays in Ancient Philosophy*, New York, 1983.

> Since you say you have never seen me distressed, you may possibly imag-
> ine that I am going to make the same pronouncement as some of the
> philosophers who hold that the sage will never suffer distress.
>
> *IND*. 70, 21,13–17 BJP

But of course he isn't, at least in his own case. His own restraint is not superhuman. Moreover, the implication is pretty clearly that such moral heroism is a
chimerical fantasy:

> I cannot say if there is anyone so wise that he is entirely free of affec-
> tions; but I have a precise knowledge of the degree to which I am such.
> I do not care about the loss of possessions, as long as I am not deprived
> of all of them and sent to a desert island, or of bodily pain, without quite
> making light of being placed in the bull of Phalaris. What will distress me
> is the ruination of my homeland, or a friend being punished by a tyrant,
> and other similar things ... So since nothing like this has happened to me
> until now, you thus have never seen me distressed (71–2, 21,17–22,7).

Not for him the Stoic sagely ideal, even if it is merely an ideal, or Epicurus'
claim that the wise man will be happy even on the rack, even while scream-
ing and groaning (DL 10.118, = 22Q(4) LS). Equally, he will not actually wel-
come material disaster, unlike Stoics such as Musonius (cf. the story of Zeno:
above, §1). He prays for health, mental and physical, while trying to prepare
himself to meet disaster with moderation. He himself is not superhuman: he
could not maintain his equanimity in the face of total destitution, or in the
case of pain severe enough to render conversations with friends an impossibility (73–6, 22,7–23,1).[38]

Finally, it is worth quoting the following:

> If someone regards all of these things as of little value, why should he
> worry about them or be worried by them? ... Someone who supposes that
> he has been deprived of something big must always be distressed and

---

38   This looks like another dig at the Epicureans, for whom the pleasures of friendship were
the primary good: *VS* 23, 28, 34, 39, 62, 66, 58, 66, 78 (= 22D, F LS); *KD* 27–8 (= 22D LS);
cf. 22G, H, O, Q LS. Epicurus allegedly claimed in his last letter that it was recollection
of philosophical conversations that assuaged his agony; Galen pointedly retorts that too
much agony makes such things impossible. But see also Kaufman, D. H., 'Galen on the
therapy of distress and the limits of emotional therapy', 2014, pp. 284–6, esp. n 33, who
stresses the non-heroic aspects of the Epicurean attitude which would appeal to Galen.

fret, unlike the person who thinks them small and continues to despise them. (65–6, 20,17–22)

That is the summation of Galen's *metriopatheia*. Let us finally see how congruent it is with Sextus's.

7 Galen and Pyrrhonism: Comparisons and Conclusions

We may begin with Pyrrho himself. Largely legendary though his legacy no doubt is, the legends are themselves instructive insofar as they illustrate the lessons which later reporters, friendly as well as hostile, sought to derive from his example:

> They say he showed his indifference by washing a pig. Once he got enraged on his sister's behalf (her name was Philista), and he told the man who chided him for it that it was not over a weak woman that one should display indifference. When a dog rushed at him and terrified him, he responded to one who censured him for it that it was not easy entirely to strip oneself of one's humanity (*ekdunai ton anthrôpon*); but one could struggle against one's circumstances, at first by actions, and if they failed, by reason.
>
> DL 9. 66, = 1C LS [part]

So it seems that Pyrrho was not entirely successful in cultivating the sort of indifference manifested by his pig-laundering. Some things, apparently, demand an emotive response; and some things provoke it willy-nilly. The phrase *ekdunai ton anthrôpon* is striking, since it vividly expresses what is apparently an ideal, and yet in a sense a self-stultifying one, and one which someone of Galen's stripe would reject even as an ideal, although the Stoics (and perhaps also the Epicureans) would not.

The Sextan sceptic is in a similar case. Not believing pain to be really bad, he will suffer less than the normal person who does; but he will still suffer. Equally, Galen thinks that some distress is unavoidable; and he too places a comparable (albeit differently oriented) emphasis upon the importance of not thinking that certain apparent goods really are goods.

Galen is a busy, engaged man; and so too, albeit presumably less frenetically so, is the Sextan sceptic. Properly understood, scepticism does not induce *apraxia*, since the sceptic is free to follow the 'criterion' of the *phainomena* (*PH* 1.22):

> We follow a sort of doctrine (*logos*) which, in accordance with what appears, directs us to live in accordance with our inherited customs and laws and ways of life, and our own *pathê*.
>
> *PH* 1.17

Sceptics do not do away with appearances, in spite of what their opponents allege. They are swayed, albeit involuntarily, by the "affective impression (*phantasia pathêtikê*)" (19), even if on occasion they will argue against appearances as a counterweight to 'dogmatic precipitancy' (20):

> Adhering to the *phainomena*, we live in accordance with the dictates of ordinary life (*hê biôtikê têrêsis*: cf. 3.235, quoted above), but without opinion, since we cannot remain wholly inactive. And the dictates of ordinary life are apparently four in number, the direction of nature; the constraint of the *pathê*, as when hunger drives us to food and thirst to drink; the tradition of the customs and laws; ... and the instruction of the arts (*technai*).
>
> *PH* 1.23–4

That last matters. Sextus, after all, was, like Galen, a doctor; a man of action, and a benefactor of humanity (*philanthrôpos*: *PH* 3.279–80). And Galen's views on these issues are closer in some respects to Sextan Pyrrhonism than he might have been willing to allow. But then Sextan Pyrrhonism is not 'rustic',[39] and Galen could easily have thought that in many important respects it was simply a version of the sensible, non-heroic view of life,[40] albeit one couched in a pointlessly phenomenalist language (*Dig.Puls.* VIII 780–3: above, §4), although he would no doubt also have accused them of denying the appearances, precisely because it does appear that pain, for example, is actually bad. Galen often elides the differences between the contemporary representatives of the schools he attacks, and earlier, and perhaps caricatured, versions of their views

39 At least I don't think so; but the issue is controversial. For a forceful expression of the view that, Sextus's own protestations notwithstanding, it must be, see Barnes, J., 'Sextan scepticism' in D. Scott (ed.)(2007) *Maieusis: Essays in Ancient Philosophy in Honour of Myles Burnyeat* (Oxford: OUP), 2007, 322–34 (he derived his own term 'rustic' from Galen's '*agroikos*'). Compare his earlier views of 1982 and 1988; and those of Frede, M. ('Des skeptikers Meinungen', *Neue Hefte für Philosophie* 15/16, 1979, 102–129), and Burnyeat, M. 'Can the sceptic live his scepticism?', in J. Barnes, M. F. Burnyeat, and M. Schofield (eds.) *Doubt and Dogmatism* (Oxford: OUP), 1980, 20–53; all are collected in Burnyeat and Frede 1997.

40 Cf. his assimilation of Academic to Stoic – and indeed his own – epistemology: see Hankinson, R. J., 'A purely verbal dispute? Galen on Stoic and Academic epistemology', in A.-J. Voelke (ed.) *Le Stoïcisme: Revue internationale de philosophie* 45.3, 1992, 267–300.

(this is clearly the case in regard to his treatment of Methodism); and in so doing, he is no more than a representative (admittedly a flamboyant one) of the traducive tendencies of his time.

One might still object that the connection I have sketched between Galen and his sceptical rivals is a tenuous one. I have stressed the sceptical emphasis on the unavoidability of the *pathê*; but these *pathê* are apparently physical pains, rather than excessive emotional states (such as anger and grief). One minimizes their unpleasant reality not by cultivating an indifference to them, but by ridding oneself of the additional painful belief that such things are really, essentially, bad. By contrast, Galen's cognitive behavioural approach stresses the importance of reflecting on the intrinsic hideousness of the manifestations of rage, as well as its self-defeating consequences, as a means of gradually curing oneself of an addiction to it. *Metriopatheia* in this sense (again it should be stressed that Galen himself does not employ the term) is something to be cultivated, rather than simply the best one may humanly hope for.

All of these differences (and some others) are genuine. But for all that, particularly in the case of distress, *lupê*, and the appropriate response to loss of any kind, the convergences of Galen's programme and that of the Pyrrhonists are clear. Some of the prescriptions are certainly different – there appears to be no sceptical counterpart to the injunction to visualize bad possible outcomes in order to immunize yourself (partially at least) against their eventuality, and by extension against less severe setbacks. Indeed there are obvious and well-known problems with the idea of sceptics issuing injunctions of any kind. But the appeal to persuasion certainly strikes a chord; scepticism is a therapy founded centrally on the practice of argument. What goes wrong in both cases involves false (or at least toxic) beliefs, beliefs which we would be much better off without, even though ridding ourselves of them (or at least minimizing them) will not (and perhaps for Galen at least should not) involve the construction of the wholly unaffected individual as some sort of ideal, even as one which is practically unattainable, as most Stoics believed it to be. Neither for Galen nor the sceptics are emotions simply reducible to beliefs, and mistaken ones at that; they are the compulsions of a fundamentally non-rational, reactive part of the soul. Even if we are essentially rational animals, there is still a humanity there is no point in trying to strip ourselves of.[41]

41   This is a very considerably altered, written version of a talk I gave at the Warwick conference splendidly organized by Caroline Petit, on July 1st, 2014. I am grateful to the participants, many of whom were old friends, and some of whom have since become so, for their engagement with my ideas, both during the session and less formally afterwards.

References

Barigazzi, A., *Galeno, Sull'ottima maniera di insegnare. Esortazione alla medicina* CMG V 1,1 Berlin: Akademie Verlag, 1991

Barnes, J., 'The beliefs of a Pyrrhonist', *Proceedings of the Cambridge Philological Society* 28, 1982, pp. 1–29; repr. in Frede and Burnyeat, 1997, 58–91

Barnes, J.,'Scepticism and the arts', in R.J.Hankinson (ed.), *Method, Medicine and Metaphysics: Apeiron* 21.2, Supp. Vol. 19 (Edmonton, Alberta: Academic Printing and Publishing), 1988, 53–77

Barnes, J., 'Sextan scepticism' in D.Scott (ed.)(2007) *Maieusis: Essays in Ancient Philosophy in Honour of Myles Burnyeat* (Oxford: OUP), 2007, 322–34

Boudon-Millot, V., *Galien: Introduction générale, Sur l'ordre de ses propres livres, Sur ses propres livres, Que l'excéllent médecin est aussi philosophe* Texte établi, traduit et annoté par, Paris, Les Belles Lettres, 2007

Boudon-Millot, V., Jouanna, J., Pietrobelli, A., *Galien, Ne pas se chagriner*, Paris, Les Belles Lettres, 2010

Burnyeat, M. F., 'Tranquillity without a stop: Timon Frag. 68' *The Classical Quarterly*, 30.1., 1980, 86–93

Burnyeat, M. F. 'Can the sceptic live his scepticism?', in J. Barnes, M. F. Burnyeat, and M. Schofield (eds.) *Doubt and Dogmatism* (Oxford: OUP), 1980, 20–53; repr. in Burnyeat, 1983, 117–48; and in Burnyeat and Frede, 1997, 25–57

Burnyeat, M. F. '"All the world's a stage-painting": scenery, optics, and Greek epistemology', *Oxford Studies in Ancient Philosophy* 52, 2017, 33–7

Burnyeat, M. F. (ed.), *The Skeptical Tradition*, California, University of California Press, 1983

Burnyeat, M. F., and Frede, M. (eds.) *The Original Sceptics*, Indianapolis: Hackett Publishing Company, 1997

De Boer, W., *Galeni de Animi Affectuum et Peccatorum Dignotione et Curatione; de Atra Bile* CMG V 4,1,1, Berlin, Akademie Verlag, 1937

De Lacy, P. H., *Galen: On the Doctrines of Hippocrates and Plato* (3 vols., ed., trans., and comm.): *CMG* V 4,1,2, Berlin, Akademie Verlag, 1978–1984

De Lacy, P. H., 'The third part of the soul', in Manuli and Vegetti, 1988, 43–64

Diels, H. A., *Poetarum Philosophorum Fragmenta*, Berlin, Weidmann, 1901; reprint Hildesheim: Weidmann, 2000.

Diels, H. A., and Kranz, W., *Die Fragmente der Vorokratiker*, Berlin, Weidmann, 1952[6]

Dillon, J. M., '*Metriopatheia* and *apatheia*: some reflections on a controversy in later Greek ethics', in J. Anton ad A. Preus (eds.) *Essays in Ancient Philosophy*, New York, 1983

Dillon, J. M., *Alcinous: The Handbook of Platonism*, Oxford: OUP, 1993

Dillon, J. M., *Essays in Ancient Philosophy*, Minneapolis: University of Minnesota Press, 1987

Frede, M., 'Des skeptikers Meinungen', *Neue Hefte für Philosophie* 15/16, 1979, 102–129 (English version in Frede, 1987; repr. In Burnyeat and Frede, 1997, 1–24)

Hankinson, R. J., 'A purely verbal dispute? Galen on Stoic and Academic epistemology', in A.-J.Voelke (ed.) *Le Stoïcisme: Revue internationale de philosophie* 45.3, 1992, 267–300

Hankinson, R. J., *The Sceptics*, Routledge, 1995

Hankinson, R. J., 'Natural criteria and the transparency of judgement: Philo, Antiochus and Galen on epistemological justification', in B. Inwood and J. Mansfeld (eds.) *Assent and Argument: Studies in Cicero's Academic Books* (Leiden, 1997), pp. 161–216

Hankinson, R. J., 'The man and his work', in Hankinson ed., *The Cambridge Companion to Galen*, 2008, 1–33

Hankinson, R. J., 'Epistemology', in Hankinson ed., *The Cambridge Companion to Galen*, 2008, 157–83

Hankinson, R. J., 'Philosophy of nature', in Hankinson ed., *The Cambridge Companion to Galen*, 2008, 210–41

Hankinson, R. J., (ed.) *The Cambridge Companion to Galen*, Cambridge: CUP 2008

Helmreich, G., *Galeni Scripta Minora* III, Leipzig, Teubner, 1893

Helmreich, G., *Galeni de Temperamentis* Leipzig, Teubner, 1904

Helmreich, G., *Galeni de Usu Partium* (2 vols.) Leipzig, Teubner, 1907–1909

Kaufman, D. H., 'Galen on the therapy of distress and the limits of emotional therapy', *Oxford Studies in Ancient Philosophy* 47, 2014 275–96

Long, A. A., and Sedley, D. N. (1987) *The Hellenistic Philosophers* 2 vols., Cambridge, CUP, 1987

Marquardt, J., *Galeni Pergameni Scripta Minora* 1 Leipzig, Teubner, 1884

May, M. T., *Galen on the Usefulness of the Parts of the Body* 2 vols, Baltimore, Johns Hopkins, 1968

Müller, I. *Galeni Scripta Minora* II, Leipzig: Teubner, 1891

Nagel, T., 'Death', *Nous* 4.1, 1970, 73–80; repr. in Nagel, 1979, *Mortal Questions*, Cambridge, CUP, 1979, 1–10

Nutton, V., *Galen: On Prognosis* (edition, translation, commentary), CMG V 8,1, Berlin, Akademie Verlag, 1979

Nutton, V., *Galen: On my own Opinions* (edition, translation, commentary), CMG V 3.2, Berlin, Akademie Verlag, 1999

Singer, P., *Galen: Selected Works*, Oxford: OUP, 1997

Singer, P., *Galen: Psychological Writings*, Cambridge, CUP, 2013

Sedley, D. N., 'The motivation of Greek skepticism', in Burnyeat, 1983, 9–29

Striker, G., 'Ataraxia: happiness as tranquillity', *The Monist* 73.1, Hellenistic Ethics, 1990, 97–110

CHAPTER 7

A New Distress: Galen's Ethics in Περὶ Ἀλυπίας and Beyond

P. N. Singer

In this chapter I consider how the new material from the περὶ ἀλυπίας (*Ind.*) contributes to our understanding of Galen's ethics. As is the case with Galen's discussions of his own books, I here suggest that helpful results are derived from the laying of the new text alongside the most relevant previously-known ones.

1   Position in Galen's *Oeuvre*

Where does περὶ ἀλυπίας sit within Galen's writings on ethics and moral psychology, and what does it add to the picture? Galen's contribution to moral psychology and ethics was previously known mainly from *Affections* and *Errors* (*Aff. Pecc. Dig.* 1 and 2). There is also highly relevant information in the admittedly problematic (because both abridged and to some extent distorted in the Arabic version) *Character Traits* (*Mor.*), and in some passages from *The Soul's Dependence on the Body* (*QAM*) and *De placitis Hippocratis et Platonis* (*PHP*). The latter two, however (to simplify two highly complex texts), are concerned mainly with certain theoretical propositions, and in particular with aspects of the relationship of soul to body. *Affections and Errors* and *Character Traits*, meanwhile – both of which he lists, in his own account of his writings, alongside περὶ ἀλυπίας in the category of works giving his views on ethical philosophy[1] – bear a much clearer affinity to that work. All three belong within a genre of practical or popularizing works of moral philosophy intended for a non-specialist audience; they offer both theory and practical advice in the areas of ethics, education and personal development.

---

1   *Lib. Prop.* 15 [12] (XIX.45 K. = 169,13–17 Boudon-Millot; for references to *Lib. Prop.* I print the new chapter number, resulting from the full text now available from Vlatadon 14, followed by the previous chapter number in square brackets). The three works, as well as a considerable number of others which are now lost, are introduced with the phrase περὶ τῶν τῆς ἠθικῆς φιλοσοφίας ἐζητημένων ὅσα μοι δοκεῖ (although an actual chapter heading, Περὶ τῶν τῆς ἠθικῆς φιλοσοφίας βιβλίων, was an addition of Müller's).

The closest similarity that περὶ ἀλυπίας has with another work in the Galenic corpus is, indeed, with *Affections*; and I should like now to spend a little time exploring both that similarity and what, specifically, *Peri alupias* adds to the other work. Both works are designed to help the reader or listener on the path to ethical improvement. According to ancient distinctions both of genre and of stage of personal development, works of 'protreptic' – encouraging the reader or listener to embark on the process of virtue acquisition in the first place – may precede a subsequent phase of instruction in which detailed guidance is given about the actual process.[2] Employing that broad categorization, one would have to situate *Peri alupias* in this subsequent phase too.

Affections and Errors has as its topic or aim the control of affections (*pathē*) and errors (*hamartēmata*) in general; περὶ ἀλυπίας has the specific focus of the elimination of distress (*lupē*). Some have linked περὶ ἀλυπίας to the genre of *consolatio*; and other recent work has explored both the philosophical and the literary relatives of the work, and aspects of Galen's self-presentation within it. There are similarities between the text and others in the tradition of popular ethical writing; it has been suggested that Plutarch's *De tranquillitate animi* provides the closest parallel.[3]

---

2   Galen explicitly puts *Aff. Pecc. Dig.* in the latter class: 'For it [*sc.* the present argument] is not one designed to convert people (προτρεπτικός) to virtue, but rather to show (ὑφηγητικός) those who are already converted the way by which it may be achieved', *Aff. Pecc. Dig.* 1.6 (v.34 K. = 23,14–16 DB). There may be a relevance here of a threefold scheme, 'protretpic, therapy, advice', which had been outlined by Philo of Larissa (Stobaeus, *Ecl.* 2.39.20–41.25); see Singer, P. N. (ed.) (2013). *Galen: Psychological Writings*, 206–7 and 240 n. 13 for discussion of this distinction and further references.

3   See especially Gill, C. (2010). *Naturalistic Psychology in Galen and Stoicism*, who draws out the similarities between each of these ethical *opuscula* and other works of practical ethics in the Graeco-Roman tradition; also Singer, *Galen: Psychological Writings*, esp. 205–32, for discussion of Galen in his ethical context. For περὶ ἀλυπίας as a *consolatio* see the introduction to Boudon-Millot, V. and Jouanna, J. (2010). *Galien, Oeuvres, 4: Ne pas se chagriner*, and contra Kotzia, P. (2012). 'Galen *Peri alupias*: Title, Genre and Two Cruces', in Manetti, D. (ed.) *Studi sul De indolentia di Galeno*, 69–91, pointing out specific differences between the content of *Peri alupias* and other ancient *consolationes* and drawing attention to a specific category of works, now lost to us, entitled περὶ ἀλυπίας. See also Rosen, R. (2012). 'Philology and the Rhetoric of Catastrophe in Galen's *De indolentia*', in, Rothschild, C. K. and Thompson, T. W. (eds) *Galen's* De indolentia, 159–74.; Asmis, E. (2012). 'Galen's *De indolentia* and the Creation of a Personal Philosophy', in ibid., 127–42; Kaufman, D. H. (2014). 'Galen on the Therapy of Distress and the Limits of Emotional Therapy', *Oxford Studies in Ancient Philosophy* 47, 275–96, highlighting features in Galen's therapy of distress which he considers to be taken directly from Stoic and Epicurean sources. Kaufman's paper appeared too late to be taken into consideration in the original version of the present chapter; but, without space to engage with all his interesting suggestions, a couple of points may be made. First, as well discussed by Gill, both Stoic and Epicurean therapeutic approaches may be seen as part of a shared repertory

There is, I believe, more to be said, both about the interesting overlaps and differences between *Affections and Errors* and περὶ ἀλυπίας and about the distinctive understanding of *lupē* that arises from a consideration of both texts in conjunction. Such an approach is attractive both because *Affections and Errors* is a fascinating but in many ways frustrating text, unclear in a number of aspects of its organization and in particular giving a quite uneven discussion, and no clear typological categorization, of the different *pathē* of the soul;[4] and also because it does, however, have quite a lot to say about *lupē* which may usefully be placed alongside the new material from περὶ ἀλυπίας.

2   *Lupē* in *Affections and Errors*

There are, in fact, passages in *Affections and Errors* which seem to present *lupē* as, not just as one *pathos* amongst many, but in some sense an overarching category. In chapter 7 of *Affections*, in what it is admittedly a not unproblematic passage textually, it is suggested that there are subspecies of distress, of which envy is one.

> ὀνομάζω δὲ φθόνον, ὅταν τις ἐπ᾽ἀλλοτρίοις ἀγαθοῖς λυπῆται. πάθος μέν ἐστι καὶ λύπη πᾶσα, χειρίστη δὲ ὁ φθόνος ἐστίν, εἴτε ἓν τῶν παθῶν εἴτε λυπῆς ἐστὶν εἶδος πλησιάζον δέ πως αὐτῇ,

> By envy I mean becoming distressed at what others enjoy. All distress is an affection, but envy is the worst distress, whether it is an affection in itself or a subspecies of distress, somehow approximate to it ...
>
> *Aff. Pecc. Dig.* 1.7 (v.35 K. = 24,13–16 De Boer)[5]

---

of techniques, also incorporated in this period by a Platonist author such as Plutarch; and such an analysis seems to me more convincing than that of a strong direct influence from Epicureanism. Secondly, while Kaufman's point (282) about the input from Posidonius, especially on Galen's view of the *praemeditatio malorum*, is well taken (on the passage in question see further n. 19 below), the relevance of the 'belief-based methods associated ... with the early Stoics' (283) seems less clear, since the importance of the rational component (corresponding to correct beliefs) alongside non-rational ones is well justified by Galen's own explicitly proposed Platonist theory of the soul. My own argument in what follows also suggests a clear connection with the Stoic and Epicurean philosophical alternatives, but in a somewhat different sense.

4   There are two short lists of *pathē*, which however do not seem to aim at exhaustiveness, and within them no clear principle of classification. The point is discussed at greater length by Singer, *Galen: Psychological Writings*, 220–1.

5   The translation of this text (here and subsequently) is that of Singer, *Galen: Psychological Writings*, who also discusses the problems of the text ad loc.

Moreover, distress or grief assumes a central role for a major part of the text, chapters 7–9.

I digress for a moment to clarify a point of terminology. For the sake of consistency, I translate *ania* and cognates with 'grief' and cognates, and similarly *lupē* with 'distress'; however, the two sets of terms seem, in the ethical context, to be regarded as virtual synonyms. Though it is arguable that the former gives, at times, a slightly intensified sense, it seems wrong to insist on a clear distinction. The verbal form ἀνιώμενος is used, for example, of the young man at *Aff. Pecc. Dig.* 1.7 (v.37 K. = 25,15 de Boer), and the verb is also used of Galen's own mother who 'would suffer grief at the smallest occurrence' (ἀνιωμένην ... ἐπὶ σμικροτάτοις, 1.8, v.41 K. = 28,6 de Boer). But the progress of the discussion, in 1.8 (from v.43 K. = 29,15 de Boer), makes it clear that *lupē* is regarded as the relevant overall heading.[6] In what follows I shall therefore treat Galen's discussion of cases of *ania* and *lupē* as referring to the same psychological–ethical phenomenon.

In chapters 7–9, then, we gain the impression that the eradication or lessening of *lupē* is an absolutely central strand in the fight against the affections. The discussion revolves around anecdotal reference to, quotation of and direct address to individuals amongst Galen's most intimate circle of friends and family. First, at *Aff. Pecc. Dig.* 1.7 (v.37 K. = 25,15 de Boer), Galen introduces the character of a young man who came to him because of the excessive grief he suffered over small matters. The argument continues to be addressed to this individual's problem up to the end of chapter 9 – albeit with some major digressions, in particular on the relationship between nature and nurture and on the ethical model offered by Galen's own parents, and his own philosophical upbringing. But both the digressions and the material directly related to the young man serve to bring out the importance, and multifarious ramifications, of distress. First, Galen attributes to his father a contrast between universally admired virtues – justice, self-control, courage and discernment – on the one

---

6 A further note of caution should be sounded in relation to the temptation to see such words as 'technical terms', and so ignore their potential fluidity: it seems to me (*pace* Nutton) that Galen uses the verb *anian* in a passage of *De methodo medendi* (*MM*) in a completely different, non-technical sense. At *MM* 7.1 (x.456–7 K.) Galen is – in line with the 'reluctant author' persona discussed in my 'New Light and Old Books', in this volume – giving reasons for his not having written the work earlier. To his standard argument, that he never wrote to advance his reputation, he adds another: he was too busy. The words there, ἡμᾶς ... πολλάκις ἀνιωμένους ἐπὶ τοῖς ἐνοχλοῦσιν οὕτω συνεχῶς ἐνίοτε χρόνον ἐφεξῆς πόλυν, ὡς μηδ᾽ ἅψασθαι συνηθῆναι βιβλίου, in this context demand the interpretation that Galen is too pressed upon by urgent duties to be able to engage in literary activity as he would like, not that he is too depressed to read. One might here translate 'troubled', 'bothered', or even 'irritated' or 'annoyed'; but surely the term carries none of the 'technical' sense of *ania* or *lupē*, with their problematic and dangerous ethical dimension, in περὶ ἀλυπίας and *Affections*.

hand, and freedom from distress, on the other. The point is that people wish to *appear* to have the former virtues, but they want actually to *be* free from distress:

> ... φαίνεσθαί γε πειρῶνται τοῖς ἄλλοις ἀνδρεῖοι καὶ σώφρονες καὶ φρόνιμοι καὶ δίκαιοι, ἄλυποι μέντοι κατ᾽ ἀλήθειαν εἶναι, κἂν μὴ φαίνωνται τοῖς πέλας· ὥστε τοῦτο μέν σοι πρῶτον ἁπάντων ἀσκητέον ἐστὶ τὸ σπουδαζόμενον ἅπασιν ἀνθρώποις μᾶλλον τῶν ἀρετῶν.

> ... they wish to *appear* to others brave, self-controlled, discerning and just, while they actually want to *be* free from distress, even if it is not apparent to those around them. And this should therefore be what you cultivate first of all, since it is sought after by all people in preference to the virtues.

> *Aff. Pecc. Dig.* 1.8 (v.43 K. = 29,8–12 de Boer)

The practice of freeing oneself from *lupē* is here presented as the practical, chronological starting-point of one's ethical progress, on the commonsense grounds that this absence of suffering is something that all people actually seek. We shall see how this perception of Galen's father's surfaces again in *Peri alupias*. Galen also talks of the model his parents provided specifically in terms of their experience of distress. His father 'never appeared distressed at any setback', while his mother 'would suffer grief at the smallest occurrence'. The terms 'distress' and 'grief' are here clearly being used to apply to one's reactions to a very wide range of everyday events which are liable to upset one: thus, *lupē* (or *ania*) here can be seen as to some extent co-extensive with irritation or anger, even though this, in its more violent manifestations, was dealt with explicitly earlier in the work.

In the part of the text addressed more closely to the young man who wishes to be freed from distress, too, the term turns out to have a very broad reference. One may, for example, suffer *lupē* not just as a result of personal loss, but in the anxiety over possible future loss, including not just of possessions but of status. Although, as mentioned, Galen does not explicitly give us any categorization of the *pathē* or account of which are the most fundamental, we are reminded of the fact that *lupē* is, indeed, an overarching category, an 'Über-*pathos*', in some Stoic sources.[7] Getting rid of *lupē*, then, begins to look rather like the Stoic drive for *apatheia*. Reference to the Stoic relatives of Galen's thought in

---

7   There is a Stoic division of *pathē* into four broad categories: distress (*lupē*), fear (*phobos*), desire (*epithumia*), pleasure (*hēdonē*); see Diogenes Laertius, *Vit. Phil.* 7.110, Stobaeus, *Ecl.*

this area leads us to another relevant consideration: the absence of the tripartite soul at this point in the discussion. The earlier phase of discussion, based strongly on that Platonic distinction of the drives of the non-rational soul into those of spirited (*thumoeides*) and desiderative (*epithumētikon*), clearly implies that any *pathos* will be a *pathos* of one of these two – that this distinction will be of fundamental significance throughout. And, as already suggested, the examples that the text dwells on at length seem to be chosen as examples of the malfunction of the spirited – that is to say, of uncontrolled rage.

Yet the discussion of *lupē* which we have just been considering is interesting precisely because it seems to follow from this broader conception of *lupē* that it cuts across the spirited–desiderative distinction.[8] This is supported both by the range of examples of *lupē* – distress at financial loss, distress caused by fear of loss, distress at perceived lack of status – and by the subsequent argument that the cause of all susceptibility to *lupē* is – an even more over-arching category – acquisitiveness (*pleonexia*). For such acquisitiveness or greed may be directed at personal possessions or luxury (surely, in Platonic terms, aims of the desiderative soul), but also at status and perceived position in society (those of the spirited).

3   *Lupē* and Its Control in περὶ ἀλυπίας

The discussion in περὶ ἀλυπίας contributes to the same picture. Here the Platonic tripartite soul does not, in fact, appear at all. Rather, removing or reducing one's susceptibility to *lupē* appears as a procedure which is absolutely fundamental to ethical well-being. Much of the argument proceeds through models: the positive ones of Aristippus and of Galen's own father, the negative ones of his mother and of the literary man whose distress led to his ultimate demise. Again, *alupia* seems to amount to something very similar to what a Stoic might call being unaffected by externals – or at least, to being affected by them as little as possible (we shall return to this point).

We might like to say that the two works are complementary: περὶ ἀλυπίας continues, and develops in more detail, particular themes outlined in *Affections and Errors*.[9] But in drawing attention to this complementarity, it is important

---

2.7.10, Cicero, *Fin.* 3.35. Cf. also the detailed categorization of the probably Stoic text, pseudo-Andronicus, *Peri pathōn*, which lists 24 species of *lupē*.

8   On this point see also Singer, *Galen: Psychological Writings*, esp. 220–1.

9   This formulation is not intended to imply anything about the relative dates of the two works, for discussion of which see Nutton in Singer, *Galen: Psychological Writings*, 45–47, arguing (against Jouanna) for a dating of *Aff. Pecc. Dig.*, as well as *Mor.*, after περὶ ἀλυπίας. (But see

to re-emphasize the point: the more general work *Affections and Errors* is, to a considerable extent, itself a work about the reduction or elimination of distress. On the other hand, περὶ ἀλυπίας introduces perspectives on *lupē* that are not to be found in *Affections and Errors*, or found there much less clearly; and I turn to two of these now, before returning to a consideration of their complementarity and attempting to summarize the findings that accrue from considering the texts conjointly.

The first such 'new' feature of *lupē* in περὶ ἀλυπίας is its potentially severe physical consequences.

> ... Φιλίδης μὲν ὁ γραμματικὸς ἀπολλυμένων αὐτῷ τῶν βιβλίων κατὰ πυρκαϊὰν ἀπὸ δυσθυμίας καὶ λύπης διέφθαρη συντακείς
>
> ... Philides the literary man, when his books were destroyed in the fire, wasted away as a result of low spirits and distress, and died.
>
> *Ind.* 7 (4,6–8 BJP)[10]

In fact, this Galenic aspect of *lupē* is not by any means a finding new to *Peri alupias*, even if it is not mentioned in *Affections and Errors*. The medical, including potentially fatal, consequences of distress (as also of worry, *phrontis* and *agōnia*), as part of a disease pattern involving the connected phenomena of sleeplessness, dryness, heat and fever, is attested in a wide range of passages in Galen's medical writings.[11] Indeed, the specific anecdote that Galen brings forward here about the literary man whose distress over losses similar to Galen's did indeed prove fatal appears elsewhere, in Galen's *Commentary on Hippocrates' 'Epidemics VI'*.

Such medical consequences are not the *direct* subject matter of *Peri alupias*, which is concerned rather with its prevention. The medical understanding of *lupē*, however, should be borne in mind as an important element in the

---

also Singer, *Galen: Psychological Writings*, 34–41, as well as 'New Light and Old Books', p. 123 n. 45 and p. 125, for methodological caution on the dating of Galen's works.).

10   Translations from *Peri alupias* are my own. On the identity between the person mentioned here and that referred to in *Hipp. Epid. VI* (discussed below), on the problem of the form of his name, and on the chronological relationship between *Peri alupias* and *Hipp. Epid. VI*, see Nutton in Singer, *Galen: Psychological Writings*, 79 n. 15. I translate γραμματικός with the vague term 'literary man'; the term has a semantic range which includes a kind of secondary-level teacher and a person with broad expertise in the analysis of literary texts.

11   See now Singer, P. N. (2017). 'The Essence of Rage: Galen on Emotional Disturbances and their Physical Correlates', in Seaford, R., Wilkins, J. and Wright, M. (eds). *Selfhood and the Soul: Essays on Ancient Thought and Literature in Honour of Christopher Gill*, 161–96, drawing attention to a range of such texts.

intellectual background. For the medical context provides a framework within which *lupē* is, for Galen, a distinct and observable physical phenomenon. Whether someone is suffering from *lupē* is thus, in a sense, an objective fact – an affection of the *psuchē* which – just like those well-known affections of the *psuchē* in Galen's anecdotes in *Prognosis* – is accessible to medical diagnosis.[12] It is not irrelevant here, either, to consider the criterion of a pathological state given in *De sanitate tuenda*: so long as the person is not *distressed* by an imperfect physical state, that state still counts as healthy.[13] For Galen *lupē* is a concrete, distinct – and potentially a medical – state. It is not a vague characterization of the phenomenon of becoming slightly upset at events.

Another area in which περὶ ἀλυπίας seems to depart from *Affections and Errors*, or at least to give greater clarity, is in relation to the question – already touched on – of how complete an elimination of *pathē* is required or desirable. As a number of previous discussions have highlighted, *Affections* seems practically to align itself with a Stoic approach whereby *pathē* are in their nature purely negative, and something very close to their complete elimination is the aim. It has also been pointed out that this appears to conflict with his Platonism, or to be more precise with what one might expect at this period from an author indebted strongly to both Plato and Aristotle in his ethical thinking, and in particular that the term *metriopatheia* – the 'moderation of the *pathē*' – which appears in some 'Middle Platonist' authors is not mentioned by Galen.[14]

It is, of course, true that, within the Platonic tripartite model which is of such importance to Galen, including in *Affections*, anger – the righteous indignation of the *thumoeides* which checks the wild desires of the *epithumētikon* – has a positive, indeed an important, role, in a way which is quite contrary to Stoic thinking. For Galen, however, though this internal dynamic within the soul is important to his analysis, anger when functioning in this way apparently does not come under the heading of *pathos*. *Pathos*, for Galen, seems, in the ethical context, to be a purely negative term: that much he has taken over from Stoic usage, however bitterly he opposes the broader intellectual framework within which that usage arose. That is to say: there is, for Galen, a legitimate role for the non-rational parts of the soul, but *pathos* arises only in these non-rational parts and only when they are *not* behaving legitimately; for

12   Relevant here is the analysis of Mattern, S. P. (2006). 'Galen's Anxious Patients: *Lypē* as Anxiety Disorder', in Petridou, G. and Thumiger, C. (eds) *Homo Patiens – Approaches to the Patient in the Ancient World*, 203–23, which however in my view over-emphasizes one particular, medicalized interpretation of *lupē* throughout the corpus.

13   *San. Tu.* 1.5 (VI.13 K. = 8,19–20, Koch; VI.19 K. = 10,29–34 Koch).

14   On this point see Donini, P. L. (2008). 'Psychology', in Hankinson, R. J. (ed.) *The Cambridge Companion to Galen*, 194; Singer, *Galen: Psychological Writings*, 208–9.

the Stoics, meanwhile, there is no such positive role for the non-rational parts of the soul, which indeed, properly speaking, do not exist: it is rather errors of rationality which lead to or constitute behaviour in *pathos*. Thus, Galen shares with Stoic thought the negative definition of *pathos*, while having a different understanding, not only of how *pathos* comes about and where it is located in the soul, but also of where *pathos* fits into the broader scheme of non-rational drives.

So we might say that even if Galen does acknowledge a positive role for some of (what the Stoics would call) *pathē*, this would not mean that he is advocating *metriopatheia*: for Galen, *pathē* are in their nature negative, and when anger (say) is functioning positively on behalf of the person that is not a case of *pathos*, not even of moderated *pathos*. Thus, an Aristotelian understanding of proper ethical/emotional response as consisting in some mean between opposites – that is, the exactly correct sort of *pathos* – seems to be absent from Galen's thinking in his ethical writings.[15]

But there is a further question, or complication. Even if Galen (a) takes there to be a positive role for some emotions, but (b) does not refer to positive manifestations of emotions as *pathē*, and therefore (c) does not advocate the concept of *metriopatheia*, there remains a further question: is the total elimination of those emotions which *are* regarded as purely negative – those ones which Galen and the Stoics would both call *pathē* – required? Galen's 'official' answer seems to be no – again, in keeping with a fundamentally Platonic–Aristotelian model (albeit one without the terminology of *metriopatheia*) – although, as discussed above, one can certainly gain the impression, throughout much of *Affections* and *Peri alupias*, that total elimination is indeed what is being advocated. In this context, it is also relevant to consider that Galen at least arguably (if one accepts a particular emendation of the text) allows also a moderate level of emotional attachment to societal status and political power, and even wealth. As elsewhere in Galen's work, excessive preoccupation with status or reputation is, to be sure, considered a great evil. But on Garofalo's emendation

---

15   A version of a theory of virtues as means does, however, appear in *Mixtures*, where the context is the assertion that a person with the best bodily mixture – conceived as a balance between extremes – will also have the right balance between ethical extremes: τῷ μὲν σώματι τοιοῦτος ὁ εὐκρατότατος ἄνθρωπος· ὡσαύτως δὲ καὶ τῇ ψυχῇ μέσος ἀκριβῶς ἐστι θρασύτητός τε καὶ δειλίας, μελλησμοῦ τε καὶ προπετείας, ἐλέου τε καὶ φθόνου. εἴη δ᾽ ἂν ὁ τοιοῦτος εὔθυμος, φιλόστοργος, φιλάνθρωπος, συνετός (*Temp.* 2.1, 1.576 K. = 42,16–20 Helmreich). This seems to be clearly in line with Aristotle's approach to virtues in *Eth. Nic.*; but such an analysis of ethical response in terms of a mean is not followed through in his ethical work, except in the sense that there is emphasis on the diet, training and the best physical nature as preconditions for ethics (esp. in *QAM* and *Mor.*); certainly individual virtues are not, on the Aristotelian model, so analysed.

of sections 80–81 (see further below), freedom from distress is equated with the possession of only a *moderate* level of attachment to these aims.

The desirability of elimination of *lupē* again points to its special status. Unlike *thumos* or *epithumia*, for example, it has no positive role. One might indeed be tempted, following the analysis outlined above, to suggest that this is precisely what *lupē* is for Galen: the negative or *pathological* manifestation of non-rational drives which (as we have seen) are not in themselves necessarily *pathē*. *Lupē*, then, like *pathos* in general, has no positive role for Galen. Does that mean that we should aim for or require its complete removal? In spite of what I have referred to as hints of a Stoic-style *apatheia, Peri alupias* gives us something the other text does not, or at least gives us much less explicitly: a specific affirmation that one *cannot* always be unaffected by circumstances.

Addressing the issue directly (in sections 70–76), Galen explicitly denies the proposition that a person – or at least that he personally – can remain free from distress in every eventuality. In contradistinction to the extreme Stoic and Epicurean claims on unaffectedness, Galen prefers a more common-sense position. He knows his own limitations; he does not, like Musonius the Stoic, ask to be tested by every possible adversity; he does not accept that one can be happy inside that notorious philosophical example of torture, the bull of Phalaris; and he mentions specific circumstances that he knows *would* cause him distress (the destruction of his home city, the persecution of a friend by a tyrant). So, the text of περὶ ἀλυπίας makes it clearer and more explicit than that of *Affections* that, in spite of the desirability of freeing oneself from *lupē* as much as one can, total indifference to, or unaffectedness by, externals cannot in all circumstances be expected. It is just that we should aim for much higher expectations and achievement in this area than are normally the case. Quite how high a level of achievement he expects, or (for he is more explicit on this point) attributes to himself, is a somewhat complex question. A very high level of impassivity to the vicissitudes of fate will be termed *megalopsuchia*;[16] and Galen does indeed attribute this quality to himself. At other points he emphasizes that his failure to succumb to distress, at least in response to most of

---

16   Galen's use of *megalopsuchia* here seems to provide another point of contact with Aristotle, for the understanding of the term seems importantly similar to the Aristotelian one. Although there are also different aspects of Aristotle's analysis of *megalopsuchia* (in particular in regard to the level of honour enjoyed by its possessor), he takes it to be a virtue that involves indifference, or at least a moderate reaction, to extremes of good or bad fortune (*Eth. Nic.* 4.3, 1124a12–15) and, interestingly also one which is in some sense a crown or adornment to the other virtues, enhancing them but impossible without them (*Eth. Nic.* 4.3, 1124a1–2). I am grateful to Matyáš Havrda for pointing out to me this similarity; see also Kotzia, P. (2014). 'Galen, *De indolentia*: Commonplaces, Traditions, and Contexts', in Rothschild, C. K. and Thompson, T. W. (eds), *Galen's* De indolentia, 91–126.

his losses, was 'no big thing'. The argument of the text functions, of course, by constantly emphasizing the enormity of his losses in order to highlight the distinctiveness of his reaction – a reaction of refusing to consider those losses to be enormous.[17] He is 'not at all moved', 'not now distressed, cheerfully carrying out my usual tasks as before', 'bearing without distress', 'not distressed, even with all such things touching me'; 'I bore it very easily, not moved in the least', 'none of these things distressed me', 'I was not distressed as others, but bore the event very easily, after losing such a great variety of possessions, any one of which on its own would have been most distressing to others'.[18]

Before returning to a final consideration of the complementary nature of the text and of the overall picture of *lupē* that emerges, I consider one more specific area in which περὶ ἀλυπίας seems to diverge, or offer something distinct from, *Affections and Errors*, this time in the sphere of practical advice. First, the central policy recommended in the latter work – that of finding a neutral advisor to monitor and report to one about one's faults – does not appear in *Peri alupias*. Conversely, the main technique which the latter work *does* prescribe, the *praemeditatio malorum* – that is to say, a sustained daily practice of anticipation of the worst, a practice which may include the internal or actual repetition of certain texts or propositions – does not appear, at least not explicitly, in *Affections and Errors*. A regular mental practice, involving recitation – specifically, of the Pythagorean *Carmen aureum* – is recommended in *Affections*, along with a process of self-interrogation whose rational force will affect one's ethical behaviour. This practice, however, is based rather on the daily examination of one's *previous* actions. περὶ ἀλυπίας gives us a further dimension of the use of text recitation for ethical or psychological purposes. A quotation from Euripides is central to the text's message on the *praemeditatio malorum*. (Interestingly, the same text appears in *De placitis Hippocratis et Platonis*, there in support of a theoretical argument about how to conceptualize the *process* of *praemeditatio* within the soul.[19]) It is perhaps noteworthy that there is no appeal here to the use of *philosophical* texts in one's daily exercise – a fact that one may relate to Galen's insistence that his father's successful moral

---

17   For a helpful discussion of the progress of Galen's argument in relation to this, and the consistency or otherwise of his view of *alupia* in the text, see Rosen, 'Rhetoric of Catastrophe'.

18   ἔφης αὐτὸς ἑωρακέναι με μηδὲ ἐπὶ βραχὺ κινηθέντα (2, 2,11–12 BJP); μηδὲν νῦν ἀνιαθῆναί με φαιδρόν τε καὶ τὰ συνήθη πράττοντα καθάπερ ἔμπροσθεν... ἀλύπως ὤφθην φέρων (3–4, 3,1–6 BJP); τὸ γὰρ μηδὲ τῶν τοιούτων πάντων ἀπτομένων ἀνιαθῆναι θαυμασιώτερον ἐδόκει σοι... πάνυ ῥᾳδίως ἤνεγκα τὸ πρᾶγμα, μήτε βραχὺ κινηθείς (11, 5,5–9 BJP); τούτων οὖν οὐδὲν ἠνίασέ με (29, 10,24–25 BJP); ἀπολέσας τοσαύτην ποικιλίαν κτημάτων ὧν ἕκαστον αὐτὸ καθ᾽ ἑαυτὸ λυπηρότατον ἂν ἐγένετο τοῖς ἄλλοις ἀνθρώποις, οὐκ ἠνιάθην ὡς ἕτεροί τινες, ἀλλὰ πάνυ ῥᾳδίως ἤνεγκα τὸ συμβάν (38, 13,4–8 BJP).

19   *PHP* 4.7 (v.417–18 K. = 282,11–23 De Lacy).

education, described as similar to his own, was achieved 'without arguments from philosophy' and that he 'did not frequent philosophers in youth'.[20] One may, indeed, connect this with Galen's sceptical attitude towards the discipline of philosophy, certainly as generally practised in his own time.[21]

4   Practical Ethics and Life Aims in περὶ ἀλυπίας and *Affections and Errors*

But let us consider some further aspects of the complementary nature of περὶ ἀλυπίας and *Affections and Errors*. In *Peri alupias*, we again meet Galen's father, and in a similar context. It is not just that his father was a model in his freedom from distress – that is, his ability not to be affected by adverse events. Rather, here too a specific perception is attributed to his father, one which matches that reported in *Affections and Errors*. Let us look at the passage, which may be compared with that cited above. (I follow the text of BJP, and excerpt what seem to me the most relevant phrases from a fairly long passage.)

> οὐ γὰρ ἄλλος ἀνθρώπων τις οὕτως ἀκριβῶς ὡς καὶ οὗτος ἐτίμησε δικαιοσύνην τε καὶ σωφροσύνην... οἶδα δέ μου τὸν πατέρα καταφρονοῦντα τῶν ἀνθρωπί-νων πραγμάτων ὡς μικρῶν... τοὺς ἥδιστα βεβιωκότας οὐδὲν ἔσχε πλείω τῶν οἰωνῶν τούτων οὓς κατὰ τὴν τῶν Ῥωμαίων πόλιν ὁρῶμεν ὑπὸ τῶν δεσποτῶν περιαγομένους ἕνεκα τοῦ τὰς θηλείας ὀχεύειν ἐπὶ μισθῷ· τοὺς δὲ τῶν τοιούτων ἡδονῶν καταφρονοῦντας, ἀρκουμένους δὲ τῷ μήτε ἀλγεῖν μήτε λυπεῖσθαι τὴν ψυχήν, οὐδέποτε ἐπήνεσεν ἀπομαντευόμενος μεῖζον τι καὶ κρεῖττον ὂν τὸ ἀγα-θὸν ἰδίαν ἔχον φύσιν, οὔτε ἐν μόνῳ τῷ μήτε ἀλγεῖν μήτε λυπεῖσθαι περιγραφό-μενον. ἀλλ᾽ ἐὰν καὶ τούτων τις ἀποχωρήσας ἐπιστήμην θείων καὶ ἀνθρωπίνων πραγμάτων ἡγήσηται τὸ ἀγαθὸν ὑπάρχειν, ἐλαχίστου μορίου τούτου ὁρῶ τοὺς ἀνθρώπους μετέχοντας... ὁ γὰρ ἐν τῷ καθόλου μὴ γινώσκων ὁποῖα τά τε θεῖα καὶ τὰ ἀνθρώπινα πράγματά εἰσιν, οὐδ᾽ ἐν τῷ κατὰ μέρος οὐδ᾽ ἐπιστημονικῶς τι ἑλέσθαι καὶ φυγεῖν δύναται.

---

20   χωρὶς τῶν ἐκ φιλοσοφίας λόγων. οὐ γὰρ ὡμίλησε φιλοσόφοις ἐν νεότητι, *Ind.* 58–9 (19,2–3 BJP).

21   On this point see further Singer, P. N. (2014). 'Galen and the Philosophers: Philosophical Engagement, Shadowy Contemporaries, Aristotelian Transformations', in Adamson, P., Hansberger, R. and Wilberding, J. (eds) *Philosophical Themes in Galen*, 7–38. Kaufman, 'Galen on the Therapy', argues that διαλεχθῆναι at 78, 24,7 BJP means 'philosophical conversation', but this seems to me a considerable over-translation, supported only by the doubtful contention that Galen is here echoing a specific passage of Epicurus. A more natural reading is surely that Galen is simply referring in a general way to conversations with friends.

For no other man esteemed justice and self-control as completely as he ...
I know that my father despised human affairs as trivial things ... he valued those who live a life devoted to pleasure no more highly than those
birds we see being taken round Rome by their masters to service females
for a price. But those who despise such pleasures, and are content with
neither experiencing pain nor distress in their souls, he never praised. He
declared that the good was something bigger and more powerful than
that, something which possessed its own nature rather than being defined only in terms of not suffering pain or distress. But if someone de-
parts from these and holds that the good is a knowledge of matters both
human and divine, I see that human beings possess only a very small
part of this ... For someone without even general knowledge of matters
human and divine cannot choose scientifically in individual matters, either, what to choose and what to avoid.

> *Ind.* 58–64 (18,22–20,10 BJP)

The refusal to praise those who are *satisfied* with being free from distress can
surely be placed alongside the remark in *Affections* suggesting the attempt to
attain *alupia* as a crucial, but not sufficient, stage in ethical progress.[22] This feature of the *Peri alupias* argument – that it does not present a straightforward
rejection of Epicurean *aochlēsia* and/or Stoic *apatheia*, but rather a statement
of their *insufficiency* – seems to me a vital one. The two passages are, in fact, of a
piece: both are suggesting the drive towards *alupia* as a practical starting-point
in the attempt at ethical self-improvement; and both are asserting that *alupia*
is necessary, but by no means sufficient, for virtue. If we wish to talk of ends
or goals, we must mention 'knowledge of things human and divine' – however
imperfectly we may attain to that.[23]

    As both this passage and that immediately following makes clear: (a) human
affairs are to be despised; (b) freedom from distress is valuable; but (c) it is not
sufficient, as there are higher human aims. These are reasserted a few lines later

---

22   The caution should be made that the verb 'praised' in the above text represents a conjec-
      ture (BJP's ἐπῄνεσεν for the MS ἔπεισεν); it is, however, a very plausible one, and it seems
      that the text must in any case be advancing *some* contrast between mere satisfaction with
      alupia on the one hand and higher goals on the other.
23   The precise progress of the argument in this passage is not straightforward, and it is pos-
      sible to interpret differently the attitude towards the notion of 'knowledge of the human
      and divine' that Galen is here presenting. I take it that Galen is expressing the extreme
      difficulty of gaining knowledge in this area, but not rejecting such knowledge altogether
      as a goal; rather, *some* effort in this direction will be of ethical value. See the discussions
      of this same passage in this volume by both Chris Gill and Jim Hankinson.

in the words 'wishing to be actively engaged in both mind and body', πάντα ... ἐνεργεῖν ... βουλόμενα καὶ κατὰ σῶμα καὶ κατὰ ψυχήν, 68, 21,7–8 BJP. (One must acknowledge, here, that this is presented as not merely a human aim, but in fact also that of 'all animals', the word πάντα here referring back to οὔτε ἐμαυτὸν οὔτε ἄλλον ἄνθρωπον οὔτε ζῷον τι – and in doing so one must also acknowledge that there an anti-Epicurean rhetoric at work here which has arguably taken Galen to a slightly unusual place in his argument, as made clear by the pejorative mention of *aochlēsia* and, indeed, by the explicit reference to other writings in which he attacks Epicurus.)[24] There is also a similarity between the two texts in the way in which these 'higher-level', or intellectual, aims are presented – and perhaps above all in the vagueness with which they are presented. If we turn to the relevant discussion in *Errors* – the part of that text devoted to the rational soul as opposed to the non-rational – two things seem striking in this context. One is Galen's apparent slipperiness when it comes actually to defining 'the goal of life';[25] the other is that, whatever the precise answer on that, he is more interested in persuading one to engage in rational training and rational scientific activity than in any goal which would more obviously be defined as ethical.

One might even say that rational or intellectual activity of the correct kind, in that text, provides an answer that seems to stand in place of the answer to 'the goal of life'; and that, perhaps, corresponds (at least as far as human beings are concerned) to what Galen describes here as 'being actively engaged in both mind and body'. Galen (or his father) seems to have developed an interesting practical-ethics approach here. We might summarize the two-step approach as follows:

(i)   Ethical improvement must start with the identification of something that causes one actual distress, *lupē*. Once one has achieved that identification, the desire to make a change allows the possibility, at least, that one will make some progress. One is no longer in denial, at this stage, and may seek practical interventions to lessen one's susceptibility. If one then succeeds in radically reducing one's susceptibility to *lupē*, this is a necessary, but by no means sufficient, condition of virtue.

---

24   A list of nine works engaging with Epicurean philosophy is given at *Lib. Prop.* 19 [16]; it is, relatedly, interesting to speculate, though we can do no more, as to how important this emphasis on 'active engagement' may have been in these lost works.

25   On this point see the discussion of Donini, P. L. (1988). 'Tipologia degli errori e loro correzione secondo Galeno', in Manuli, P. and Vegetti, M. (eds) *Le opere psicologiche di Galeno: Atti del terzo Colloquio Galenico internazionale, Pavia, 10–12 settembre 1986,* 65–116 and Singer, *Galen: Psychological Writings,* 229–32.

(ii)   While it is difficult to define precisely the goal in this higher realm – that
       of the rational soul – some things are clear. In particular, (a) the aims
       pursued by most people – political ambition, accumulation of wealth –
       are to be despised; and (b) some kind of mental engagement, or direct-
       ed activity, is essential to human life. Fairly clearly, too, the type of such
       activity strongly preferred by Galen (and his father) is that aimed at the
       acquisition of knowledge, especially (as far as possible) knowledge of a
       mathematically reliable kind.

In relation to step (ii), and in particular the definition of 'the goal', there is, as
already suggested, some vagueness – though we should here acknowledge the
limitations of our sources, since a considerable list of Galen's ethical writings
is lost to us. But it also seems at least possible that Galen is deliberately vague
in this context, preferring a strong argument in favour of intellectually rigorous
and mathematically-based mental activity to a conventional definition of virtue of the sort approved by any of the established philosophical schools. The
above talk of a two-step approach should not, however, be taken to deny the
interconnectedness of the phases. The removal, or reduction, of one's liability
to distress is for Galen intimately related to the adoption of appropriate life
aims, or to which things in life we take to be valuable or not valuable. The
early education mentioned above simultaneously instils appropriate notions
of what counts as good *and* habituates one to appropriate reactions and behaviour: the rational (evaluative) and non-rational (habituated) responses go
hand in hand. This connectedness is particularly reinforced, in περὶ ἀλυπίας,
in sections 80–81, where the absence of distress is closely correlated with an
appropriate assessment of the aims of honour, wealth, reputation and political
power. (And especially so if we adopt the reading of this passage suggested by
Garofalo, whereby 'those who do not suffer distress as the many do' are equated
with 'those who have a moderate attachment to honour, etc.')[26] Here again, it
seems, the taking of the two texts, *Affections and Errors* and περὶ ἀλυπίας, alongside each other, has helped to form a picture of Galenic thinking in this area.

A final point is worth our consideration: what range of emotional reactions
is admissible within *alupia*? For Galen, as we have already suggested, *lupē* is a
quasi-medical category. The usual context for its mention is in consideration
of predisposing causes that can lead to physical ailments of various kinds.
The example of the literary man dying of grief should not, perhaps, from
this perspective, be seen as an extreme one. This, Galen seems to suggest, is
within normal medical experience: it is the sort of thing that *lupē* can do, or
rather lead to. Galen's boast is that he was seen to be 'not moved at all', 'not

---

26   See in this volume Singer, 'Note on MS Vlatadon 14', text (t).

distressed', that he 'bore it easily'; and scholars have not been slow to point to both the boastfulness and the apparently unrealistic nature of the claim. But what exactly is meant here? It seems to me that Galen is not, in fact, presenting some other-wordly, saint-like behaviour. The point rather is that he is able to go about his daily business; he does not succumb; he does not allow his life to be ruined.

The terms used for what does *not* happen to Galen – *kinēthenta, aniathēnai* – seem to me perfectly consistent with the notion that one experiences *some* negative emotional reactions; what is crucial is that they are controlled, not allowed to dominate. And such control is a perfectly possible – Galen quite plausibly argues – as a result of the right kind of training in childhood in combination with ethical discipline, involving a consideration of how small such setbacks are in the scheme of things, in adulthood. The social aspect of one's reaction, too, is relevant to this discourse. Galen uses a range of expressions to describe the visual or outward aspect of his behaviour: you *saw* that I was not moved, I was *observed* bearing it easily; the reaction is described as wonderful; it is compared with that of others; the term *phaidron*, too (literally 'bright', 'radiant'), refers to an outward demeanour or impression. The observable, outward aspect must be considered; self-control includes a competitive element: one is judged by one's ability publicly to rise above the normal reaction. But there must, surely, be a range of negative emotions which a person may experience without being defined as falling into *lupē*.

By *lupē*, in short, Galen means something more dramatic and more specific – and, in medical terms, far more dangerous – than a controllable feeling of sadness or annoyance. It is a negative emotion whose control is central to the ethical project of self-improvement, and which if uncontrolled can have disastrous medical consequences. In both contexts, the ethical and the medical, Galen develops the concept in a distinctive and original way. A way which, above all, attempts to do justice to the realities, the challenges and the dangers of lived experience.

Acknowledgements

The author gratefully acknowledges the financial support of the Wellcome Trust and the Alexander von Humboldt-Stiftung during the research and writing of this paper. Heartfelt thanks go also to the editor, Caroline Petit, for her invitation to participate in the conference from which this chapter arose, and especially for her very helpful advice and encouragement during its subsequent development. The faults which it retains are, of course, my own.

References

Secondary Literature

Asmis, E. 'Galen's *De indolentia* and the Creation of a Personal Philosophy'. In *Galen's De indolentia*, ed. C. K. Rothschild and T. W. Thompson, 127–42. Tübingen: Mohr Siebeck, 2014.

Boudon-Millot, V. 'Un traité perdu de Galien miraculeusement retrouvé, le *Sur l'inutilité de se chagriner*: texte grec et traduction française'. In *La science médicale antique: nouveaux regards (Études réunies en l'honneur de Jacques Jouanna)*, ed. V. Boudon-Millot, A. Guardasole and C. Magdelaine, 73–123. Paris: Éditions Duschesne, 2007.

Boudon-Millot, V. (ed., trans. and notes) *Galien, Tome I*, Paris: Les Belles Lettres, 2007.

Boudon-Millot, V. and Jouanna, J. (ed. and trans.), with A. Pietrobelli, *Galien, Oeuvres, 4: Ne pas se chagriner*. Paris: Les Belles Lettres, 2010.

Donini, P. L. 'Tipologia degli errori e loro correzione secondo Galeno'. In *Le opere psicologiche di Galeno: Atti del terzo Colloquio Galenico internazionale, Pavia, 10–12 settembre 1986*, ed. P. Manuli and M. Vegetti, 65–116. Naples: Bibliopolis, 1988.

Donini, P. L. 'Psychology'. In *The Cambridge Companion to Galen*, ed. R. J. Hankinson, 184–209. Cambridge: Cambridge University Press, 2008.

Gill, C. *Naturalistic Psychology in Galen and Stoicism.* Oxford: Oxford University Press, 2010.

Hankinson, R. J. (ed.) *The Cambridge Companion to Galen*. Cambridge: Cambridge University Press, 2008.

Kaufman, D. H. 'Galen on the Therapy of Distress and the Limits of Emotional Therapy', *Oxford Studies in Ancient Philosophy* 47 (2014), 275–96.

Kotzia, P. 'Galen *Peri alupias*: Title, Genre and Two Cruces'. In *Studi sul De indolentia di Galeno*, ed. D. Manetti, 69–91. Pisa and Rome: Fabrizio Serra Editore, 2012.

Kotzia, P. 'Galen, *De indolentia*: Commonplaces, Traditions, and Contexts'. In *Galen's De indolentia*, ed. C. K. Rothschild and T. W. Thompson, 91–126. Tübingen: Mohr Siebeck, 2014.

Kotzia, P. and Sotiroudis, P. Γαληνοῦ *Peri alupias*, *Hellenica* 60 (2010), 63–148.

Kraus, P. 'Kitāb al-Akhlāq li-Jālinus', *Bulletin of the Faculty of Arts of the Egyptian University* 5.1 (1937/9), 1–51.

Manetti, D. (ed.) *Studi sul De indolentia di Galeno*, Pisa and Rome: Fabrizio Serra Editore, 2012.

Manuli, P. and Vegetti, M. (eds). *Le opere psicologiche di Galeno: atti del terzo Colloquio Galenico Internazionale, Pavia, 1986*. Naples: Bibliopolis, 1988.

Mattern, S. P. 'Galen's Anxious Patients: *Lypē* as Anxiety Disorder'. In *Homo Patiens*, ed. G. Petridou and C. Thumiger, 203–23. Leiden and Boston: Brill, 2016.

Nutton, V. (ed. and trans.) *Galen: De propriis placitis*, Berlin: Akademie Verlag (CMG V 3,2), 1999.

Rosen, R. 'Philology and the Rhetoric of Catastrophe in Galen's *De indolentia*'. In *Galen's* De indolentia, ed. C. K. Rothschild and T. W. Thompson, 159–74. Tübingen: Mohr Siebeck, 2014.

Singer, P. N. *Galen: Selected Works*. Translation with introduction and notes. Oxford: Oxford University Press, 1997.

Singer, P. N. (ed.) *Galen: Psychological Writings: Avoiding Distress, The Diagnosis and Treatment of Affections and Errors Peculiar to Each Person's Soul, Character Traits and The Capacities of the Soul Depend on the Mixtures of the Body*, translated with introduction and notes by V. Nutton, D. Davies and P. N. Singer, with the collaboration of Piero Tassinari. Cambridge: Cambridge University Press, 2013.

Singer, P. N. 'Galen and the Philosophers: Philosophical Engagement, Shadowy Contemporaries, Aristotelian Transformations', in *Philosophical Themes in Galen*, ed. P. Adamson, R. Hansberger and J. Wilberding, Bulletin of the Institute of Classical Studies Supplement 114, 7–38. London: Institute of Classical Studies, 2014.

Singer, P. N. 'The Essence of Rage: Galen on Emotional Disturbances and their Physical Correlates'. In *Selfhood and the Soul: Essays on Ancient Thought and Literature in Honour of Christopher Gill*, ed. R. Seaford, J. Wilkins and M. Wright, 161–96. Oxford: Oxford University Press, 2017.

Vegetti, M. *Galeno: nuovi scritti autobiografici*. Rome: Carocci, 2013.

Texts: Editions, Translations and Abbreviations

ps.-Andronicus

Peri pathōn

Aristotle

Eth. Nic. = Nicomachean Ethics

Cicero

Fin. = De finibus

Diogenes Laertius

Vit. Phil. = Vitae Philosophorum

Galen

Texts of Galen are cited by volume and page number in Kühn's edition, followed where available by page and line number in the most recent critical edition.

K. = C. G. Kühn, *Claudii Galeni Opera Omnia*, 22 vols. Leipzig, 1821–1833.

CMG = Corpus Medicorum Graecorum, Leipzig and Berlin, 1908–.

Aff. Pecc. Dig. 1 and 2 = *De propriorum animi cuiuslibet affectuum dignotione et curatione* and *De animi cuiuslibet peccatorum dignotione et curatione* (*Affections and Errors of the Soul*). [K. v]. Ed. W. de Boer. Berlin and Leipzig: Teubner, CMG V 4,1,1, 1937; trans. in Singer, *Galen: Psychological Writings*.

Hipp. Epid. VI = *In Hippocratis Epidemiarum librum* VI (*Commentary on Hippocrates 'Epidemics VI'*). [K. XVIIA–B (partial)]. Ed./German trans. E. Wenkebach and E. Pfaff. Berlin: Akademie Verlag, CMG V 10,2,2, 1956.

Ind. = *De indolentia* (*Peri alupias*). [Not in K.] Ed. V. Boudon-Millot and J. Jouanna, with the collaboration of A. Pietrobelli: *Ne pas se chagriner*. Paris: Les Belles Lettres, 2010 (BJP); trans. by V. Nutton in Singer, *Galen: Psychological Writings*.

Lib. Prop. = *De libris propriis* (*My Own Books*). [K. XIX]. Ed. V. Boudon-Millot. Paris: Les Belles Lettres, 2007; trans. in Singer, *Galen: Selected Works*.

MM = *De methodo medendi.* (*The Therapeutic Method*). [K X]. Trans. I. Johnston and G. H. R. Horsley. Cambridge, Mass.: Harvard University Press (Loeb), 2011.

Mor. = *De moribus.* (*Character Traits*). [Not in K.]. Ed. Kraus, 'Kitāb al-Akhlāq', trans. D. Davies in Singer, *Galen: Psychological Writings*.

Ord. Lib. Prop. = *De ordine librorum propriorum* (*The Order of My Own Books*). [K. XIX]. Ed. V. Boudon-Millot. Paris: Les Belles Lettres, 2007; trans. in Singer, *Galen: Selected Works*.

PHP = *De placitis Hippocratis et Platonis* (*The Doctrines of Hippocrates and Plato*). [K. v]. Ed. and trans. P. De Lacy, 3 vols. Berlin: Akademie Verlag, CMG V 4,1,2, 1978–84.

Praen. = *De praenotione ad Epigenem.* (*Prognosis*). [K. XIV]. Ed. and trans. V. Nutton. Berlin: Akademie Verlag (CMG V 8,1), 1979.

QAM = *Quod animi mores corporis temperamenta sequantur.* (*The Soul's Dependence on the Body*). [K. IV]. Ed. I. Müller, in *C. Galeni Scripta Minora*, 2. Leipzig: Teubner, 1891; trans. in Singer, *Galen: Psychological Writings*.

San. Tu. = *De sanitate tuenda.* (*Matters of Health*). [K. VI]. Ed. K. Koch. Berlin and Leipzig: Teubner, CMG V 4,2, 1923.

Temp. = *De temperamentis.* (*Mixtures*). [K. I]. Ed. G. Helmreich. Leipzig: Teubner, 1904.

'Pythagoras'

Ed. J. C. Thom, *The Pythagorean Golden Verses*. Leiden, New York and Cologne: Brill, 1995.

Stobaeus

Ecl. = *Eclogae*

CHAPTER 8

Wisdom and Emotion: Galen's Philosophical Position in *Avoiding Distress*

Teun Tieleman

1 Introduction

Soon after its recovery in 2005, Galen's *Avoiding Distress* (περὶ ἀλυπίας) was recognized as an extremely important new source of information on its author's
life and times. Writing shortly after the murder of the emperor Commodus (192
CE) Galen provides intriguing glimpses of the latter's reign of terror, at least
as experienced by members of the imperial court and the senatorial circles in
which he moved (esp. §§ 54–57; cf. 50). In addition, scholars were intrigued
by what Galen tells us about his collection of books and the libraries of Rome
which had been destroyed by the great fire that struck Rome at the end of 192
CE. This 'cultural catastrophe' (in Vegetti's apt phrase)[1] is presented as the immediate occasion for the writing of the tract: a long-standing friend of Galen's
from his native Pergamum (who however remains anonymous) has sent him a
letter asking how Galen managed to cope with this terrible blow, which not only
involved books by himself and other authors but also drugs, recipes for drugs
as well as medical instruments. In particular, the friend is curious to know how
Galen had avoided succumbing to distress (λύπη). *On Avoiding Distress* (hereafter
Ind.), a 'letter-treatise,'[2] is Galen's reply and clearly a very personal kind of docu-
ment. At the same time, it clearly stands in a literary and philosophical tradition.
Christopher Gill[3] has pointed out that it invites comparison with Plutarch's *On
Tranquillity of Mind* (Περὶ εὐθυμίας), another letter-treatise aimed at helping its

---

1 Vegetti, M., *Galeno. Nuovi scritti autobiografici. Introduzione, traduzione e commento di –.*
Carocci editore, 2013, p. 254.

2 On this ancient genre see Stirewalt, L.M., *Studies in Ancient Greek Epistolography*, SBL
Resources for Biblical Study 27. Atlanta, GA, Scholars Press, 1993, pp. 18–19; cf. *eiusd*. 'The
Form and Function of the Greek Letter-Essay,' in K.P. Dornfried, *The Romans Debate. Revised
and Expanded Edition*, Peabody Mass., Hendrickson Publishers, 1991, pp. 147–171 (p. 152). Cf.
Kotzia, P., 'Galen περὶ ἀλυπίας: title, genre and two cruces,' in Manetti, D. ed., *Studi sul De
Indolentia di Galeno*, 2012, pp. 69–92 (p. 69).

3 Gill, C., *Naturalistic Psychology in Galen and Stoicism*, Oxford, 2010, p. 262. We may also compare Cicero, *Tusculans* book III.

readers avoid or at least moderate distress (465a, 465d). But in fact tracts entitled Περὶ λυπῆς and written by philosophers from various schools are attested from the Hellenistic period onwards, a line comparable to that devoted to other emotions such as the *On Anger* literature.[4] Galen's treatise, then, should be considered against the backdrop of ancient philosophical therapeutics with which it shares some of its arguments and *exempla*, as has been shown by others. In fact, Galen had read and worked on Chrysippus' celebrated *Therapeutics* (the fourth book of the latter's *On Emotions*). His refutation of its moral psychology in *PHP* books IV and V some thirty years before the writing of *Ind.* did not keep him from referring to Chrysippus' work as a well-known and useful moral guide in *On Affected Parts* III, 1 (VIII, p. 138 K. = *SVF* III, 457). Just as doctors belonging to different medical schools concurred in prescribing particular therapies of proven efficacy, so too the philosophical therapist may be pragmatic about the arguments and exercises he recommends, regardless of their original provenance. This is illustrated by Galen above all.

As has been noted by Nutton, Asmis and others, Galen in *Ind.* shows himself to be both pragmatic and independent in working out his position on the basis of his philosophical education as well as his own experience, both personal and medical.[5] But more can and should be done to gauge Galen's acquaintance with philosophical sources and to determine how exactly he uses them to develop his own point of view. Here of course different options were open to Galen. In fact, his position has been associated with the ideal of the moderation of emotion (*metriopatheia*) and the Aristotelian tradition in particular.[6] I want to redress the balance in favour of the Stoic by highlighting what I believe are instances of his discriminating and creative use of Stoic concepts. It is clear that Galen has strong doubts about the possibility of eradicating, in himself and others, all emotions, i.e. the Stoic ideal of complete freedom from emotion, *apatheia* (ἀπάθεια). He also distances himself from the moral heroics of the kind exemplified by Stoics such as Musonius (§ 73). Yet Galen's reminders

---

4   For some examples see Kotzia, P., 'Galen περὶ ἀλυπίας: title, genre and two cruces,' 2012, p. 74.

5   Nutton, V., *Galen, Avoiding Distress* (translation and introduction) in P. N. Singer *et al.* (eds.) *Galen. Psychological Writings*, Cambridge, CUP, 2013, p. 66; Asmis, E. 'Galen's *De indolentia* and the Creation of a Personal Philosophy,' in Rothschild & Thompson eds., *Galen's* De indolentia. *Essays on a newly Discovered Letter*, 2014, esp. 128–129 ("personal philosophy"); Kaufman, D. H., 'Galen on the Therapy of Distress and the Limits of Emotional Therapy,' *Oxford Studies in Ancient Philosophy* 47, 2014, pp. 275–296 (p. 294).

6   On the moderation vs. eradication debate in antiquity see Dillon, J., '"Metriopatheia and Apatheia": Some Reflections on a Controversy in later Greek ethics,' in J.P. Anton & A. Preuss (eds.) *Essays on Ancient Greek Philosophy*, vol. II, 1983, 508–517; Sorabji, R., *Emotion and Peace of Mind. From Stoic Agitation to Christian Temptation*, Oxford, 2000, pp. 194–210; S. Weisser, *Eradication on modération des passions. Histoire de la controverse chez Cicéron et Philon d'Alexandre*, *Monothéismes et Philosophie*, forthcoming from Brepols (Turnhout) (*non vidi*).

of our human weakness and vulnerability and the limits of emotion therapy[7] should not distract us from the fact that he does find a use for several Stoic ideas and arguments. It is not as if the Stoics were content to hold out the distant ideal of the sage: they had developed a complete therapeutics address-ing the needs of all those still very much prone to emotion.[8] But Galen also claims that he feels no emotion whatsoever at least in regard to certain things that most people would experience as extremely painful. This again looks like *apatheia* rather than all-round *metriopatheia*. How should we explain this po-sition and how coherent is it?

2   The Status of Philosophy

It useful first to take stock of the attitude to philosophy taken by Galen in these pages. The treatise opens with a reference to the letter of his friend requesting him to disclose which training or which arguments or which doctrines had caused him never to experience distress.[9] Some translators show a distinct reluctance to render the third option (δόγματα) through a term such as 'doc-trines' or 'creeds' let alone 'dogmas' as too specific and suggestive of sectarian affiliation.[10] Although the sentence purports to give the phrasing of Galen's old friend, the latter must have been aware that Galen avoided association with any philosophical school in particular and so did not imply any affiliation on Galen's part. But this seems over-cautious. The dramatic situation implies a long separation between Galen and his friend, who had remained in far-off Pergamum, and now wonders how Galen had succeeded in responding to his great losses with such enviable equanimity. Apart from that, the term in the sense of philosophical doctrine does not commit Galen to the acceptance of all doctrines of any particular school, which would amount to the sectarian atti-tude he denounces elsewhere. Of course, Galen avoids doctrines unsupported by experience and may use the term in rejecting dogmatism of the speculative

---

7   On which see further Kaufman, D. H., 'Galen on the Therapy of Distress and the Limits of Emotional Therapy,' *Oxford Studies in Ancient Philosophy* 47, 2014, pp. 275–296.

8   Stoic therapy starts from the needs and possibilities of the person in the grip of emotion; cf. *infra*, n. 45.

9   *Ind.* 1, p.2.3–5 BJP: "Ἔλαβόν σου τὴν ἐπιστολὴν ἐν ᾗ παρεκάλεις μοι δηλῶσαί σοι τίς ἄσκησις ἢ λόγοι τίνες ἢ δόγματα <τίνα> παρεσκεύασαν με μηδέποτε λυπεῖσθαι.

10   Nutton renders 'considerations' (explained in n.3), Boudon and Jouanna's French has 'conceptions,' Lami and Garofalo, however, translate, correctly I think, 'dottrine' and so does Vegetti. Similarly λογοί is rendered 'discours' by Boudon and Jouanna and 'discorsi' by Lami and Garofalo and by Vegetti. Nutton here translate, more precisely, 'arguments.' See also Kotzia, P., 'Galen, *De indolentia*: Commonplaces, Traditions, and Contexts,' 2014, pp. 96–97.

kind. But he freely ascribes them to his heroes Hippocrates and Plato, as in the title of his *PHP*, which pertains to doctrines in moral psychology, elementary theory and methodology.[11] So in Galen's case too, asking about his doctrines comes as a natural question, especially among educated people who look to philosophy for moral guidance.[12] Elsewhere in *Ind.* and other works Galen refers to education (παιδεία) and nature (φύσις) as sources of mental strength and of the ability to avoid distress.[13] For members of his social class (as his own biography illustrates) this education included philosophy. By opening his tract in this particular way, then, Galen effectively announces that his answer to his friend's question will address his relation to philosophy and philosophical schools, as indeed we find him doing later on.[14]

The linking of doctrines, arguments and training invites comparison with *An. Dig.* 6.7, p.25.15–19 DB (= V, p. 37 K.), where a young man who is troubled by small matters asks Galen how it is possible that he is not even affected by big ones, "either through training or particular doctrines or natural make-up."[15] The situation clearly runs parallel to the opening passage of *Ind.* Here Galen omits mention of natural capacity – only to stress it more forcefully in the later parts of *Ind.* (§§ 57–59).[16] This may be a particular emphasis of Galen's. Other authors just give the pair of doctrines and training.[17] Likewise at *An. Dig.* 3.14–4.1, p.12–16 De Boer (V, p.4 K.) Galen says that even the person with the best natural aptitude (εὐφυεστατος)[18] and finest moral education

11   Cf. *PHP* 3.1.33, 4.7.23. At *Loc. Aff.* VIII, 191 K Galen distinguishes common notions (κοιναὶ ἔννοιαι) and doctrines (δόγματα), the latter forming the subject of debates among philosophers and physicians.

12   For the linking found at *Opt. Doct.* 100, l.9 Barigazzi (I, 47 K.): ἐν φιλοσοφίᾳ καὶ δόγμασι.

13   They are often linked this way: see *Ind.* 51, p.16.17–20; *ibid.* 57, p.18.17–18, 79, p. 24.12–15 BJP. *Loc. aff.* VIII, p. 301 K.

14   §§ 62–68, on which see *infra*, pp. 208–211.

15   *An. dig.* V. 37: ἡ λύπη δ᾿ ἅπασι φαίνεται κακόν, ὥσπερ ὁ πόνος ἐν τῷ σώματι. καί τις τῶν συνηθεστάτων ἐμοὶ νεανίσκων ἐπὶ σμικροῖς ἀνιώμενος, ἐς ἑσπέραν ποτὲ κατανοήσας τοῦτο, παραγενόμενος πρός με <κατὰ> βαθὺν ὄρθρον ὅλης ἔφη τῆς νυκτὸς ἀγρυπνῶν ἐπὶ τῷδε τῷ πράγματι μεταξύ πως εἰς ἀνάμνησιν ἀφικέσθαι μου μηδ᾿ ἐπὶ <τοῖς> μεγίστοις οὕτως ἀνιωμένου, ὡς ἐπὶ τοῖς μικροῖς αὐτός. ἠξίου <δ᾿ οὖν> μαθεῖν, ὅπως μοι τοῦτο περιεγένετο, πότερον ἐξ ἀσκήσεως ἢ τινων δογμάτων ἢ φύντι τοιούτῳ.

16   Cf. Kaufman, D. H., 'Galen on the Therapy of Distress and the Limits of Emotional Therapy,' 2014, p. 291.

17   For the linking of philosophical doctrines (δόγματα) and training (ἄσκησις) see Celsus *ap.* Origenes, *Contra Celsum* 1.2, l. 4; Hippolytus, *Ref.* 9.13.6, 9.27.2.

18   The idea of a natural aptitude of souls for virtue (εὐφυΐα) appears to have been a particularly Stoic concern. Already Cleanthes devoted a tract to it: *SVF* I, 481 (p.107, l.15). Another testimony (*SVF* III, 366, from Stobaeus) aligns aptitude with being well-born or nobility (εὐγενεία) understood in a philosophically purged, moral sense (cf. Seneca, *Ep.* 44) but also refers to a debate among Stoics about the relative contributions towards virtue

remains fallible so that we remain in need of training (ἄσκησις) throughout life. Conversely, training is useless for those with no natural aptitude or without an excellent education (Ind. 57, p.18 BJP). The method of training he recommends is imagining that one's worst fears come true, i.e. the technique of 'dwelling in advance' (προενδημεῖν), which was recommended by Stoics and other philosophers.[19] According to Galen

> The wise man (σοφὸς ἀνήρ) constantly reminds himself of everything he might possibly suffer, but someone who is not wise (σοφός), provided that he does not live like an animal, is in some way also stimulated to a knowledge of the human condition by the realities of daily life (§ 53, translation Nutton, slightly altered).[20]

Obviously, the wise person as the embodiment of an ideal was never meant to leave the non-wise any excuse for not undertaking the effort of self-improvement. But Galen's point seems to be that this piece of wisdom is not

---

by nature and training. Further, εὐφυία and its opposite ἀφυία are classed as preferred and not-preferred indifferents respectively: SVF III, 127, 135, 136. The Stoic sage will fall in love with young men who show their aptitude for virtue through their countenance: SVF III, 716. Further evidence closer in time to Galen comes from educational contexts in Epictetus: Diss. 1.29.35, 2.16.17, 2.24.28, 3.6.9 (= Musonius fr. 46), 3.6.10 (education reinforces natural aptitude), 3.23.14, 4.10.3; similarly Musonius Rufus: Frs. 46, Diss. 1, l.35, 13b, l.10. Passages such as the ones just listed show that the Stoics, like e.g. Aristotle before them, recognized that people are born with different capacities for moral virtue; hence this is not peculiar to Galen. Modern scholars however tend to stress the egalitarian nature of Hellenistic therapy, e.g. Kaufman, D. H., 'Galen on the Therapy of Distress and the Limits of Emotional Therapy,' 2014, p. 293: "Epicurean and Stoic therapy [...] are [...] fully applicable to anyone at all, whatever their nature and upbringing."

19 Cic. Tusc. 3.28–31 (with particular reference to distress) ascribes the idea to the Cyrenaics (cf. ibid. 59), but says at 3.52 that Chrysippus the Stoic was of the same opinion. Cf. also Seneca, Ad Marciam 9.1–10; 11.1. See Sorabji, R. Emotion and Peace of Mind, 2000, p. 236 for discussion and further references. On the technique in Ind. See Kotzia, P., 'Galen, De indolentia: Commonplaces, Traditions, and Contexts,' 2014, p. 107–114.

20 Galen at § 52 cites a passage from an otherwise lost play by Euripides (fr. 814 Mette, fr. 964 Nauck) in which the speaker – Theseus – says that he learned from a wise man to imagine constantly disasters that might hit him, so that if one were to occur it would not be novel and affect his soul. He cites it again at § 77. If the reading ὑπέρ (p. 23.6 BJP) is correct Galen takes Theseus to speak on behalf of Euripides himself, who had reportedly studied with the philosopher Anaxagoras, a tradition recorded by Cicero, Tusc. 3.30. See also Nutton ad loc. (n. 114). For the same quotation see PHP 4.7.10–11 (Posid. F165 EK) where he takes it from the Stoic Posidonius and also refers to Anaxagoras who famously said when he was told about his son's dead: 'I knew I had begotten a mortal.'

something elevated but lies for grabs for anyone with a bit of sense and some experience of life.

3   Magnanimity

In *Ind.* the virtue, or excellence, enabling us to cope with the blows dealt by fate and so avoid becoming distressed is 'greatness of soul' or magnanimity (μεγαλοψυχία).[21] Thus at *Ind.* 50–51, p.16.10–19 BJP Galen says:

> Not to be distressed (μὴ λυπηθῆναι) at the loss of all my drugs, all my books, and, besides, the recipes of major drugs, as well as the writings on them I had prepared for publication along with many other treatises [...], that is already a prime display of nobility (γενναῖον) and nigh on magnanimity (μεγαλοψυχίας). What led me to such magnanimity you already know first because you were brought up with me from the start and educated alongside me (translation Nutton's).

Galen goes on to explain that in addition to upbringing and education he had profited from his observations of political life in Rome, which had driven home to him the need to remind oneself of everything one might possibly suffer, i.e. use the technique of 'dwelling in advance' (προενδημεῖν) as a form of training (§ 52–53). Once again we find the same sources of moral success which Galen often links and stresses: upbringing, education, training (see section 2 above). For our present purposes it may be observed that the magnanimity Galen has in mind is the mental or moral strength which results when these factors work to one's advantage so that one is not, or not to the same extent, distressed because of trouble. Further, it may be noted that Galen does not claim to have reached the state of magnanimity but something close to it. A related passage *On Affected Parts* VIII, pp. 301–302 K. links Galen's notion of magnanimity as invulnerability to distress to that of tension:

> In those in whom the vital tension is weak and who experience strong psychic affections from lack of education, the substance of the soul is

---

21   Already Gill, *Naturalistic Psychology in Galen and Stoicism*, 2010, p. 264 has pointed out that Galen characterizes magnanimity in Stoic terms rather than Aristotelian ones; he was followed by Kotzia, P., 'Galen, *De indolentia*: Commonplaces, Traditions, and Contexts,' 2014, p. 107. Nutton, *Galen, Avoiding Distress*, 2013, p. 92 n. 94 refers to the Epicureans alongside the Stoics.

easily dissoluble. Of people of this kind some have indeed died from distress, albeit not instantly [...]. But no magnanimous man ever met his death either as a result of forms of distress or other affections stronger than distress, for the tension of their soul is strong and its affections small.[22]

It is interesting to note that Galen here seems to ascribe a crucial role to education rather than natural endowment, but he may take this for granted. What this passage adds is the notion of the soul's tension (τόνος), which is best known from Stoic moral psychology: good tension (εὐτονία) is based on the right balance of the psychic pneuma enabling the soul to withstand the impact of incoming impressions, whereas lack of tension (ἀτονία) is linked to mental weakness (ἀκρασία) and a soul prone to emotion.[23] It is especially the second scholarch Cleanthes who seems to have stressed the notion of mental strength in relation to moral excellence.[24] For him and other Stoics these notions refer to corporeal realities, in particular the tension of the psychic pneuma. Galen does not subscribe to the Stoic theory of a pneumatic soul and is reluctant to pronounce upon the substance (οὐσία) of the soul, to which he nonetheless refers in the above passages. But what may have weighed a great deal for him is the fact Plato too speaks of the soul's tension (and relaxation) in *Republic* III, in a passage dealing with the impact of particular forms of education on the souls of the prospective guardians (411e–412a; cf. 411a), which may in fact have inspired the Stoics to introduce the idea in the corporealist psychology they developed.[25]

---

22 ὅσοις γὰρ ἀσθενής ἐστιν ὁ ζωτικὸς τόνος, ἰσχυρά τε πάθη ψυχικὰ πάσχουσιν ἐξ ἀπαιδευσίας, εὐδιάλυτος τούτοις ἐστὶν ἡ τῆς ψυχῆς οὐσία· τῶν τοιούτων ἔνιοι καὶ διὰ λύπην ἀπέθανον, οὐ μὴν εὐθέως ὥσπερ ἐν τοῖς προειρημένοις· ἀνὴρ δ' οὐδεὶς μεγαλόψυχος οὔτ' ἐπὶ λύπαις οὔτ' ἐπὶ τοῖς ἄλλοις ὅσα λύπης ἰσχυρότερα θανάτῳ περιέπεσον· ὅ τε γὰρ τόνος τῆς ψυχῆς αὐτοῖς ἰσχυρός ἐστι τά τε παθήματα σμικρά.

23 On the soul's τόνος and related terms ee esp. the verbatim fragments from Chrysippus' *On Affections* preserved by Galen, *PHP* IV.6 and printed by Von Arnim as *SVF* III, 473.

24 See esp. Plut. *Stoic. Rep.* 7, p.1034d (*SVF* I Cleanthes 563): ὁ δὲ Κλεάνθης ἐν ὑπομνήμασι φυσικοῖς εἰπὼν ὅτι πληγὴ πυρὸς ὁ τόνος ἐστί, κἂν ἱκανὸς ἐν τῇ ψυχῇ γένηται πρὸς τὸ ἐπιτελεῖν τὰ ἐπιβάλλοντα, ἰσχὺς καλεῖται καὶ κράτος, ἐπιφέρει κατὰ λέξιν, "ἡ δ' ἰσχὺς αὕτη καὶ τὸ κράτος, ὅταν μὲν ἐν τοῖς φανεῖσιν ἐμμενετέοις ἐγγένηται, ἐγκράτειά ἐστιν· ὅταν δ' ἐν τοῖς ὑπομενετέοις, ἀνδρεία· περὶ τὰς ἀξίας δὲ δικαιοσύνη· περὶ τὰς αἱρέσεις καὶ ἐκκλίσεις σωφροσύνη.

25 On Galen's notion of mental tension and the Platonic and Stoic backdrop see Trompeter, J. 'Die gespannte Seele: Tonos bei Galen.' *Phronesis* 61.1, 2016, pp. 82–109; cf. also Vegetti M., 'I nervi dell'anima,' in J. Kollesch & D. Nickel (eds.) *Galen und das hellenistische Erbe. Verhandlungen des 4. Internationalen Galen-Symposiums*, Stuttgart, Franz Steiner Verlag, 1993, pp. 63–77.

Galen links magnanimity to another notion as well: contempt, viz. of possession or what he elsewhere in *Ind.* calls human matters. Here contempt means
looking down on them as small or unimportant, that is to say, have the correct
view on their true value. This fortifies the soul so that it can deal with their loss.
The idea is also in the background of Galen's exchange with the troubled young
man as recounted in *An. dig.* (see above, p. 202): the young man is kept from
his sleep by small things, whereas Galen is not even troubled by big ones. In
Ind. Galen's own father provides an example of this attitude.[26] This can also be
expressed as the ability of rising above them so that they look small. But again
Galen makes it clear that he himself cannot rise above all forms of adversity.
Thus he would not make light of the prospect of being roasted in the bull of
Phalaris (as the Epicurean and Stoic varieties of the sage were supposed to
do).[27]

The notion of magnanimity at issue here is Stoic rather than Aristotelian,
even if present-day students may be more familiar with Aristotle's magnanimous person as portrayed in *Nicomachean Ethics* IV.3: the not entirely likeable
character who is conscious of his own worth and acts accordingly. The Stoic notion, however, is not so much concerned with pride and self-esteem but closely
related to courage. Galen in one passage from *PHP* seems turn the Stoic notion
against the Stoic Chrysippus and so must have been fully conscious of its provenance.[28] Magnanimity (μεγαλοψυχία,) is classed as a subspecies of courage
(ἀνδρεία) in early Stoic texts, viz. "the knowledge that makes us rise above those
things that are of such a nature that they happen to wise and non-wise alike."[29]
This clearly refers to the fated, unavoidable events of the potentially frighten-
ing and distressing kind, depending on whether one is capable of assessing

---

26   Gal. *Ind.* 49, p. 16.3 BJP: [...] καταφρονήσαντι παντοδαπῆς ἀπωλείας κτημάτων [...]; *ibid.* 61,
      p.19.13–15: Οἶδα δὲ μου τὸν πατέρα καταφρονοῦντα τῶν ἀνθρωπίνων πραγμάτων ὡς μικρῶν.
      Ibid. 71, 22.1–2: [...] μέχρι τοῦ μὴ καταφρονεῖν [...] τοῦ Φαλάριδος ταύρου. Cf. 62, 19.20, 78.24.3.
27   Gal. *Ind.* 78b, p. 23.14 BJP: Οὐ μὴν ὑπεράνω πασῶν [*scil.* ἀνιαρὰς περιστάσεις] εἰμι... *Ibid.* 71,
      22.1–2: [...] μέχρι τοῦ μὴ καταφρονεῖν [...] τοῦ Φαλάριδος ταύρου. Cf. 62, 19.20, 78.24.3.
28   *PHP* 3.2.18 De Lacy (cf. *SVF* II, 906, p. 254, 1–18): Galen sarcastically speaks of the magna-
      nimity of the Stoic Chrysippus as proven from his undeterred attitude in citing poetic
      lines that actually tell against the Stoic cardiocentric doctrine of the soul he has set out to
      defend. Galen here uses a Stoic virtue to bestow mock-praise on a Stoic.
29   *SVF* III, 264 (Stobaeus) τὴν δὲ ἀνδρείαν περὶ τὰς ὑπομονάς· [...] τῇ δὲ ἀνδρείᾳ [*scil.* ὑποτετάχθαι]
      καρτερίαν, θαρραλεότητα, μεγαλοψυχίαν, εὐψυχίαν, φιλοπονίαν [...] μεγαλοψυχίαν δὲ ἐπιστήμην
      ὑπεράνω ποιοῦσαν τῶν πεφυκότων ἐν σπουδαίοις τε γίνεσθαι καὶ φαύλοις. Identical definition
      at *SVF* II, 269 (ps. Andronicus). Cf. *SVF* III, 265 (Diog. Laert. 7.92): τὴν δὲ μεγαλοψυχίαν
      ἐπιστήμην <ἢ> ἕξιν ὑπεράνω ποιοῦσαν τῶν συμβαινόντων κοινῇ φαύλοις τε καὶ σπουδαίοις.

their value correctly (i.e. as indifferents).[30] This, then, is the notion with which we find Galen operating in *Ind.* The prominence it is given here may reflect the fact that well before Galen's time magnanimity was upgraded vis-à-vis courage, a move that may perhaps be associated with the name Panaetius of Rhodes (ca. 185–109 BCE) and, at least as its status is concerned, reflect Aristotelian influence.[31] Thus Cicero in his *On Duties*, presumably drawing on Panaetius' work of the same title, presents magnanimity among the four main or generic excellences as that which resides in the "greatness and strength of an elevated and invincible mind" marked by a "contempt for human matters."[32] Had the early Stoics already typified magnanimity as the ability of rise above human life's ups and downs as inconsequential, the idea is now also expressed in terms of holding them in contempt or despising them, as in Galen's text. Panaetius' associate Hecato of Rhodes (who may have lived on well into the first century BCE) made the further step of classing courage, alongside mental health, strength and beauty, among a new class of excellences or virtues, viz. the non-theoretical ones, which unlike the theoretical ones do not involve assent and, according to the report given by Diogenes Laertius, could even be possessed by the non-wise.[33] Like the innate aptitude for moral progress towards excellence, good mental qualities of this sort had been acknowledged by the early Stoics, who classed them as preferred indifferents.[34] Hecato's move may have been motivated by his wish to integrate the qualities in question more completely into the Stoic ethical system.[35] For our purposes suffice it to note that Hecato retained the link between theoretical and non-theoretical excellences, de-scribing them as supervening on the theoretical ones: thus health is said to be co-extensive with and attendant upon temperance.[36] This then must also have been the relation between magnanimity, a theoretical virtue, and courage. But

---

30   As is clear from the definition of courage, the generic concept: SVF II, 262 (Stob.): ἀνδρείαν
      δὲ ἐπιστήμην δεινῶν καὶ οὐ δεινῶν καὶ οὐδετέρων. Philo, *Leg. all.* 67 (SVF II, 263): ἐπιστήμη γάρ
      ἐστιν ὑπομενετέων καὶ οὐχ ὑπομενετέων καὶ οὐδετέρων.
31   See Dyck, A., 'Panaetius' conception of μεγαλοψυχία,' *Museum Helveticum* 38, 1981, 153–161.
32   Cic. *Off.* 1, 5, 15 (= T 56 Alesse, fr. 103 vStr., part): omne quod est honestum, id quattuor par-
      tium oritur ex aliqua. Aut enim in perspicientia veri sollertiaque versitur, aut in hominum
      societate tuenda tribuendoque suum cuique et rerum contractarum fide, *aut in animi ex-
      celsi atque invicti magnitudine et robore*, aut in omnium quae fiunt und dicuntur ordine et
      modo, in quo inest modestia et temperantia. Cf. *ibid.* 1, 13 (= T 55 Alesse, fr. 98 v.Str., part)
      magnitudo animi exsistit humanarumque rerum *contemptio*; cf. III, 96 and Posidonius *ap.*
      Sen. *Ep.* 87.32, 35 (magnitudo animi) = F 170 EK.
33   D.L. 7.90 = Hecato Fr. 6 Gomoll.
34   See SVF III, 127, 136.
35   For more discussion and further references see Pohlenz (1984) 240–241, (1980) 123–124.
36   D.L. 7.90 = Hecato Fr. 6.

if theoretical virtue entails non-theoretical virtue, non-theoretical virtue does not entail theoretical virtue, since non-wise persons can have non-theoretical virtues such as courage. But how exactly the non-theoretical qualities functioned, must remain a moot point. Maybe they constituted a person's natural aptitude for moral progress and the attainment of virtue in the theoretical sense but this must remain an assumption for lack of evidence. But we do possess an argument from Hecato's second book *On Goods* on magnanimity as the basis for the Stoic thesis that virtue is sufficient in itself for happiness:

> For if, he says [*scil.* Hecato], magnanimity is sufficient for raising us above everything and magnanimity is a part of virtue, then too virtue will be sufficient in itself for happiness, despising all things that seem troublesome (transl. Hicks, slightly modified).[37]

This fragment is not only concerned with the same notion of magnanimity as is used by Galen,[38] but it makes magnanimity the key to the excellent person's invulnerability. Hecato no doubt reflects the prominence of the notion among Stoics from Panaetius onwards. This prominence itself is also reflected by Galen in his turn.

The idea of taking a bird's eye view at human affairs as a way of achieving tranquillity is of course widespread, especially in Stoic and Cynicizing literature, and not necessarily in conjunction with the specific virtue of magnanimity. There is something of this attitude in Galen too, although it neither leads to the degree of detachment from the *comédie humaine* one encounters in some Cynic and even Stoic texts, where laughing can be presented as the only adequate response of the philosopher.[39]

---

37   Hecato *ap.* D.L. 7.127–128 = fr. 3 Gomoll: εἰ γὰρ, φησίν, αὐτάρκης ἐστὶν ἡ μεγαλοψυχία πρὸς τὸ πάντων ὑπεράνω ποιεῖν, ἔστι δὲ μέρος τῆς ἀρετῆς, αὐτάρκης ἔσται καὶ ἡ ἀρετὴ πρὸς εὐδαιμονίαν καταφρονοῦσα καὶ τῶν δοκούντων ὀχληρῶν.

38   Cf. Gal. *Ind.* 78b, p. 23.14 BJP: Οὐ μὴν ὑπεράνω πασῶν [*scil.* ἀνιαρὰς περιστάσεις] εἰμι… 49, p. 16.3 BJP: […] καταφρονήσαντι παντοδαπῆς ἀπωλείας κτημάτων […]; *ibid.* 61, p.19.13–15: Οἶδα δέ μου τὸν πατέρα καταφρονοῦντα τῶν ἀνθρωπίνων πραγμάτων ὡς μικρῶν. *Ibid.* 71, 22.1–2: […] μέχρι τοῦ μὴ καταφρονεῖν […] τοῦ Φαλάριδος ταύρου.

39   Even the Stoic Seneca can speak like this: *Ep.* 41.5: vis isto divina descendit; animum excellentem, moderatum, omnia tamquam minora transeuntem, quidquid timemus optamusque ridentem … Cf. *ibid.* 78.18 (laughing while under torture), 80.6 (laughing in spite of poverty). For a bird's eye passage in his work see also the beginning of the second book of the *Natural Questions*.

4   Wisdom

Despising human affairs as of little value – a moral attitude Galen attributes to his father and says he has adopted himself in his old age (*Ind.* § 61; cf. 65) – saves one from distress: one no longer supposes that one has been deprived of something big (§ 66). This of course raises the question of where true value lies. What is the real good? In what follows at §§ 62–68 Galen considers the positions of two philosophical schools: Epicureanism and Stoicism. Having said that his father rejected common, non-philosophical hedonism, Galen adds that he never praised those who were satisfied with being free from pain or distress in their souls – a clear reference to the Epicureans (§ 62): Galen's father felt that the good must be of its nature something bigger than just being free from something (ibid.). Here it is to be understood that Galen follows his father. At the end of the section (§ 68), speaking now on his own behalf, he adds an argument against the Epicurean ideal of remaining undisturbed: this goes against the observable fact human beings and indeed all animals want to be active in both mind and body, as he had established earlier in his work (now lost) *Against* (or *On*) *Epicurus*.

In §§ 63 and 64 he considers the position of those who take the good to be "knowledge of matters both human and divine:"

> (63) If someone will [...] hold that the good is a knowledge of matters both human and divine, then I see that mankind possesses only a very small part of this, and that, if it is so very small, we cannot have a precise knowledge of everything else also. (64) But someone who has not even a general knowledge of matters human and divine can neither make even in part or scientifically a decision on what to choose and what to avoid (translation Nutton's).[40]

Commentators have been quick to identify the definition of the good as Aristotelian.[41] However, they have been unable to produce sound textual support fort his identification. In fact we have to look elsewhere, to Stoicism. Thus

---

40   *Ind.* 63–64, p.20.2–10: Ἀλλ᾽ ἐὰν καὶ τούτων [scil. the Epicurean doctrines] τις ἀποχωρήσας ἐπιστήμην θείων καὶ ἀνθρωπίνων πραγμάτων ἡγήσηται τὸ ἀγαθὸν ὑπάρχειν, ἐλάχιστου μορίου τούτου ὁρῶ τοὺς ἀνθρώπους μετέχοντας. εἰ δὲ τοῦτο ἐλάχιστον, δῆλον ὅτι καὶ τῶν ἄλλων ἁπάντων ἀκριβῆ γνῶσιν οὐκ ἔχομεν· ὁ γὰρ ἐν τῷ καθόλου μὴ γινώσκων ὁποῖα τά τε θεῖα καὶ τὰ ἀνθρώπινα πράγματα εἰσὶν, οὐδ᾽ ἐν τῷ κατὰ μέρος, οὐδ᾽ ἐπιστημονικῶς τι ἑλέσθαι καὶ φυγεῖν δύναται.

41   Thus Boudon-Jouanna *ad loc.* ("La terminologie est clairement Aristotélicienne"), Nutton *ad loc.* (n. 104), citing Arist. *Met.* VI.1, 1026a18–32; XI.7, 10641–4, following Hankinson, R.J., *Galen, On the Therapeutic Method, Books I and II*, 1991, p. 82, who cites them in connection

we encounter the same definition with explicit attribution tot he Stoics in the proem to the Aëtian *Placita*: "The Stoics have said that wisdom is the knowledge of things human and divine, whereas philosophy is the exercise of expertise in utility."[42] And Sextus Empiricus borrows the same definition from his dogmatist opponents, who, here as elsewhere, are to be identified as the Stoics: "Philosophy is the pursuit of wisdom, and wisdom is the knowledge of things divine and human."[43]

As we have seen, Galen objects to this conception of the good that it lies beyond the reach of mankind. Our knowledge is limited and imprecise – which means that we cannot makes decisions about what to choose and what to avoid on the basis of knowledge (ἐπιστημονικῶς). Leaving aside for a moment the question whether this is a fair piece of criticism of Stoicism and a strong argument, it is worth noting that in addition to the definition of the good we have here another echo of a Stoic definition, viz. that of moderation as the knowledge of what to choose and what to avoid, as can be attested by several sources.[44]

Having established that Galen is engaging with the Stoics, we may now take a closer look at his argument. As we have seen, he presents Stoicism as requiring general knowledge of an impossibly broad range of subjects. This is unattainable so we are left empty-handed in regard to the decisions we have to make in particular situations also. In fact, our knowledge is very limited.

---

with the same definition of philosophy as distinguished from the liberal arts used by Galen at *MM* I.2, X p. 2 K.

42 Aëtius, *Placita I. Prooem.* 2 (*SVF* II, 35): οἱ μὲν οὖν Στωϊκοὶ ἔφασαν τὴν μὲν σοφίαν εἶναι θείων τε καὶ ἀνθρωπίνων ἐπιστήμην, τὴν δὲ φιλοσοφίαν ἄσκησιν ἐπιτηδείου τέχνης· ἐπιτήδειον δὲ εἶναι μίαν καὶ ἀνωτάτω τὴν ἀρετήν, ἀρετὰς δὲ τὰς γενικωτάτας τρεῖς, φυσικὴν ἠθικὴν λογικήν· δι' ἣν αἰτίαν καὶ τριμερής ἐστιν ἡ φιλοσοφία, ἧς τὸ (5) μὲν φυσικόν, τὸ δὲ ἠθικόν, τὸ δὲ λογικόν· καὶ φυσικὸν μὲν ὅταν περὶ κόσμου ζητῶμεν καὶ τῶν ἐν κόσμῳ, ἠθικὸν δὲ τὸ κατησχολημένον περὶ τὸν ἀνθρώπινον βίον, λογικὸν δὲ τὸ περὶ τὸν λόγον, ὃ καὶ διαλεκτικὸν καλοῦσιν.

43 Sextus, *M* IX, 13 (= *SVF* II, 36): τὴν φιλοσοφίαν φασὶν ἐπιτήδευσιν εἶναι σοφίας, τὴν δὲ σοφίαν ἐπιστήμην θείων τε καὶ ἀνθρωπίνων πραγμάτων. Cf. *ibid.* IX 123 = *SVF* II, 1017.

44 Stobaeus *Ecl.* II 59, 4 W. (*SVF* III, 362): φρόνησιν δ' εἶναι ἐπιστήμην ὧν ποιητέον καὶ οὐ ποιητέον καὶ οὐδετέρων ἢ ἐπιστήμην ἀγαθῶν καὶ κακῶν καὶ οὐδετέρων φύσει πολιτικοῦ ζώου (καὶ ἐπὶ τῶν λοιπῶν δὲ ἀρετῶν οὕτως ἀκούειν παραγγέλλουσι). σωφροσύνην δ' εἶναι ἐπιστήμην αἱρετῶν καὶ φευκτῶν καὶ οὐδετέρων· δικαιοσύνην δὲ ἐπιστήμην ἀπονεμητικὴν τῆς ἀξίας ἑκάστῳ· ἀνδρείαν δὲ ἐπιστήμην δεινῶν καὶ οὐ δεινῶν καὶ οὐδετέρων. Cf. *SVF* III, 263, 274. Plut. *Stoic. Rep.* 7, p.1034d (*SVF* I Cleanthes 563, for which fr. See also *supra*, n. 24): "ἡ δ' ἰσχὺς αὕτη καὶ τὸ κράτος [...] περὶ τὰς αἱρέσεις καὶ ἐκκλίσεις σωφροσύνη." Galen, *PHP* VII 2 (208. 591 M.) (= *SVF* I Ariston 374): νομίσας γοῦν ὁ Ἀρίστων μίαν εἶναι τῆς ψυχῆς δύναμιν, ᾗ λογιζόμεθα, καὶ τὴν ἀρετὴν τῆς ψυχῆς ἔθετο μίαν, ἐπιστήμην ἀγαθῶν καὶ κακῶν. ὅταν μὲν οὖν αἱρεῖσθαί τε δέῃ τἀγαθὰ καὶ φεύγειν τὰ κακά, τὴν ἐπιστήμην τήνδε καλεῖ σωφροσύνην· ὅταν δὲ πράττειν μὲν τἀγαθά, μὴ πράττειν δὲ τὰ κακά, φρόνησιν· ἀνδρείαν δὲ ὅταν τὰ μὲν θαρρῇ, τὰ δὲ φεύγῃ. ὅταν δὲ τὸ κατὰ ἀξίαν ἑκάστῳ νέμῃ, δικαιοσύνην.

Galen goes on to explain that this realization kept him from politics and public office, all the more so since he saw that even decent politicians could do little for people in need (§ 64). This point may reflect the Stoic injunction to take part in politics and government: so Stoicism does not equip us with workable principles for taking care of other people's lives through politics as well as leading our own lives. He goes on (§ 65) to say that "brought up in this way of thinking" he always considers "all these things" (i.e. presumably the pursuit of social and political goals) as of little worth. So how could he suppose "leisure, instruments, drugs, books, reputation and riches to be precious"? Here we have some of the items he had indeed lost in the great fire, adding a few others of what the Stoics classed as indifferents such as reputation and riches. Clearly, Galen is now back again at his task of explaining why the losses of the kind he suffered did not distress him (and nor will others in the same category might these occur in the future). But the logic of this passage is not very clear. Nutton indicates some textual uncertainties which may lie behind our difficulties. Galen's critique of Stoicism as failing to provide an attainable ideal and so a workable basis for morality and politics switches to his own limitations and difficulties when he explains why he did not enter politics. This leads to the biggest leap, viz. that Galen looks down on human affairs as of little worth. Ironically, this conclusion states what every decent Stoic would also subscribe to, namely that we should not make our well-being depend on external items such as possessions or a good reputation, for if we do we shall be distressed when we loose them.

After this Galen goes on to wind up his argument, saying that he believes that he has given a full answer to his friends question about avoiding distress (§69). However, he does not stop at this point, but presents a conclusion, first about himself (§ 69–79) and then (§ 79, end-84) mankind in general. At § 71 he summarizes his own relation to distress as follows:

> Now I cannot say if there is anyone so wise that he is entirely free from affections, but I have a precise knowledge of the degree to which I am such a one: I do not care about the loss of possessions without quite being deprived of them all and sent to a desert island, or of bodily pain without quite making light of being placed in the bull of Phalaris. What will distress me is the ruination of my homeland, or a friend being punished by a tyrant, and other similar things, and I pray to the gods that none of this should ever happen to me (translation Nutton's).

First we have a reference to Stoic *apatheia*: Galen doubts whether anyone is so wise as to have attained this ideal and be entirely free of them. But speaking for himself he makes it clear that he does not care about loss of possessions or bodily pain. The claim here is that in these cases he is free from affections, most notably distress. But there are exceptions. He goes on to give examples of extreme misfortune that will distress him: a homeland ruined, a friend punished (some of his examples surfaced earlier in connection with Commodus' tyrannical rule). From the Stoic point of view these things count as indifferent and hence, ideally, should not be allowed to trigger an emotional response either.[45] Galen does not say that a moderate emotional response is in order here. Neither here, nor elsewhere in his treatise, does he say or imply that the personal catastrophe he suffered in loosing his books, drugs and recipes, elicited distress only to a *moderate* degree. This is not his personal ideal. The final part shows that the emphasis is different. Galen says he will fortify his soul through training: without ever being able to respond like the Stoic wise man he can hope to display endurance (καρτερία, 79a). It is striking that Galen once again dwells on the method of anticipating misfortune as the only training he finds helpful against painful bad turns (§ 76–77).

As we have seen, Galen next turns to mankind in general, attributing people's unhappiness to their being immoderately (ἀμέτρως) attached to esteem, wealth, reputation and political power. Their insatiable desires will not fail to make them unhappy (81). There is also a reference to those who are only moderately (μετρίως) attached to these things, but the text is uncertain at this point: Galen probably implies that the moderate ones are best placed to avoid unhappiness, at least to some degree. In this connection Galen praises his friend for his simple lifestyle and curbing his desires.

Galen does not apply what he says here to himself, but comments on the situation in which other people find themselves. For them moderation of desire and emotional attachment is the best they can achieve. Does this place Galen in the *metriopatheia* camp?[46] I think not. The objects in question include some of those which Galen had said he does not mind loosing *at all*, most notably

---

45   As Graver points out in 'The Weeping Wise: Stoic and Epicurean Consolations in Seneca's
      99th Epistle,' in T. Fögen, ed. *Tears in the Graeco-Roman World*, Berlin-New York, De
      Gruyter, 2009, pp. 235–252 (p. 237), Stoic authors of works of consolation such as Seneca
      regularly give some leeway to grief experienced in moderation (though not to grieve at all
      would be better): see e.g. *Ep.* 63.1.

46   Cf. Hankinson, R. J., 'Actions and passions: affection, emotion and moral self-management
      in Galen's philosophical psychology,' in J. Brunschwig & M. Nussbaum (eds.) *Passions &
      Perceptions. Studies in Hellenistic Philosophy of Mind*, 1993, pp. 203–204, who, writing on
      this issue long before the discovery of *Ind.*, notes that no clear answer tot his question is to
      be found in the texts but proceeds to offer a tentative suggestion, viz. that Galen may have
      advocated extirpation only in the case of excessive and uncontrollable emotion, which is
      pathos in the sense of disease, i.e. an unnatural condition, while accepting emotion in the

possessions and political power. When he adds that he expects to be distressed by being deprived of life's barest necessities, he is just marking off his own position against the moral heroics of diehard Stoics such as Musonius Rufus (cf. § 73, where he dismisses Musonius Rufus, who had prayed to Zeus to send him *any* eventuality). But on the other hand we have seen that Galen stresses his complete indifference to *certain* bad turns or losses, which is definitely not an expression of *metriopatheia* but rather of selective *apatheia*, at least as an ideal for himself to pursue; others may get no further than respond with moderate emotion to misfortunes. One may compare Philo, *Leg. Alleg.* III, 129–132, who draws a distinction between *metriopatheia* as appropriate to the man of median virtue who is still progressing (symbolized by Aaron) and *apatheia* as proper to the accomplished sage (symbolized by Moses), as if, in John Dillon's apt words, the concepts could be accommodated on a sliding scale.[47]

Platonists could not derive from Plato's work clear and unequivocal guidance when it came to deciding on which side they should be in this controversy, which had arisen some time after Plato under the influence of Stoicism. Like Philo, Platonists of the Imperial period display a striking unwillingness or inability to keep the two competing alternatives apart.[48] Galen, not an adherent of the Platonist (or any other) school but a great admirer of Plato, also combines the two options. An emphasis peculiar to him seems to be his doubts as to whether complete *apatheia* (which may be desirable as such) is attainable in real life, given our basic needs and vulnerability as human beings.

5   **Conclusion**

I have been highlighting a few concepts that seem central to the position developed by Galen in regard to distress. Even if he stresses the role of natural aptitude, family background and upbringing, he is not averse to philosophy but on the contrary draws on philosophical concepts, arguments and debates

---

sense of the natural activity of the soul's affective part. But instead of being a compromise position this would just boil down to *metriopatheia*.

47   Dillon, J., '"Metriopatheia and Apatheia": Some Reflections on a Controversy in later Greek ethics,' 1983, p. 515. For *metriopatheia* and *apatheia* as corresponding to two different stages of moral progress see Plotinus, *Enn.* 1.2.2 (14–18) and 1.2.3 (20), who links them to ordinary 'civic' virtue and what 'purified' virtue respectively. Cf. Sorabji, R. *Emotion and Peace of Mind*, 2000, p. 203. Contrast Seneca, *Ep.* 116 for a clear statement of the difference between moderation and eradication from a Stoic point of view.

48   Dillon, J., '"Metriopatheia and Apatheia": Some Reflections on a Controversy in later Greek ethics,' 1983, pp. 515–516.

to a greater degree than sometimes has been assumed, especially in the case of Stoicism. There is the prominence given to the Stoic virtue of magnanimity. But we have found more Stoic elements. Indeed, the distinction between natural aptitude, training and philosophical education is philosophical in itself, reflecting as it does Stoic distinctions and debates. Another recurrent element is the ideal of wisdom. Here Galen demarcates his position vis-a-vis Stoicism or at least its hardline variety that peddles a form of moral heroics and an unattainable ideal of complete freedom from emotion (*apatheia*). As we have seen, the alternative developed by Galen is not aimed at moderation of emotion. Affections are to be avoided as much as possible and with regard to some objects or situation it is possible to avoid them completely, as in the case of Galen's response to the loss of his books, drugs and recipes. For many other people moderation of emotion is the most they can achieve.

References

Asmis, E. 'Galen's *De indolentia* and the Creation of a Personal Philosophy,' in Rothschild & Thompson eds., *Galen's* De indolentia. *Essays on a newly Discovered Letter*. Studien und Texte zu Antike und Christentum 88. Tübingen: Mohr Siebeck, 2014, pp. 127–142.

Boudon – Millot, V. & J. Jouanna, eds., *Galien, Tome IV: Ne pas se chagriner*. Avec la collaboration de A. Pietrobelli. Paris, Les Belles Lettres, 2010.

Deichgräber, K., 'Galen als Erforscher des menschlichen Pulses. Ein Beitrag zur Selbstdarstellung des Wissenschaftlers (De dignotione pulsuum I 1),' *Sitzungsberichte Ak. Wiss. Berlin. Kl. Sprache, Literatur und Kunst*, 1956, 3 (Berlin: Akademie-Verlag 1957).

Dillon, J., '"Metriopatheia and Apatheia": Some Reflections on a Controversy in later Greek ethics,' in J. P. Anton & A. Preuss (eds.) *Essays on Ancient Greek Philosophy*, vol. II (Albany: SUNY Press) 1983, 508–517; repr. as Study nr. VIII in J. M. Dillon, *The Golden Chain. Studies in the Development of Platonism and Christianity*, Aldershot, Variorum 1990.

Dyck, A., 'Panaetius' conception of μεγαλοψυχία,' *Museum Helveticum* 38, 1981, 153–161.

Garofalo, I. & A. Lami, eds., *Galeno. L'anima e il dolore*. De indolentia. De propriis placitis. Classici greci e latini. Milano, Bur Rizzoli, 2012

Gill, C. 'Peace of Mind and Being Yourself: Panetius to Plutarch,' *ANRW* II.36.7, 1994, 4599–4640.

Gill, C., *Naturalistic Psychology in Galen and Stoicism*, Oxford, 2010, [262–266].

Graver, M., 'The Weeping Wise: Stoic and Epicurean Consolations in Seneca's 99th Epistle,' in T. Fögen, ed. *Tears in the Graeco-Roman World*, Berlin-New York, De Gruyter, 2009, pp. 235–252.

Hankinson, R. J., *Galen, On the Therapeutic Method, Books I and II. Translated with an Introduction and Commentary*, Clarendon Press, Oxford, 1991.

Hankinson, R. J., 'Actions and passions: affection, emotion and moral self-management in Galen's philosophical psychology,' in J. Brunschwig & M. Nussbaum (eds.) *Passions & Perceptions. Studies in Hellenistic Philosophy of Mind. Proceedings of the Fifth Symposium Hellenisticum*, Cambridge, CUP, 1993, pp. 184–222.

Kaufman, D. H., 'Galen on the Therapy of Distress and the Limits of Emotional Therapy,' *Oxford Studies in Ancient Philosophy* 47, 2014, pp. 275–296.

Κοτζιά, Π. – Π. Σωτηρούδης, Γαληνού Περὶ ἀλυπίας, ΕΛΛΗΝΙΚΑ 60, 2010, pp. 63–150.

Kotzia, P., 'Galen περὶ ἀλυπίας: title, genre and two cruces,' in Manetti, D. ed., *Studi sul De Indolentia di Galeno*, 2012, pp. 69–92.

Kotzia, P., 'Galen, *De indolentia*: Commonplaces, Traditions, and Contexts,' in Rothschild & Thompson, *Galen's* De indolentia. *Essays on a newly Discovered Letter*, 2014, pp. 91–126.

Manetti, D. ed., *Studi sul* De Indolentia *di Galeno*. Vol. 4 of *Biblioteca di "Galenos"; Contributi alla ricerca sui testi medici antichi*. Pisa: Fabrizio Serra, 2012.

Nutton, V., *Galen, Avoiding Distress* (translation and introduction) in P. N. Singer *et al.* (eds.) *Galen. Psychological Writings*, Cambridge, CUP, 2013, pp. 43–106.

Pohlenz, M., *Die Stoa. Geschichte einer geistigen Bewegung*, 2. Band, Göttingen, Vandenhoeck und Ruprecht, 5. Auflage, 1980.

Pohlenz, M. *Die Stoa. Geschichte einer geistigen Bewegung*, 1. Band, Göttingen, Vandenhoeck und Ruprecht, 6. Auflage, 1984.

Rothschild, C. K. and T. W. Thompson, eds., *Galen's* De indolentia. *Essays on a newly Discovered Letter*. Studien und Texte zu Antike und Christentum 88, Tübingen, Mohr Siebeck, 2014.

Sorabji, R., *Emotion and Peace of Mind. From Stoic Agitation to Christian Temptation*, Oxford, OUP, 2000.

Stirewalt, L. M., 'The Form and Function of the Greek Letter-Essay,' in K. P. Dornfried, *The Romans Debate. Revised and Expanded Edition*, Peabody Mass., Hendrickson Publishers, 1991, pp. 147–171.

Stirewalt, L. M., *Studies in Ancient Greek Epistolography*, SBL Resources for Biblical Study 27. Atlanta, GA, Scholars Press, 1993.

Trompeter, J., 'Die gespannte Seele: Tonos bei Galen.' *Phronesis* 61.1, 2016, pp. 82–109.

Vegetti M., 'I nervi dell'anima,' in J. Kollesch & D. Nickel (eds.) *Galen und das hellenistische Erbe. Verhandlungen des 4. Internationalen Galen-Symposiums*, Stuttgart, Franz Steiner Verlag, 1993, pp. 63–77; repr. In M. Vegetti, *Dialoghi con gli antichi*. A cura de Silvia Gastaldi *et al.* (Akademia Verlag 2007) pp. 279–296.

Vegetti, M., *Galeno. Nuovi scritti autobiografici. Introduzione, traduzione e commento di –* . Carocci editore, 2013.

Weisser, S., Eradication on modération des passions. Histoire de la controverse chez Cicéron et Philon d'Alexandre, *Monothéismes et Philosophié*, forthcoming from Brepols (Turnhout) (*non vidi*).

PART 3

Galen's Περὶ Ἀλυπίας *and the History of the Roman Empire*

∵

CHAPTER 9

Galen and the Plague

Rebecca Flemming

Galen's περὶ ἀλυπίας contains two references to the great plague which characterised his times, now usually known as the 'Antonine Plague'. Neither is sustained or substantial, the new information offered is slight and somewhat slippery; but these passages make an important point none the less. Both serve to emphasise what might be called the qualitative impact of the pestilence, as distinct from its quantitative effects on the economy and population, the political integrity and resilience, of the Roman Empire. These have been the focus of much recent debate, and there is a lot at stake in the discussions, inconclusive as they have been so far; but other key issues – the personal toll of the plague, the miasmatic way in which it touched everything, became embedded in everyday life and record, even structured time – have been rather overlooked in the search for data, and the contest between models.[1] Galen's struggle against distress, in this and other areas, offers an opportunity to redress the balance somewhat, put the spotlight back on questions of what it was like to live through repeated waves of pestilence, not just as a physician, but also a man with friends and household dependents, a man located at the centre of Empire, in close proximity to imperial power.

The first move Galen makes in setting up the main premise of the περὶ ἀλυπίας – that he is a man in such admirably firm control of his response to potentially upsetting events, to a variety of losses, that he can usefully instruct others in emotional management – is in reference to the plague.[2] Its presence provides a natural frame for any such exposition, and one particular occurrence offers a good case of his exemplary conduct in this respect. For it was witnessing Galen's imperturbability despite the death of almost all the slaves he had in Rome, 'during a major outbreak of the long-lasting plague', which

---

1 Launched by R. Duncan-Jones' key article, 'The impact of the Antonine Plague', *JRA* 9 (1996), 108–136, the quantitative bibliography is now extensive. See e.g. E. Lo Cascio (ed.), *L'impato dell' 'Peste Antonina'* (Bari: Edipuglia, 2012); and most recently, Colin P. Elliott, 'The Antonine plague, climate change, and local violence in Roman Egypt', *Past and Present* 231 (2016), 3–31.

2 The introductory sequence is Gal. *Ind.* 1–7.

had initially impressed the unknown addressee of this epistolary text.[3] He had heard other stories of non-disturbance in the face of misfortune too, and, now, reports of Galen's unchanged demeanour and behaviour after an even worse disaster had reached him, generating a keen desire to discover how Galen does it. What training and teaching kept him steady following the devastation of the great fire which had consumed all the possessions he kept in the alleged safety of the substantial storehouses on the Sacred Way? Possessions which included many, many valuable, valued, and even irreplaceable books and things which had all burned, without apparently troubling Galen.

It is, indeed, in enumerating these destroyed possessions, in providing exquisite detail about the worth, the meaning, of all he has lost, that Galen makes his second reference to the plague.[4] Amongst his massive losses was perhaps the best collection of pharmacological recipes in the whole Roman world, accumulated through both active endeavour and the workings of fate. These workings had seen his fellow-citizen and student, Teuthras, obtain from another Pergemene physician – Eumenes – an outstanding compilation of remedies and then leave them to Galen, 'having died in the first outbreak of the plague' at Rome.[5] The timing of this inheritance, 'a little after' (μετ' ὀλίγον χρόνον) Galen first came to the imperial capital himself, may be significant in terms of broader pestilential chronology, but there are also more particular points to make, about both the casualness and the poignancy of this plague reference. There is a sense in which the course of this epidemic disease and Galen's career share a temporal structure, and combine to produce patterns of meaning for him.

These references are best understood, however, as part of a larger Galenic package, alongside Galen's other engagements with the 'great plague', and, indeed, against the background of more general historical descriptions of the disease, its profile and patterning. So, this is what follows, though necessarily in a targeted rather than total way. First a rough outline of the origins and spread of the 'Antonine Plague', as reported in a range of sources, including Galen, will be sketched out, then there will be further discussion of the disease itself, a topic on which Galen also has a lot to offer. Too much, indeed to cover

---

3   Gal. *Ind.* 1: κατὰ τινα τοῦ πολυχρονίου λοιμοῦ μεγάλην ἐμβολὴν (2, 6–7 BJP). Translations are my own unless noted. I have made much use of V. Nutton's translation, notes and introduction to the text, however (in P. Singer (ed.), *Galen: Psychological Writings* (Cambridge: Cambridge University Press, 2013), 43–106); as well as those in the main edition I have used: V. Boudon-Millot, J. Jouanna and A. Pietrobelli (ed., trans. and comm.), *Galien: Ne pas se chagriner* (Paris: Les Belles Lettres, 2010).

4   This sequence is Gal. *Ind.* 31–35.

5   Gal. 34–5: ἀποθανὼν ἐν τῇ πρώτῃ τοῦ λοιμοῦ καταβολῇ (12.15–16 BJP).

in this essay, the main aim here is to illustrate where Galen puts the emphasis in this respect, what is important to him about the plague as a medical event, before considering the identity of the disease in modern terms. Finally, the focus will return to the specific contributions of περὶ ἀλυπίας to this pestilential story, to the question of the emotional impact of the plague, to matters of sensibility and distress.

1   Profile of a Plague: Origins and Outbreaks

The accounts of the 'Antonine Plague' provided in surviving historical texts are both patchy and programmatic, and though there is some roughly contemporary reporting, most are much later than the events they describe. Still, they are reasonably consistent in outline.[6] The pestilence originated in the East, where Lucius Verus (co-emperor with Marcus Aurelius) was campaigning against the Parthians in the mid-160s AD. A moment of military indiscipline, probably of impiety, in a temple in Babylonia as the conflict was coming to a successful conclusion is evoked as the immediate cause in some sources; though others omit any mention of a specific trigger for disaster.[7] All agree, however, that Verus' troops brought disease back west with them on their victorious return. Rome, Italy, and the provinces were all affected, and the army was particularly badly hit; a concern with Roman manpower is thematised by many of the authors.[8] In his fourth-century summary of Roman history, for example, Eutropius asserts that the outbreak of plague following the Persian victory under Marcus Aurelius was so severe that, 'in Rome and throughout Italy and the provinces most people, and almost all soldiers in the army, were afflicted by weakness'.[9] This was especially dangerous since the empire was now facing a threat along its north-eastern frontiers, and, allegedly, had to scramble to

---

6   An outline already much discussed, see e.g. Duncan-Jones (1996); A. Marcore, 'La peste antonina. Testmonzianze e interpretazione', *Rivista storica italiana* 15 (2002), 801–819; A. Marino Storchi, 'Una rilettura della fonti storico-letterarie sulla peste di età antonina', in Lo Cascio (ed: 2012), 29–61; and D. Gourevitch, *Limos kai Loimos: A Study of the Galenic Plague* (Paris: Éditions de Bocard, 2013), 77–127.

7   Ammianus Marcellinus 23.6.24 and SHA *Verus* 8.1.1–2 both mention a temple episode; the abbreviated reference at Cassius Dio, *epit.* 71.2.4 does not; see also Luc. *Hist. Conscr.* 15.

8   On the plague's reach and military focus see e.g. Ammianus Marcellinus 23.6.24 and Orosius 7.15.5 and 27.7.

9   Eutropius, *Breviarium* 8.12: Romae ac per Italiam provinciasque maxima hominum pars, militum omnes fere copiae languore defecerint.

mobilise sufficient forces for the Marcommanic Wars which open at the end of the AD 160s.[10]

The fighting with Parthia was concluded by autumn AD 165, and Verus likely left in spring 166, arriving back in Rome by the end of the summer. Some of his army might have gone ahead of him, or, indeed, the movement of troops and disease might not have been quite so perfectly matched as the historical accounts assert, retrospectively more closely aligned than at the time; for Galen seems to claim that the plague reached Rome before the emperor. He states, in *On Prognosis*, that he brought his first (roughly four-year) stay in the imperial capital to a clandestine close before Verus' return from the East, since he feared that the emperors would then demand his attention.[11] While, in *On my own Books*, Galen asserts that his departure was, 'when the great plague began', in response to that beginning.[12] Hunain's Arabic translation fills the lacuna in the Greek after Galen left Rome for his homeland with the claim that no drug of sufficient strength could be found to combat this plague, as it spread so widely before diminishing.[13]

These statements, appearing in treatises composed perhaps two decades apart, are, like much of Galen's biographical self-reporting, inconsistent but not seriously contradictory. The events – the onset of the 'great plague', Verus' return, and Galen's departure – happened at around the same time, and one is prioritised in one account, one in the other, with some flexibility about the precise sequence. Still, rather frustratingly, this direct witness to the initial onset of pestilence in Rome is indecisive about its timing. A point further emphasised by the reference in περί ἀλυπίας already mentioned, to Teuthras' demise in the 'first outbreak of the great plague' and 'not long' after Galen's own entrance on the Roman scene. The two assertions are somewhat at odds, but, again, the best way to reconcile them is by recourse to the imprecision of Galenic memory, rather than anything more radical or determinate. Still, what is clear is that the 'great plague' did have a beginning, there was a definite first episode in the sequence; and that it was associated in Galen's mind with his own first stay in the imperial capital, and with medical challenge.

There is also the suggestion that the episode of pestilence (νόσος λοιμώδες) vividly described by the orator Aelius Aristides in his *Sacred Tales* should be

---

10   See also e.g. SHA *Marcus* 21.6 and Orosius 7.15.6.

11   Gal. *Praen.* 9.5 (118.16 CMG V 8,1). On Galen's biography generally, see S. Mattern, *The Prince of Medicine: Galen in the Roman Empire* (Oxford: OUP, 2015), with discussion of the plague at 193–205.

12   Gal. *Lib. Prop.* 1.16: ἀρξαμένου τοῦ μεγάλου λοιμοῦ (139.24–27 BM).

13   French translation at Gal. *Lib. Prop.* 1.16 (139.52–62 BM), and see notes 7 and 8 (189–190 BM).

located in the suburbs of Smyrna in the summer of AD 165.[14] If this is right, and regardless of whether Aristides' own claims to have almost followed many of his neighbours and slaves, not to mention his livestock, to the grave are to be believed, then this would indicate that the plague spread ahead of any post-war military movements.[15] So, perhaps the Parthian campaign contributed to, exacerbated, an outbreak of pestilence which was already developing in the East, and would have hit Smyrna anyway; rather than being the primary cause and driver of the epidemic. Soldiers passing through on their way to the fighting, dragging resources with them, added to some displaced civilians, would all have disruptive effects, increasing both the possibilities for transmission of and susceptibility to disease. The subsequent relocation of these troops then helped make this plague a more decisively and severely imperial affair than it would otherwise have been: both geographically and militarily.

The next outbreak of plague Galen encounters certainly fits this pattern. Imperial demand brought him back to Italy in late AD 168 (having spent only a couple of years away in Pergamum).[16] He was summoned to attend on the emperors in their winter quarters, in Aquileia, between northern campaigns against various Germanic peoples (including the Marcomanni) who had crossed the Danube and threatened Roman territory. Two new legions had been raised, from Italy, but it seems likely that troops who had fought in Parthia were also involved, they certainly would be.[17] It had been predominantly Danubian units which had been dispatched East, and were now back defending their previous patch. Galen's movements were, however, again tracked by those of epidemic disease:

> On my arrival in Aquileia the plague attacked more destructively than ever before, so the emperors fled immediately to Rome with a small force of men. For the rest of us, survival became very difficult for a long time. Most, indeed, died, the effects of the plague being exacerbated by the fact that all this was occurring in the middle of winter.[18]

---

14 Aelius Aristides, *Or.* 48.38–45. The chronology is provided by C. Behr, *Aelius Aristides and the Sacred Tales* (Amsterdam: Hakkert, 1968), 96–97, as part of his complete account of Aelius life and career, and while plausible is far from certain.

15 Gourevitch is sceptical, arguing that Aristides' eagerness to remain the centre of pathological attention cannot conceal the fact that his symptoms are a poor match for those of the plague (2013: 62–5).

16 Gal. *Lib. Prop.* 3.1 (141.17–21 BM); and see Mattern (2015), 195–7.

17 To replace legions destroyed in Parthia prior to Verus' campaign, though plague was also having an effect.

18 Gal. *Lib. Prop.* 3.3: ἐπιβάντος οὖν μου τῆς Ἀκυλίας κατέσκηψεν ὁ λοιμὸς ὡς οὔπω πρότερον, ὥστε τοὺς μὲν αὐτοκράτορας αὐτίκα φεύγειν εἰς Ῥώμην ἅμα στρατιώταις ὀλίγοις, ἡμᾶς δὲ τοὺς

Flight did not save Lucius Verus who died on the road back to Rome, re-portedly of apoplexy, and was given full funeral honours, with apotheosis, by Marcus Aurelius in the imperial capital.[19]

The earliest outbreak of this plague recorded in Jerome's *Chronicle*, the uni-versal chronology he compiled in the late fourth-century, is listed for AD 168, when, 'A plague (*lues*) took hold of many provinces, and affected Rome'.[20] Four years later things were even worse, 'There was such a great plague throughout the whole world that the Roman army was reduced almost to extinction'.[21] It is tempting to move Jerome's dating scheme forward a little, to align it with Galen's first and second episodes, but outbreaks certainly continued, at local and more regional level, for decades thereafter. The somewhat wayward narra-tives of the Marcommanic Wars provided by the later imperial biographies of the *Historia Augusta* interweave pestilence and campaigning up until Marcus Aurelius' death on the frontier in AD 180.[22] Plague is also a regular presence in Galen's prolific literary output from this period, often mentioned though never the focus of attention; and it will remain a feature of his writing at least into the 190s. Whether this 'long-lasting' plague persisted into the mid-third century AD, when further episodes of pestilence are recorded in Egypt and North Africa, Rome and the cities of Greece, or whether this was a new disease event, is open to debate.[23] Many of these Galenic references are to pestilence in general, and, even if a particular case or situation is mentioned, it is often not located in time and space. The household depredations cited in περὶ ἀλυπίας occurred in Rome, for instance, but when is not specified, the addressee was there and need not be reminded. One other major outbreak of the plague in the impe-rial capital is specifically described, in the historical narratives of Cassius Dio and Herodian, just a few years before the great fire which destroyed so many of Galen's possessions in AD 192. Both authors were recording events in their own life-times, and provide numerous interesting details, if also emphasising the programmatic nature of their historical projects as they do so. Neither had warm feelings towards Commodus, which puts a particular spin on any disas-ters which may have occurred in his reign; Dio, indeed, explicitly condemned

πολλοὺς μόλις ἐν χρόνῳ πολλῷ διασωθῆναι πλείστων ἀπολλυμένων οὐ μόνον διὰ τὸν λοιμὸν ἀλλὰ καὶ διὰ τὸ μέσου χειμῶνος εἶναι τὰ πραττόμενα (142.5–11 BM).

19   Apoplexy: SHA *Verus* 9.11; apotheosis: Gal. *Lib. Prop.* 3.4.

20   Jerome, *Chron.* Helm p.287: lues multas provincias occupavit Roma ex parte vexata.

21   Jerome, *Chron.* Helm p.288: tanta per totum orbem pestilentia fuit ut paene usque ad internecionem Romanus exercitus deletus sit.

22   SHA, *Marcus* 13.3, 17.2 and 21.6.

23   See K. Harper, 'Pandemics and passages to late antiquity: rethinking the plague of c.249–270 described by Cyprian', *JRA* 28 (2015), 223–260.

him as 'more harmful' (χαλεπώτερος) to the Romans than any disease.[24] Dio's claim that this epidemic episode was the worst he had ever come across needs, therefore, to be read with this in mind, as also his supporting statement that 'two thousand often died in a single day' in the city.[25] The additional allegation that death by disease was supplemented by large scale poisoning, performed by paid criminals equipped with sharp needles and a deadly compound, is also there for a specific purpose. The same thing happened under Domitian, Dio notes, implying, of course, a broader repetition of tyrannical rule.[26]

That there was indeed a severe plague outbreak in Rome around AD 190 is, however, confirmed by Herodian.[27] All Italy was affected, but especially Rome, on account of its populousness and openness: 'great destruction of both men and livestock resulted'.[28] Physicians advised Commodus to flee to a safer location, and advised those who remained in the city to make copious use of incense and other aromatics. This would either keep the corrupt air out of their bodies, or overcome any that did manage to enter. The tactic failed for both humans and the animals they shared their space with. The situation was made even worse by famine and a corrupt imperial freedman, Cleander, who stands in for an absent emperor in the narrative. Plagues are, of course, prime sites for moralising, and both Dio and Herodian take full advantage; but severity and periodicity are also emphasised, as well as a focus on Rome. In addition, Herodian has physicians play a role in his version of events, albeit not a particularly positive one, and, it is a more medical perspective that will be engaged with now. What kind of a disease was it that had such a devastating effect on Rome, Italy and the provinces?

2 Symptoms of a Plague

As with all the major epidemic events of antiquity, there has been much debate about the identity of the disease implicated in the Antonine plague.[29] Though the literary record is rich and diverse, and includes contributions from a medical writer – Galen – the problems in such an enterprise are acute; at least in the absence of direct archaeological evidence for the relevant pathogens, such as

---

24   Dio, *epit.* 73.15.1.
25   Dio, *epit.* 73.14.3: δισχίλιοι γοῦν πολλάκις ἡμέρας μιᾶς...ἐτελεύτησαν.
26   Dio, *epit.* 73.14.4.
27   Herodian 1.12.1–2.
28   Herodian 1.12.1: πολλή τέ τις φθορὰ ἐγένετο ὑποζυγίων ἅμα καὶ ἀνθρώπων.
29   Summarised at Gourevitch (2013), 67–71.

has been forthcoming for various later outbreaks of plague, for instance.[30] The historical accounts do not mention any symptoms, while Galen's references are scattered and unsystematic, either too specific or too general to bear much diagnostic weight. He does not provide a complete description, nor any sustained analysis, of the plague as disease anywhere in his surviving oeuvre. All ancient literary engagements with illness occur, moreover, on their own terms, shaped by both contemporary pathological interests and assumptions and the rhetorical project of the writing concerned.

Despite this, a scholarly consensus has, somewhat surprisingly, been established around the identification of the Antonine plague as smallpox, based largely on Galen's testimony, as most influentially interpreted by the Littmans in a key article of 1973.[31] There are, however, real difficulties with this proposed match, and further complications have been introduced by the most recent genomic work on the variola virus, the causative agent of smallpox, as well as new phylogenetic studies of one of the other pestilential contenders, measles. These points will be developed in the next section of this essay. The main aim here is to show the consistencies in Galen's own approach to the plague, to allow what mattered to him to come through first.

The starting point for Galen's approach is a definitional one. Plague, *loimos* in Greek, is not a disease in itself, like *phrenitis* or *podagra*, rather, as Galen himself explains, it is a term applied to an epidemic (ἐπίδημον) disease event – that is when lots of people in a single place are stricken in the same way at the same time – which is particularly sustained and deadly.[32] Plague is an extreme epidemic, caused by the condition of the air, as any illness which simultaneously affects so many sharing the same location must be: or, as Galen insists, caused by the interaction between the surrounding air and individual constitutions.[33] Such an aetiology can support a range of ailments. The ambient at-

---

30   For the initial pathogenic identifications see: K. I. Bos et al., 'A draft genome of *Yersinia pestis* from victims of the Black Death', *Nature* 478 (2011), 506–510; and M. Harbeck et al., '*Yersinia pestis* DNA from skeletal remains from the 6th Century AD reveals insights into Justinianic Plague', *PLoS Pathogens* 9, no. 5 (2013): e1003349; for some wider reflections on the intersections of genetics and history see M. H. Green (ed.), *Pandemic Disease in the Medieval World: Rethinking the Black Death. The Medieval Globe* 1 (2014).

31   R. J. and M. L. Littman, 'Galen and the Antonine plague', *AJP* 94 (1973), 243–255; followed by many since, including almost all contributors to Lo Cascio (ed: 2012), and Gourevitch (2013), 53–75; as well as more generally. 'It is widely agreed to have been smallpox', says R. Sallares: 'Ecology', in W. Scheidel, I. Morris and R. Saller (eds), *The Cambridge Economic History of the Greco-Roman World* (Cambridge: Cambridge University Press, 2007), 37.

32   Gal. *Hipp. Epid. III* 3.21–22 (*CMG* V 10.2.1 120.5–19); *HVA* 1.8 (*CMG* V 9.1 122.18–123.17).

33   Gal. *Diff. Feb.*1.6 (7. 289–90 K); and see J. Jouanna, 'Air, miasma and contagion in the time of Hippocrates and the survival of miasmas in post-Hippocratic medicine (Rufus of

mosphere, what is breathed and inhabited, can disrupt somatic balance and functioning in a host of ways.

It is this basic understanding of *loimos*, very widely shared by physicians and patients alike, which shapes Galen's fragmented literary engagement with pestilence.[34] Or, to be precise, it is the combination of this abstract notion with the concrete advent of plague in his life and world, which spreads *loimos* further, and more thickly, across his oeuvre. The pestilential presence makes his dealings with the phenomenon within the overall categorical architecture of the medical art, in its pathological, therapeutic, and prognostic spaces, more direct and pressing, while also forming part of his biography and practice. When drawing on his own experience to support his arguments about health, disease, and cure, the plague is unavoidably there, as the passage at the centre of most modern diagnostic efforts shows very clearly.

This is the most medically detailed plague episode in Galen's extant works, which appears in the fifth book of the massive *On the Method of Healing*. This book provides systematic coverage of the treatment of wounds, sores, and ulcers; that is of a particular grouping of conditions arising from the breakdown of bodily continuity, one of Galen's fundamental disease types in this text, types around which the treatise is organised. Case histories are key to the exposition within these larger categories, however, as they allow Galen to demonstrate especially vividly the therapeutic pay-off from his superior understanding of human illness and injury in all its forms.[35] The particular point of intersection between the plague and somatic discontinuity is in respect to ulcers (*helkoi*) which occur inside the larynx, trachea, and passages into the lungs, an eventuality which is serious and challenging, but, crucially, treatable. Indeed, Galen claims to have enjoyed quite considerable success in this area, following a specific incident.

> In particular, I discovered the cure of them, in that place, at the time of the great plague (would that it will at some point cease), when it first came upon us. At that time, a young man broke out in ulcers all over his whole body on the ninth day, just as did almost all the others who were saved. On that day there was also a slight cough. On the following day,

Ephesus, Galen and Palladius)', in his collected essays, *Greek Medicine from Hippocrates to Galen*, trans. N. Allies (Leiden: Brill, 2012), 122–136.

34   See also [Gal.], *Def. Med.* 153 (19.391–2 K); and, with some shifts of emphasis, the summary chapter on plague in the Greek encyclopaedic tradition, from Rufus of Ephesus: Orib. *Syn.* 6.25; Aetius 5.95; Paul of Aegina 2.35.

35   On case histories in Galen see: S. Mattern, *Galen and the Rhetoric of Healing* (Baltimore: John Hopkins University Press, 2008).

immediately after he bathed, he coughed more violently and brought up with the cough what they call a scab ...[36]

This indicated to Galen that the young man was ulcerated inside and out, including somewhere in his airways, and, though reaching those passages is always tricky, he prescribed treatment accordingly, in dialogue with the patient, himself not 'inexperienced' (ἄπειρος) in medical matters.[37] After three more days in Rome, 'where the plague still raged' (ἔνθα περ ἐλοίμωξεν), the youth boarded a sea-ward ship, disembarking four days later at Stabiae, on the Bay of Naples. There he took advantage of the wondrous local milk supply, to good effect. For, following a lengthy explanation of why the milk produced at Stabiae is so outstanding, Galen concludes the case: 'That young man who had a ulcer in the trachea from the pestilential disease became healthy, and others after him likewise.'[38] It is only here, then, that the plague passes from narrative frame to pathological cause, from a means of situating the case in time, as well as space, to aetiology.

This general pestilential theme is then further developed as the sequence continues, for Galen understands the ulceration in these cases as part of a wider set of beneficial somatic responses to the plague.

> Those easily restored to health from the plague seem to me to have been previously dried and purged in respect to the whole body, for vomiting occurred in some of them and the stomach was disturbed in all. And, in the same way, in those already purged who were going to be saved, dark pustules (*exanthemata*) appear clearly over the whole body, in most ulcerous, in all dry. And it was obvious to the observer that, what was left of the blood which had been putrefied during these fevers, had, like a kind of ash, been forced through the skin by nature, just like many other superfluities.[39]

---

36 Gal. *MM* 5.12 (II 84 Loeb): εὕρομεν δὲ μάλιστα τὴν θεραπείαν αὐτῶν ἐνθένδε κατὰ τὸν μέγαν τοῦτον λοιμόν, ὃν εἴη ποτὲ παύσεσθαι, πρῶτον εἰσβάλλοντα. τότε νεανίσκος τις ἐνναταῖος ἐξήνθησεν ἕλκεσιν ὅλον τὸ σῶμα, καθάπερ καὶ οἱ ἄλλοι σχεδὸν ἅπαντες οἱ σωθέντες. ἐν τούτῳ δὲ καὶ ὑπέβηττε βραχέα. τῇ δ᾽ ὑστεραίᾳ λουσάμενος αὐτίκα μὲν ἔβηξε σφοδρότερον, ἀνηνέχθη δ᾽ αὐτῷ μετὰ τῆς βηχὸς ἣν ὀνομάζουσιν ἐφελκίδα....

37 Gal. *MM* 5.12 (II 86 Loeb).

38 Gal. *MM* 5.12 (II 92 Loeb): ἐκεῖνος μέν γε οὖν ὁ νεανίας ἐκ τῆς λοιμώδους νόσου κατὰ τὴν ἀρτηρίαν ἕλκος ἔχων ὑγιὴς ἐγένετο καὶ ἄλλοι μετ᾽ αὐτὸν ὁμοίως.

39 Gal. *MM* 5.12 (II 92–4 Loeb): οἱ δ᾽ ἐκ τοῦ λοιμοῦ ῥᾳδίως ὑγιάζεσθαί μοι δοκοῦσι τῷ προεξηράνθαι τε καὶ προκεκαθάρθαι σύμπαν τὸ σῶμα· καὶ γὰρ ἔμετός τισιν αὐτῶν ἐγένετο καὶ ἡ γαστὴρ ἅπασιν ἐταράχθη. καὶ οὕτως ἤδη κεκενωμένοις τοῖς σῴζεσθαι μέλλουσιν ἐξανθήματα μέλανα διὰ παντὸς τοῦ σώματος ἀθρόως ἐπεφαίνετο· τοῖς πλείστοις μὲν ἑλκώδη, πᾶσι δὲ ξηρά. καὶ ἦν εὔδηλον ἰδόντι

These pustules, or eruptions, required no treatment, were indeed part of the healing process. If ulcerous they formed scabs, which dropped off leaving the patient close to health, if not they were dry and itchy, then fell off like scales, from which all became healthy. For, in plague, drying, roughening, and scabbing have already occurred, that is the aim of any medicament that might be applied has been achieved.[40]

These generalisations are about those who have, or will, recover from the plague, rather than all afflicted, but skin eruptions feature in another sustained pestilential discussion, with reference to the 'most long-lasting plague' (πολυχρονιωτάτῳ λοιμῷ) now occurring.[41] Galen quotes from Thucydides' description of the Athenian Plague which had such devastating effects during the Peloponnesian War in this respect:

> On the outside the body was not hot to the touch, nor was there pallor; the skin was rather red, livid, and broke out into small blisters and ulcers (*helkoi*).[42]

Fever and various other gastrointestinal issues – including loss of appetite, loose bowels, and bloody or black stools – are also symptoms associated with the present *loimos* elsewhere in Galen's oeuvre.[43] Most frequently emphasised, however, is that those suffering from this pestilence did not recognise 'themselves or their friends', another Thucydidean symptom, as is explicitly noted.[44] This is not a failure of the faculty of memory itself, but rather the disease produces interference in access to that faculty, like a cataract does in the case of sight.

Galen worried about the predictive powers of the pulse in the present 'great plague' (μεγάλας λοιμός), indeed, he worried about the wider diagnostic and prognostic challenges of pestilential disease, its confounding characteristics for physicians and laymen alike.[45] Its corrosive inner heat is deceptive, the

---

τοῦ σεσηπότος ἐν τοῖς πυρετοῖς αἵματος εἶναι τοῦτο λείψανον, οἷον τέφραν τινὰ τῆς φύσεως ὠθούσης ἐπὶ τὸ δέρμα, καθάπερ ἄλλα πολλὰ τῶν περιττῶν.

40   Gal. *MM* 5.12 (II 94 Loeb).

41   Gal. *Hipp. Epid. VI* 1.29 (*CMG* V 10.2.2 53.16–19).

42   Thuc. 2.49.5: καὶ τὸ μὲν ἔξωθεν ἁπτομένῳ σῶμα οὔτ᾽ ἄγαν θερμὸν ἦν οὔτε χλωρόν, ἀλλ᾽ ὑπέρυθρον, πελιτνόν, φλυκταίναις μικραῖς καὶ ἕλκεσιν ἐξηνθηκός. At *CMG* V 10.2.2 52.3–7 and 53.19–54.1.

43   Gal. *MM* 10.11 (10.733 K), *Hipp. Aph.* 4.21 (17B.682–3 K), *Hipp. Epid. III* 3.59–60 (*CMG* V 10.2.1 144.21–145.11).

44   Gal. *QAM* 5: ἀγνοῆσαι διὰ νόσημα σφᾶς τ᾽αὐτοὺς καὶ τοὺς ἐπιτηδείους (*SM* 2 49.3–11); *Diff. Symp.* 3.4 (7.62 K) and *Caus. Symp.* 3.2.7.1 (7.201K); Thucydides, 2.49.8.

45   Gal. *Praes. Puls.* 3.3 and 4 (9.341–2 and 357–9 K).

hectic fevers it engenders are slippery and dangerous, and, of course, there is the sheer volume of cases, the thousands (μύριοι) affected in this 'long-lasting plague' (πολυχρόνιος λοιμός). This volume is a conceptual as well as a practical problem, a technical as well as a social issue, for ancient medicine is essentially about individuals not populations. To be able to operate most effectively, a physician needed knowledge of the patient's specific constitution, their healthy base-line, in order to understand both what is wrong and how best to treat it, to return the sick person to their previous state of health. There are established short-cuts. Some generalisations can be made based on age and sex, for instance, in respect to geography and environment, the seasons and weather, but these are rough guides which require calibration in every case.[46] Plague makes that impossible.

The kind of sustained engagement Galen enjoyed with the young man with the pestilentially ulcerated trachea, the complex individualised therapy he is able to dispense, and the patient himself actively participates in, cannot be extended to so many sufferers. It is the process not the prescription which requires repetition, and there is just not the time available to do so. The point had been underlined by Galen's insistence that it is the interaction between individual constitutions, particular somatic states, and putrefying air which produces plague, which engenders disease in many people, but not all, and not all the same in terms of severity and symptoms. Those whose bodies are well-balanced, unobstructed, and unburdened by excess or superfluities, especially moistures, are less susceptible, more likely to recover quickly, through purging and drying.[47] Generalised remedies will always be touted in such circumstances, but there is no such thing. Those who drank a draught of Armenian earth in the recent plague, for instance, were either cured immediately or died; and Galen makes no mention of the stories about Hippocrates bringing health to pestilential cities by burning a range of sweet smelling substances across the area, designed to combat the putrid qualities of the atmosphere.[48] Stabian milk, for example, is highly beneficial for a range of diseases, and completes, rather than comprises, the therapeutic package for the young man.

---

46   See e.g. Gal. GMM 1.1 (11.1–6 K).

47   Gal. Diff. Resp. 1.6 (7.291–2 K).

48   Gal. SMT 9.1 (12.191 K). This is taking Robert Leigh and Véronique Boudon-Millot to be correct in their recent editions, with translations (into English and French respectively) and commentaries, of On Theriac to Piso, Attributed to Galen (Leiden: Brill, 2016), 61, and (Paris: Les Belles Lettres, 2016), lii–lxxiv, that the work (which does mention Hippocrates curing the plague: Ther. 16) is not by Galen. On these stories more generally see J. Rubin Pinault, Hippocratic Lives and Legends (Leiden: Brill, 1992), 35–60.

The situation is not as bleak as depicted by Thucydides. In the Athenian Plague, he claimed, physicians were useless, ignorant of how to treat the disease, and particularly vulnerable as a result, but no other human art (ἀνθρωπεία τέχνη) was any more help, nor were appeals to the divine; all were eventually abandoned by the afflicted populace, despair dominated.[49] Galen has knowledge and understanding, but not the necessary capacity. There is a sense in which pestilence, such as the one he lived through, inherently exceeded the medical art. But though there was some confusion amongst the profession, Galen does not emphasise either their errors or their susceptibility. His friend Teuthras is the only medical casualty he notes, and, while all his slaves in Rome succumbed, as also most of the men over-wintering in Aquileia, Galen himself seems not to have been affected. There may be reasons why he would not have mentioned it, however, even if he had fallen ill. Immunity from, rather than empathy with, others' ailments is the preferred position of the classical physician.[50] Their authority was vested more in their own health and integrity than in any shared experience of suffering.

Still, the appeal of Thucydides here, the way his plague narrative is the main frame of reference for Galen's own pestilential engagements, as also for others in antiquity and after, is not just about the stature of the author and his text.[51] It is not just about the vividness and detail of Thucydides' account, which Galen contrasts with a certain Hippocratic sparseness on at least one occasion.[52] It is also, and primarily, about the way pestilence extends beyond medicine: is essentially a collective, communal phenomenon, a historical as much as a medical event. The repetition of some symptoms helps strengthen the connection, but should not be mistaken for any kind of assertion that the disease involved was the same, that is a claim which would make little sense to Galen; rather, the Athenian plague is the only meaningful precedent for the scale and severity of what he experienced overall.

---

49   Thuc. 2.47.4.

50   B. Holmes, 'In strange lands: Disembodied authority and the physician role in the Hippocratic Corpus and beyond', in M. Asper (ed.), *Writing Science: Medical and Mathematical Authorship in Ancient Greece* (Berlin: de Gruyter, 2013), 431–472.

51   See F. Kudlien, 'Galens Urteil über die Thukydideische Pestbeschreibung', *Episteme* 5 (1971), 132–3; other Thucydidean episodes include: Lucr. 6.1139–1286; Lucian, *Hist. Conscr.* 13; and Procopius, 2.22–33.

52   Gal. *Diff. Resp.* 2.7 (7.850–851 K).

3   Identifying the Plague

The Littmans do not mention the loss of memory, the loss of self and family, but are otherwise content that all the symptoms and signs Galen described in the Antonine epidemic, 'are consistent with smallpox'.[53] Putting it more strongly, though his account is incomplete, and serves his own purposes, it is sufficient 'to enable firm identification of the disease as smallpox because of the excellent description of the most important diagnostic sign, the exanthema.' It is the passage in *On the Method of Healing* which is most decisive here, rendering both bubonic plague and typhus, the two other possibilities they considered, 'unlikely', and conforming especially closely to haemorrhagic smallpox. The ulceration and scabbing of the pustules in this sequence is key, characteristic of smallpox rather than any other acute feverish diseases involving skin eruptions. Bubonic plague is something of an outlier, but modern typhus, measles, and smallpox all begin with fevers and an assortment of aches, pains, and general un-wellness, followed by rashes that often start on the face (may be in the mouth and throat, which are also otherwise affected) and spread over the whole body (more or less).[54] Except in smallpox, these rashes tend to stay flat, or, at least, remain flatter; the eponymous buboes of bubonic plague are rather different.[55]

   There are, of course, questions about how conclusive any historical diagnosis of this kind can ever be, and opinions vary on exactly how close the match of symptoms asserted by the Littmans really is. Much seems to rest on quite precise interpretations of terms often used vaguely and interchangeably, such as *exanthema* and *helkoi*. Two larger difficulties with the identification of the Antonine Plague as smallpox have also been noted, including by its supporters. In her recent survey of the topic, Danielle Gourevitch considers it, 'safe to suggest that this Galenic and fearful epidemic was due to a virus of the *Poxviridae* family (genus *Orthopoxvirus*) which are responsible for smallpox and other related diseases', that is, it was very similar to, but not necessarily identical with, modern smallpox (eradicated in 1979).[56] But she admits that the omission of any reference to the indelible scarring, the disfiguring facial pockmarks, which

53   R. J. and M. L. Littman (1973), 252.

54   See, for example, the relevant chapters in K. F. Kiple (ed.), *The Cambridge World History of Human Disease* (Cambridge: Cambridge University Press, 1993): 871–5 (measles); 1008–13 (smallpox); and 1080–4 (typhus).

55   And buboes – glandular swellings – do feature in general discussions of somatic swellings and surface eruptions in classical medicine, including by Galen (e.g. *MM* 13.5: III 328 Loeb), but not in his descriptions of the 'great plague'.

56   Gourevitch (2013), 72–5.

became the disease's signature is problematic in this respect. She adds a further challenge too, drawing attention to the concurrence of human and animal sickness and death in the plague accounts of Aelius Aristides and Herodian, two of the more contemporary witnesses to events, already cited. Smallpox is exclusively human. There are more or less closely related poxviruses which affect many other species, including livestock, some of which are zoonotic – that is transferable to people – but these infections are generally mild, localised and poorly transmissible among humans; indeed, most animal poxes are not very virulent.[57] In modern terms, therefore, there is no single poxvirus which could produce the Antonine plague as described in the ancient sources.

The absence of references to the scarring characteristic of modern smallpox has been explained in various vague and unsatisfactory ways in the scholarship. Such an omission does not, of course, prove that this important feature was not part of the pestilential scene in the Roman Empire of the second century AD, but there are a number of reasons to think that if it had been, the sources would have recorded the fact. Visibly disfiguring diseases were a popular theme among Roman writers, for instance, redolent with moral meaning, and remedies for removing scars and facial blemishes were standard in the pharmacological repertoire, a reliable earner for any physician it can be assumed. Pliny the Elder makes the most of nasty (*foedus*) facial, or facially focused, afflictions as markers of imperial excess with his stories of the arrival of *lichena* and *elephantiasis* on Italian shores in the *Natural History*.[58] While the obviously punitive deaths recounted for figures such as Sulla, Herod the Great, and Galerius involve, amongst other unpleasant details, an inner putrefaction which is manifest on the surface, as the whole skin itches unbearably and flesh turns into lice or worms, which cannot be washed away.[59] Galen himself covered recipes for a range of growths, tumours, pustules, and scars on the face in his voluminous collection of compound medicaments organised according to the somatic location affected.[60] This included many compounds to treat *lichena*, some of which specify that they overcome the eruptions without ulceration or scarring, though others excoriate the skin, and should be followed by a restorative plaster.

It has been suggested that the variability of the virus, differences of population and environment, might have led to less scarring in the Roman context.

---

57   S. L. Haller et al., 'Poxvirus and the evolution of host range and virulence,' *Infection, Genetics and Evolution* 21 (2013), 15–40.

58   Plin. *NH* 26.1–11; and see R. Flemming, 'Pliny and the pathologies of Empire', *Papers of the Langford Latin Seminar* 14 (2010), 1–24.

59   Plut. *Sulla* 36.2–3; Josephus, *BJ* 1.656; Lactantius *DMP* 33.

60   Gal. *Comp. Med. Loc.* 5.3 (12 822–48 K).

This is certainly possible. Recent genomic work on poxviruses has emphasised their variation and adaptability: milder, so called 'minor' strains of the variola virus, the causative agent of smallpox, have repeatedly emerged, may indeed be the original form in humans, though it is calculated that the more virulent 'major' strain developed at least three thousand years ago, so before the period under scrutiny here.[61] However, while severe facial pockmarks follow recovery from variola minor much less frequently than recovery from variola major, in about 7% rather than 75% of cases in the most systematic modern study, this accompanies a fatality rate of less than 1% (in contrast to 10%–30% for the major strains).[62] So, to depress the scarring rates to a level where it is plausible that this would not be reported as part of the course of the disease would, according to the available information, not be compatible with the heavy mortality experienced during pestilential outbreaks at Rome and Aquileia. There is a larger methodological question at stake here too. What does it mean to identify the Antonine Plague as smallpox if that move is based on the historical variability of the disease, is reliant on the fact that pathogens and their interactions with their hosts change significantly over time?

Gourevitch's explanation for the human and animal nature of the pestilence is a rhetorical one. It is, she readily confesses, an argument of last resort, but the dying livestock have been recruited for dramatic emphasis, to increase the emotional impact of these accounts.[63] There are precedents. The mules and hounds of the Achaeans are the first targets of Apollo's pestilential arrows in the opening sequence of the *Iliad*, while the order of mortality is reversed, and animals play a more complex role, in Thucydides' plague narrative.[64] Though bodies were lying around unburied, signalling the high toll exacted by the disease on both human life and social organisation, carrion eating birds and beasts avoided them, or died after tasting their flesh. The absence of carrion birds was notable, while the presence of domestic dogs allowed these lethal results to be witnessed directly. This latter point was further embellished by the Epicurean poet Lucretius, who, towards the end of the Roman Republic reworked the

61   Haller et al. (2014), 18–19 and 34; see also C. Smithson, J. Imbery and C. Upton. 'Re-
      assemby and analysis of an ancient variola virus genome', *Viruses* 2017, 9, 253 (doi:10.3390/
      v9090253).
62   Z. Jezek, W. Hardjotanojo and A. G. Rangaraj, 'Facial scarring after varicella: A compari-
      son with variola major and variola minor', *American Journal of Epidemiology* 114 (1981),
      798–803.
63   Gourevitch (2013), 74–5.
64   Homer, *Iliad* 1.50–52; Thuc. 2.50.1–2.

Thucydidean plague to close his epic *On the Nature of Things*.[65] The suffering of man's faithful canine companions was displayed on the streets, like the unburied corpses, as the power of the disease dragged the life from their limbs.[66]

The references to dying livestock in Aelius Aristides and Herodian seem perfunctory in comparison. They add to the destructive footprint of the *loimos* they describe, but the real emotional and political work is done elsewhere in these accounts. There is a closer resemblance to a couple of plague reports in the Roman annalistic tradition. The Augustan historian Livy records a severe and sustained *pestilentia*, lasting for about five years from 436 BC, which brought death to city and countryside, killing 'man and livestock' (*hominum pecorumque*) alike, and while he had a plague outbreak in cattle succeeded by one among people in the years 175–4 BC, the later excerptor of Republican prodigies, Julius Obsequens, brutally compressed the whole episode.[67]

> During a serious pestilence affecting humans and cattle, corpses lay unburied, for Libitina was overwhelmed, but no vultures appeared.[68]

The Thucydidean echoes are obvious, here and in Livy, but if the 'man and livestock' phrase had become one topos among many routinely deployed on these occasions, it is more sparingly used than most, and perhaps more specifically.

The possibility that pestilential outbreaks involving humans and livestock were a specific phenomenon in the Roman world is given some credence by recent genomic work on one of the other diseases referred to so far – measles – and by the reported recurrence of such events in the early middle ages.[69] So, though the timing is still somewhat uncertain, new techniques and methods are under development, require further calibration, it has been established that the measles virus appeared much later than had been previously assumed.[70] It, and its close relative the rinderpest virus, the causative agent of rinderpest, an epidemically very virulent and lethal disease of cattle (and other ungulates), until eradicated in 2011, only went their separate ways sometime between the

65   David Sedley, *Lucretius and the Transformation of Greek Wisdom* (Cambridge: Cambridge University Press, 1991), 160–165.

66   Lucr. 6.1222–5.

67   Livy 4.25.4 and 41.21.5–7.

68   Obs. 10: Gravi pestilentia hominum boumque cadavera non sufficiente Libitina cum iacerent, vulturius non apparuit.

69   T. P. Newfield, 'Human-bovine plagues in the early middle ages', *Journal of Interdisciplinary History* 48 (2015), 1–38.

70   See generally on method: R. Bick et al., 'Measurably evolving pathogens in the genomic era', *Trends in Ecology and Evolution* 30 (2015), 306–313.

ninth and twelfth centuries AD.[71] Before that, the common ancestor morbillivirus could have infected humans and cattle, with the only available guide to its effects coming from modern measles and rinderpest respectively. The Antonine Plague, like its Republican predecessors and medieval successors, might demonstrate the point. Certainly, whatever human sickness this now extinct archaeovirus generated cannot, on the current state of knowledge, be ruled out of the pathological picture for Galen's great *loimos*.

This is, of course, all pretty speculative, but so, in the circumstances, is the smallpox diagnosis for the Antonine Plague. Here too the relationship between modern smallpox and any ancient disease has been thrown into deeper uncertainty by recent genomic studies. The variola virus genome isolated from a mummified child who lived in mid-seventeenth century Lithuania turned out to be ancestral to all twentieth century strains. Modern smallpox is, then, just that, the evolutionary history of the virus prior to that point, with all the possible variations in virulence and the wider set of interactions between pathogen and host, has become more distant than it once was.[72] There is one more resource that can, and should, be brought to bear on the problem, however, that is the voluminous Arabic writings of the great Persian physician of the medieval Islamic world, Abū Bakr Muḥammad ibn Zakarīyā al-Rāzī, commonly known in the Anglophone world by his latinised name, Rhazes. He is the medical figure commonly credited with mutually distinguishing smallpox and measles, and providing the first 'scientific' description of the latter, if not the former, around AD 900.[73] While his contribution is not nearly so straightforward as is often assumed or asserted, Rhazes' engagement with Galen is

---

71   Combining the estimates in A. Furuse, A. Suzuki and H. Oshitani, 'Origin of measles virus: Divergence from rinderpest virus between the 11th and 12th centuries', *Virology Journal* 7: 52 (2010); and J. O. Wertheim and S. L Kosakovsky Pond, 'Purifying selection can obscure the age of viral lineages', *Molecular Biology and Evolution* 28 (2011), 3355–65.

72   A. T. Duggan et al, '17th Century variola virus reveals the recent history of samllpox', *Current Biology* 26 (2016), 3407–412. See also: P. Pajer et al., 'Characterization of two historic smallpox specimens from a Czech museum', *Viruses* 2017, 9, 200 (doi: 10.3390/v9080200) with A. Porter et al., 'Comment: Characterization of two historic smallpox specimens from a Czech museum', *Viruses* 2017, 9, 276 (doi: 10.3390/v9080276); and Smithson, Imbery and Upton (2017).

73   This is often asserted in specific and general histories of disease – e.g. D. R. Hopkins, *The Greatest Killer: Smallpox in History* (Cambridge: Cambridge University Press, 2002), 27; and W. H. MacNeill, *Plagues and Peoples*, rev. edn. (New York: Random House, 1998), 131 – as well as being more or less assumed in much of the genomic literature about pathogen evolution, e.g. A. Furuse, A. Suzuki and H. Oshitani (2010); Wertheim and Kosakovsky Pond (2011), 3363.

certainly worth discussing in this context, as also various other aspects of his treatment of the diseases *jadari* and *hasbah*, which have been construed as terms for smallpox and measles respectively.

In the preface to his short treatise dedicated to *jadari* and *hasbah*, Rhazes explains that his focus will be on the former.[74] It is *jadari* which has yet to receive a thorough textual treatment, an omission his discourse rectifies. It is not, however, that the disease has been entirely overlooked by previous medical authors, rather that these discussions remain incomplete, especially in respect to the causes and cure of the complaint. Indeed, Rhazes opens his disquisition with a defence of Galen against charges of having failed to mention this affliction. He cites four passages to prove his case, from the first book of *On Compound Drugs according to Kind*, the fourteenth book of the great work *On Pulses* (that is book two of *Prognosis from the Pulse*), the ninth book of *On the Usefulness of the Parts*, and the fourth book of his commentary on Plato's *Timaeus*.[75] The term *jadari* appears in all these excerpts, taken from the Arabic translations of these works, in contexts which are broadly in line with Rhazes' understanding of the disease.[76] That it is produced by the putrefaction and fermentation of the blood, which generates fever, inflammation and the eruption of superfluities through the skin, amongst other effects.[77]

William Alexander Greenhill, who carefully translated the treatise into English from the original Arabic in the mid-nineteenth century, did not have access to these Arabic versions of Galen's works. Still, he diligently compared the quotes in Rhazes with the surviving Greek, as far as possible, and concluded that *jadari* most probably renders *ionthos* and *herpes* in these passages,

---

74 The Arabic text remains unedited and unpublished, so I have had to rely on the English translation of W. A. Greenhill – Abu Becr Mohammed ibn Zacariya Ar-Razi, *A Treatise on the Small-Pox and Measles* (London: Sydenham Society, 1847), 22–73 – with its rich annotations and Arabic index. References will be, therefore, to that translation. The volume (abbreviated here as *TSM*) also includes translations, from Arabic and Latin, of passages from other works of Rhazes which cover these diseases, with considerable consistency, not to say repetition.

75 Rhazes, *Kitab fi al-jadari wa-al-hasbah* (*KJH*) 1,1–2 (*TSM* 27–28). Galen's many treatises on the pulse were combined on the syllabus of the medical schools of late antique Alexandria, and thereafter.

76 Rhazes makes it clear later in the same chapter (1.2: *TSM* 28) that he worked with Arabic material, and asked those familiar with Greek and Syriac whether he had missed anything. There is broader discussion about his competence in these languages, see O. Kahl, *The Sanskrit, Syriac and Persian Sources in the* Comprehensive Book *of Rhazes* (Leiden: Brill, 2015), 5–7.

77 As stated at e.g. *KJH* 1.6 (*TSM* 29–30).

that is words for tumours and pustules themselves.[78] Certainly none of these excerpts are at all plague related, nor does Rhazes make the connection more generally, for either *jadari* or *hasbah*. Though his knowledge of Galen's oeuvre was very extensive, and there is indeed a lengthy plague sequence in the next book of *Prognosis from the Pulse*, as has been noted. Part of the explanation may be that, for Rhazes, both *jadari* and *hasbah*, the latter being essentially a more bilious variant of the former, are common childhood diseases, rarely fatal.[79] This presumption was shared, moreover, by the assortment of other medical writers, mostly from the eighth and ninth centuries AD, whose views on the subject he collected in his compendious *Kitab al-Hawi*.[80] *Jadari* and *hasbah* are rarely avoided on the road to adulthood, but while they can kill, they usually do not. These are everyday diseases, dangerous in some forms; but not the stuff of plagues.

The modern understanding of smallpox and measles makes sense of this disjunction. One of the key features of these diseases, as well as another acute feverish illness involving skin eruptions, that is scarlet fever, and, to a lesser extent typhus, is that they endow those who survive their depredations with immunity (as also rinderpest and animal poxes). For mortality to be as high as reported for the Antonine Plague, at least in Rome and various military encampments, and for adults to be hit as hard as Galen indicates, this has to have been a 'virgin soil epidemic' involving one of these diseases.[81] In such cases, where smallpox or measles were previously unknown, or last encountered long ago, as in medieval Japan, and early modern Spanish America, for example, the effect on communities lacking resistance can be devastating.[82] Whereas,

---

78   *TSM* 141–150.

79   *KJH* 3.2: bilious nature of *hasbah*; 1.6: childhood diseases (*TSM* 35 and 29–30).

80   Rhazes noted down passages from all the medical texts he read, and organised them together with his own views on the subject and some relevant case histories under appropriate headings, this compilation seems to have been essentially for his own use, but was then published after his death, and indeed rendered into Latin (as the *Continens*): see e.g. Kahl (2015), 3–5. Greenhill translated the passages (*TSM* 101–130) from an Arabic manuscript in the Bodleian (Marsh 156).

81   Though the notion of the 'virgin soil' is sometimes construed more broadly and problematically, see e.g. D. S. Jones, 'Virgin soils revisited', *William and Mary Quarterly* 60 (2003), 703–742.

82   On Japan see e.g. A. B. Jannetta, *Epidemics and Mortality in Early Modern Japan* (Princeton: Princeton University Press, 1986); and W. W. Farris, *Population, Disease and Land in Early Japan* (Cambridge, MA: Harvard University Press, 1985); the literature on the Americas is more extensive, see e.g. S. A. Alchon, *A Pest in the Land: New World Epidemics in Global perspective* (Albuquerque: University of New Mexico Press, 2003); and N. D. Cook and

in circumstances where the environment and population allow the pathogens to establish a permanent presence, that is where these conditions become endemic, they are largely restricted to children, to the not yet immune. This then is the situation Rhazes and his recent predecessors described for *jadari* and *hasbah*, in a geographical region that includes the area in which Verus campaigned. The new Abbasid capital of Baghdad was founded just a little north of the old Parthian and Sassanian centre of Ctesiphon, and about 80 km north of Babylon. Rhazes spent time in Baghdad, as did most of his sources, even if they, like him, often originated further east, deeper in Persia.[83]

This is, of course, over half a millennium after the Antonine Plague, long enough for a disease like smallpox to become endemic even if it had reached Mesopotamia at the same time as Verus did.[84] This was not Rome's first Parthian expedition, after all, and the eastern boundaries of the Empire were porous and flexible in many ways. The point, however, is a more general one about the patterning of the diseases under scrutiny here, that while Rhazes' failure to place *jadari* and *hasbah* in a lineage which goes back to Galen's 'great plague', his preference for vaguer, non-epidemic ancestry for at least the former is noteworthy, this is what might be expected if these were modern smallpox and measles. So how good is the fit between Rhazes descriptions of these two diseases and their proposed modern counterparts more broadly? Obviously any discrimination between, individuation of, acute feverish diseases involving skin eruptions is a move in the right direction, but there is more to it than that.

Three points are worth making in this regard. The first is that, amongst the very long, and mostly generic, list of early signs of *jadari* and *hasbah*, back pains are more particular to the former, whereas nausea and anxiety are more prevalent in the latter.[85] Modern textbooks include back pain as a typical symptom of smallpox, but not measles, while being pretty indifferent about the rest.[86] The second is the assertion made apparently in Rhazes' own voice in the *Hawi*, as well as by one of the recent authorities he cites, a member of the Syro-Persian Nestorian family of physicians from Gondeshapur who shared

---

W. G. Lowell (eds.), *Secret Judgements of God: Old World Disease in Colonial Spanish America* (Norman: University of Oklahoma Press, 2001).

83   For Rhazes' biography see e.g. TSM 137–141; Kahl (2015), 1–2.

84   In Japan, smallpox, which probably arrived from China in the sixth century AD, but is more clearly identified in a massive epidemic of 735, seems to have become endemic by the twelfth century, while measles did not: Jannetta (1986), 65–70 and 108–117.

85   KJH 3 (TSM 34–35).

86   See e.g. Kiple (ed: 1993), 1009.

the name Bokhtishu, that the pustules in *jadari* are raised, whereas the rash in *hasbah* stays flat.[87] Though, otherwise, discussion of the skin eruptions occurs more in a prognostic than diagnostic setting, and often along similar lines in both diseases, though with some specific variations.[88] Third is the clear division between *jadari* and *hasbah* in respect to what happens on the somatic surface in the aftermath of these affections. In the treatise dedicated to them there is a chapter on removing the marks and scars of *jadari*, which includes a number of recipes for applications to remove marks on the eyes, face and elsewhere on the body.[89] It is also suggested that frequent bathing, rubbing, and growing fat and fleshy will help fill in and smooth over the pockmarks. Many of the other authors excerpted in the *Hawi* also offer such medicaments and advice, but only for *jadari, hasbah* is not mentioned in this context.[90]

It does, therefore, seem that the *jadari* of Rhazes and his recent predecessors is a reasonably good match for modern smallpox, but that is less clearly the case for *hasbah* and measles. It is worth mentioning that, in Greenhill's day (and beyond), the Arabic term *hasbah* mostly signified scarlet fever.[91] Smallpox had been distinguished from other acute feverish diseases involving skin eruptions, with *hasbah* designating the rest. The Antonine Plague, as described by Galen and others, appears to align more with this blurred remainder than the more determinate *jadari*, however, as it crucially lacks the scarring, the facial marks, which are so intrinsic to the tradition.[92] The consensus around smallpox needs to be challenged and questions of identification re-opened. Further genomic and historical work will certainly help shed light on the matter, even if no appropriate ancient DNA is forthcoming.[93]

---

87   *Hawi* 47 and 71 (*TSM* 113 and 121).

88   *KJH* 14 (*TSM* 71–73).

89   *KJH* 11 (*TSM* 60–63).

90   *Hawi* 22, 36–39, 44, 48, 50, 53, and 76–9 (*TSM* 106, 110–111, 112–113, 114, 116, and 124).

91   *TSM* 136.

92   Pockmarks are even noted by native reporters of early outbreaks of smallpox in Mexico, were noticeable on initial encounter, see R. McCaa, 'Spanish and Nahuatl views on smallpox and demographic catastrophe in Mexico', *Journal of Interdisciplinary History* 25 (1995), 423.

93   Though the evidence of second century Roman epidemic mortality presented in P. Blanchard et al, 'A mass grave from the catacomb of Saints Peter and Marcellinus in Rome, second-third century AD', *Antiquity* 81 (2007), 989–998, may be less straightforward than first suggested, a DNA from the skeletons could still produce interesting results. The international historical smallpox project just launched by the Mütter Research Institute is also promising.

4 Conclusions

To return to Galen, however, and his efforts to avoid, or at least to control, distress, the distress which inhered in the pestilential age he inhabited. For the 'great plague' reached Rome – the imperial capital and centre of Galen's career – not long after he did, and it met him again in Aquileia, where it temporarily inserted itself between him and the persons of the emperors. It ebbed and flowed thereafter, but was characterised by persistence and longevity, this was 'the most long-lasting plague' (would that it would end!). Time was both structured by the epidemic, so that locating an event 'in the first outbreak of the great plague' became an obvious move to make, and un-structured by its continuity, by the uncertainty of its end.

Galen lost a whole household of slaves to the plague, though he seems to have considered them as possessions, not people, in his accounting of damage due to fire and pestilence in περὶ ἀλυπίας. He also lost his friend Teuthras. He claims to have witnessed the death of most of the army gathered at Aquileia, and saw 'thousands' afflicted by the epidemic in Rome. Those presented as his patients, however, individuals with whom he interacted, rather than the un-differentiated masses of city dwellers and soldiers who may or may not have received his therapeutic attentions (he does not say), fared rather better. Galen identified and concentrated on the group with good prospects, who could be saved, with the correct approach.

The great plague was medically challenging, tricky and misleading, violent and dangerous, but the body was not defenceless, and medicine could align itself with, assist and support, its inherent purgative responses. It was also socially challenging – friends and family were no longer recognised as such by sufferers – but there is no suggestion of a collapse of the moral order, as is so central to Thucydides' plague narrative. Issues of Roman manpower and famine emphasised in other sources were of little concern to Galen. He recorded the loss of troops, but Marcus Aurelius headed north to deal with the Germanic incursions just a couple of sentences later, apparently untroubled by these depredations. The sense that *loimos* is not just a medical matter, exceeds the capacity of the art, spills over into other domains, is always present, but never fully articulated. This hinterland is glimpsed, sporadically, across Galen's oeuvre, its painful depths revealed momentarily, as in περὶ ἀλυπίας, but rarely explored. What is medically manageable receives more discussion, and pushes back against the uncontrollable aspects of pestilence to some extent, but without taming them. That Galen's engagement with the plague is piecemeal and uneven, is thus an integral part of the phenomenon; the picture is patchy and incomplete because it has to be.

Acknowledgements

My thanks to the audience at the Warwick Conference, and those at a Classics Department seminar in the University of Princeton, for their comments and suggestions.

References

Alchon, S. A., *A Pest in the Land: New World Epidemics in Global perspective* (Albuquerque: University of New Mexico Press, 2003)

Behr, C., *Aelius Aristides and the Sacred Tales* (Amsterdam: Hakkert, 1968)

Bick, R, et al., 'Measurably evolving pathogens in the genomic era', *Trends in Ecology and Evolution* 30 (2015), 306–313

Blanchard P. et al, 'A mass grave from the catacomb of Saints Peter and Marcellinus in Rome, second-third century AD', *Antiquity* 81 (2007), 989–998

Bos K. I., et al., 'A draft genome of *Yersinia pestis* from victims of the Black Death', *Nature* 478 (2011), 506–510

Boudon-Millot, V., Jouanna, J., and Pietrobelli, A. (ed., trans. and comm.), *Galien: Ne pas se chagriner* (Paris: Les Belles Lettres, 2010)

Cook N. D., and Lowell W.G. (eds.), *Secret Judgements of God: Old World Disease in Colonial Spanish America* (Norman: University of Oklahoma Press, 2001)

Duggan A.T. et al, '17th Century variola virus reveals the recent history of samllpox', *Current Biology* 26 (2016), 3407–412

Duncan-Jones R., 'The impact of the Antonine Plague', *JRA* 9 (1996), 108–136

Elliott, C. P., 'The Antonine plague, climate change, and local violence in Roman Egypt', *Past and Present* 231 (2016), 3–31

Farris, W.W., *Population, Disease and Land in Early Japan* (Cambridge, MA: Harvard University Press, 1985)

Flemming, R., 'Pliny and the pathologies of Empire', *Papers of the Langford Latin Seminar* 14 (2010), 1–24

Furuse, A., Suzuki, A. and Oshitani, H., 'Origin of measles virus: Divergence from rinderpest virus between the 11th and 12th centuries', *Virology Journal* 7: 52 (2010)

Gourevitch, D., *Limos kai Loimos: A Study of the Galenic Plague* (Paris: Éditions de Bocard, 2013), 77–127

Green M. H. (ed.), *Pandemic Disease in the Medieval World: Rethinking the Black Death. The Medieval Globe* 1 (2014)

Haller S. L. et al., 'Poxvirus and the evolution of host range and virulence,' *Infection, Genetics and Evolution* 21 (2013), 15–40

Harbeck M. et al., '*Yersinia pestis* DNA from skeletal remains from the 6th Century AD reveals insights into Justinianic Plague,' *PLoS Pathogens* 9, no. 5 (2013): e1003349

Harper, K., 'Pandemics and passages to late antiquity: rethinking the plague of c.249–270 described by Cyprian', *JRA* 28 (2015), 223–260

Holmes, B., 'In strange lands: Disembodied authority and the physician role in the Hippocratic Corpus and beyond', in M. Asper (ed.), *Writing Science: Medical and Mathematical Authorship in Ancient Greece* (Berlin: de Gruyter, 2013), 431–472

Jannetta, A. B., *Epidemics and Mortality in Early Modern Japan* (Princeton: Princeton University Press, 1986)

Jezek, Z., Hardjotanojo W. and Rangaraj, A. G., 'Facial scarring after varicella: A comparison with variola major and variola minor', *American Journal of Epidemiology* 114 (1981), 798–803

Jones, D. S., 'Virgin soils revisited', *William and Mary Quarterly* 60 (2003), 703–742

Jouanna, J., 'Air, miasma and contagion in the time of Hippocrates and the survival of miasmas in post-Hippocratic medicine (Rufus of Ephesus, Galen and Palladius)', in his collected essays, *Greek Medicine from Hippocrates to Galen*, trans. N. Allies (Leiden: Brill, 2012), 122–136

Hopkins, D. R., *The Greatest Killer: Smallpox in History* (Cambridge: Cambridge University Press, 2002)

Kahl, O., *The Sanskrit, Syriac and Persian Sources in the* Comprehensive Book *of Rhazes* (Leiden: Brill, 2015)

Kiple, K. F. (ed.), *The Cambridge World History of Human Disease* (Cambridge: Cambridge University Press, 1993)

Kudlien, F., 'Galens Urteil über die Thukydideische Pestbeschreibung', *Episteme* 5 (1971), 132–3

Littman, R. J. and M. L., 'Galen and the Antonine plague', *AJP* 94 (1973), 243–255

Lo Cascio, E. (ed.), *L'impato dell' 'Peste Antonina'* (Bari: Edipuglia, 2012)

MacNeill, W. H., *Plagues and Peoples*, rev. edn. (New York: Random House, 1998)

Marcore, A., 'La peste antonina. Testmonzianze e interpretazione', *Rivista storica italiana* 15 (2002), 801–819

Marino Storchi, A., 'Una rilettura della fonti storico-letterarie sulla peste di età antonina', in Lo Cascio (ed: 2012), 29–61

Mattern, S., *The Prince of Medicine: Galen in the Roman Empire* (Oxford: OUP, 2015)

Mattern, S., *Galen and the Rhetoric of Healing* (Baltimore: John Hopkins University Press, 2008)

McCaa, R., 'Spanish and Nahuatl views on smallpox and demographic catastrophe in Mexico', *Journal of Interdisciplinary History* 25 (1995), 423

Newfield, T. P., 'Human-bovine plagues in the early middle ages', *Journal of Interdisciplinary History* 48 (2015), 1–38

Pajer P., et al., 'Characterization of two historic smallpox specimens from a Czech museum', *Viruses* 2017, 9, 200 (doi: 10.3390/v9080200)

Porter A. et al., 'Comment: Characterization of two historic smallpox specimens from a Czech museum', *Viruses* 2017, 9, 276 (doi: 10.3390/v9080276)

Sallares, R., 'Ecology', in W. Scheidel, I. Morris and R. Saller (eds), *The Cambridge Economic History of the Greco-Roman World* (Cambridge: Cambridge University Press, 2007)

Sedley, D., *Lucretius and the Transformation of Greek Wisdom* (Cambridge: Cambridge University Press, 1991), 160–165

Singer P. (ed.), *Galen: Psychological Writings*, Cambridge: CUP, 2013

Smithson, C., Imbery J. and Upton, C., 'Re-assembly and analysis of an ancient variola virus genome', *Viruses* 2017, 9, 253 (doi:10.3390/v9090253)

Wertheim J.O. and Kosakovsky Pond, S.L., 'Purifying selection can obscure the age of viral lineages', *Molecular Biology and Evolution* 28 (2011), 3355–65

CHAPTER 10

Galen and the Last Days of Commodus

Matthew Nicholls

Posterity's impression of the emperor Commodus has been almost universally negative. From Herodian and Dio to the lurid accounts in the 4th C *Historia Augusta*, to Machiavelli and the modern age, he is decried as a monstrous tyrant, enslaved to his own ungovernable passions and an enemy to all virtue.[1]

The chief literary sources for Commodus' reign are not without their limitations. Dio, Herodian, and the *Historia Augusta* present accounts that are partially transmitted and/or highly dramatised, and veer towards cliché; each later account seems to build to some extent directly on its predecessor(s), limiting their collective usefulness as independent testimony.

Cassius Dio was, like Galen, a Greek contemporary of Commodus, well placed as a senator to observe his reign at close quarters. However, the part of his history which covers the reign of Commodus survives only in the 11th century summary of Iohannes Xiphilinus. What remains conveys an unremittingly critical, if somewhat scattered, impression of Commodus; Dio's loathing for the emperor is self-evident and is often attributed to his concern for the erosion of the senate's prestige and dignity (including his own experience of Commodus' dangerous and humiliating reign), and the personal fates of many of his senatorial peers. This may well be so, though it is worth remembering also that Dio's work, like Tacitus' a century earlier, was written under a new regime with an interest in portraying the rule of its predecessor, from whose violent downfall it had profited, as a period of disharmonious tyranny. There is also an element of historiographical convention in the work of a Dio or an Herodian; the age of Tacitus and Pliny had established senatorial utility and liberty as one important standard by which an historian might judge a reign, and write about it (Suetonius added other criteria including building works which, as we will see, also play a part in accounts of Commodus).

Herodian, a slightly later contemporary, characterises Commodus as a tyrant whose youthful elevation to power as the first emperor born 'in the purple' to a reigning father set an unhappy pattern for the child-emperors Herodian saw in the third century. The reliability of Herodian's account is also questionable;

---

1   Herodian 1.48; Dio 73.1.1, 73.4.1; SHA *Comm.* passim and esp. 1.7–8.

he is obviously hostile to Commodus, portraying him as an archetypal bad, autocratic emperor, and his account is highly dramatised.[2]

The pro-senatorial agenda evident in Dio – or the emphasis of an anti-senatorial stance as a short-hand for tyranny – is amplified in the *Vita Commodi* of the *Historia Augusta*, a late 4th C AD set of imperial biographies whose unreliability is so infamous that there is little need to rehearse it here, but whose accounts of otherwise scarcely documented reigns nonetheless draw reluctant historians like moths to a flame. The *HA*'s Commodus is a one-dimensional monster, a conflation of every bad-emperor trope. He is personally venal, susceptible to bad advisers, jealous of virtue, hostile to the entire senatorial order, in love with arena sports and harlots, given to driving chariots, and flirts outrageously with the idea of his own divinity: "*saevior Domitiano, impurior Nerone*".[3] After a while the accounts of his turpitude start to sound hollow as the *HA* author casts around for ever stranger proofs of his wickedness ("He displayed two misshapen hunchbacks on a silver platter after smearing them with mustard");[4] the only remotely positive characteristic attributed to him in the entire Life is an ability to dance and whistle, which is then condemned as unbecoming to an emperor.[5]

There is, then, much to suspect in the literary record. It reads at points like an aggregation of clichés; it is evidently shaped by its authors' own agendas and is, especially in the case of the earlier two writers, the product of an age which had various types of interest vested in looking back critically at the end of the Antonine dynasty.

An account of the period from a well-placed contemporary, with interests that were not necessarily the same as those of Dio's senatorial order, would therefore be valuable. Galen's περὶ ἀλυπίας (or 'On Avoidance of Grief'; henceforward *PA* or in references '*Ind.*', as elsewhere in this volume, for the Latin title *De Indolentia*) provides such a source, and though the direct testimony it offers is limited, it does offer contemporary witness to events at Rome in the last year of Commodus, and something of an immediate initial judgement on his reign. It is not an entirely disinterested account: Galen was, or had been, a member of the Antonine court, and I will suggest that his comments are probably intended

---

2   Hekster, O. (2002). *Commodus: An Emperor at the Crossroads*, 6; Kolb, F. (1972). *Literarische Beziehungen zwischen Cassius Dio, Herodian, under der Historia Augusta*, 160–1; Alföldy, G. (1971) 'Bellum Desertorum', *Bonner Jahrbuch* 171 (1971), 367–76.

3   "More savage than Domitian, fouler than Nero": SHA *Comm.* 19. All translations from Greek and Latin are by the author.

4   SHA *Comm.* 11.

5   SHA *Comm.* 1, which also says that he was able to fashion goblets and "play the gladiator or jester".

to be in some sense self-exculpatory. However, since Galen is emphatically not writing, like Dio, with the benefit of longer hindsight, or from the perspective and with the agenda of a senatorial historian, and unlike our other sources has the dubious benefit of having experienced Commodus' reign at first hand, the *PA* does, I think, offer useful new insight into this period.[6]

Firstly, we can be confident that the *PA* was written very shortly after the events it describes, and is therefore considerably earlier than any other surviving testimony. This does not in itself guarantee a superior insight into Commodus' reign: events were still unfolding, and Galen is cautious rather than explicit in his account, not wanting to risk leaving himself exposed. On the other hand, the negative verdict of posterity on Commodus had not yet had time to crystallise, lending extra weight to this early testimony.

The date of the *PA* is reasonably well established. The text principally concerns the fire at Rome in AD 192, the year on whose last day Commodus was assassinated. Galen discusses the fire as a very recent event. It had happened, he writes, "at the end of winter" and "two months" before Galen had intended to move some of his lost books to Campania "at the beginning of summer" (*Ind.* 23a, 20), so a date in the late winter or early spring of 192 seems right. However, later on the *PA* implies that Commodus is no longer emperor (*Ind.* 54–5, discussed below, whose criticisms of Commodus would have been fatally indiscrete were he still alive and in power),[7] which implies that Galen is writing perhaps a year or so after the fire, some time in 193. This interval of time fits with other details in the text: Galen tells us that he has returned to Rome from Campania after the fire; also, since news of the fire has reached his anonymous correspondent via a messenger, and a letter from him has come back to Galen, to which the *PA* is ostensibly a reply (*Ind.* 1–3), we also have to allow time for this epistolary exchange to have taken place.[8]

Secondly, Galen's propinquity to the Antonine court adds to the importance of his account. He knew Commodus (from well before his principate) and his father personally; his service as an imperial physician brought him at times into unusual intimacy with the most powerful people in the empire, and he must have been able to observe elements of court life at close hand. His return to Italy and then to Rome was precipitated by an imperial summons to military service in Aquileia and the flight of the imperial court back to Rome after an

---

6 As e.g. Boudon-Millot notes: "pour les historiens, ce nouveau témoignage est important. C'est le réquisitoire le plus ancien qu'on possède contre la tyrannie de Commode": Boudon-Millot, V. and Jouanna, J., with Pietrobelli, A. (2010). *Galien. Ne pas se chagriner*, 145.

7 cf. Rothschild, C. K. 'The Apocolocyntosis of Commodus' in ead. and Thompson, T. W. (2014). *Galen's De Indolentia*, 175–202, at 176 n.7.

8 cf. Nutton, V. (2012). *Ancient Medicine*, 232.

outbreak of plague.[9] Galen won the confidence of Marcus Aurelius by treating him on campaign in Germany,[10] making a substantial reputation for himself and becoming an imperial protégé. Released from further military service by Marcus Aurelius in 169, Galen returned to Rome and found there all he needed to embark upon a protracted period of research and writing. He looked after the young Commodus on his father Marcus Aurelius' orders and had earned praise from Annia Faustina for treating him for a fever while the emperor was away at war between AD 172 and 175.[11] He was thus at pains, in happier times, to indicate his continuing relationship with the imperial house: one that was never wholly attractive to him, but which brought undeniable benefits of material comfort and professional prestige (one fruit of this relationship, for example, was that many of the works he wrote during this time were deposited in the imperial library of the Templum Pacis, surely a mark of favour).[12]

Galen is generally reticent on the subject of contemporary politics, whether through conviction, expediency, or the fact that his authorial interests lay elsewhere.[13] However, the PA is markedly more politically engaged. As Rothschild points out, it adds, though relatively short, three more references to Commodus to the previous total of six in Galen's entire extant corpus, three of which refer to the medical care of the young Commodus and only one of which seems to offer criticism of the adult emperor, for discarding valuable stores of theriac.[14] The comments in the PA, by contrast, are all directly critical of Commodus' tyranny, as if the events of 192 had prompted Galen to a much more explicit political position than he had adopted hitherto. What we have, then, is a text by a well-placed insider, someone with personal knowledge of the late emperor, who was in or near Rome during the dynasty's dramatic last year and who felt

---

9   Galen *Libr. Prop.* 1.15, 2.18 (XIX.14 and XIX.17–18 K.); cf Nutton, V. (1973). 'The Chronology of Galen's Career', *Classical Quarterly* 23 no. 1, 158–71.

10   Galen *Praen.* 11 (XIV.660 K.).

11   See below n.14.

12   *Libr. Prop.* 2.19 (XIX.19 K.). Cf the similar honouring of Josephus, who received Titus' autograph imprimatur for his work (Josephus *Vit.* 363): Eusebius *Hist. eccl.* 3.9.2, Jerome *De vir. ill.* 13.1.

13   For Galen's political comments elsewhere, see Hankinson, R. J. 'The Man and his work' in id. ed. (2008). *The Cambridge Companion to Galen*, 1–33.

14   *Ant.* XIV.65.3 K.; the other passages regarding Galen's medical care of the young Commodus are *Praen.* XIV.650K.; *Praen.* XIV.657 K.; *Praen.* XIV.661K.; *Lib. Prop.* XIX.18–19K. See also Nutton, V. (1979). *Galen: On Prognosis*, 218. *Hipp Epid.* XVIIB.150.7 K. is about the paternity of Commodus. cf. Rothschild *Apocolocyntosis*, 178 with n.20. There is also Galen's account of the ability of Perennis' slaves to resist torture, an episode which implies criticism of the regime's abuses. It is preserved in the Arabic epitome of the lost *On Moral Character*; see Hankinson 'The Man and His Work', 21.

moved by the fall of Commodus to make relatively direct political remarks. What can this add to our understanding of the period?

The passages in which Galen directly refers to court life under Commodus in the *PA* come in a cluster in paragraphs 49, 50a and 54–55, just over half way into the text. Paragraph 49 is a straightforward testimony to Galen's unwilling participation in the life of the Antonine court:

> Ὥστε οὐδ'ἐμοὶ μέγα τι πέπρακται καταφρονήσαντι παντοδαπῆς ἀπωλείας κτημάτων, ὥσπερ τῆς ἐν αὐλῇ μοναρχικῇ διατριβῆς ἣν οὐ μόνον οὐκ ἐπεθύμησα τότ'ἔχειν, ἀλλὰ καὶ τῆς τύχης βιαίως εἰς αὐτὴν ἑλκούσης ἀντέσχον οὐχ ἅπαξ οὐδὲ δὶς ἀλλὰ καὶ πολλάκις.

> It was no great matter for me to scorn the loss of all my possessions, as I scorned also my time in the imperial court, which I not only did not want, but when Fate forcefully drew me towards it, I resisted not once, or twice, but many times.

> *Ind.* 49[15]

This claim is particularly convenient to Galen in the aftermath of Commodus' downfall; he made it again in e.g. *Libr. Prop.* XIX.18 K. where the phrase ἐξ ἀνάγκης echoes the βίαιως of the *PA*. To be fair, a reluctance to serve in the imperial court (at least an affected one) also colours other mentions of Galen's imperial connections.[16]

Galen's claim that he was a reluctant member of the court is amplified by the immediately following statement that he had many enemies there:

> οὐδὲ γὰρ οὐδὲ τοῦτο μέγα μὴ μανῆναι τὴν μανίαν πολλῶν τῶν ἐν αὐλῇ βασιλικῇ κατηγορησάντων.

> It was not even a great matter to avoid falling into madness despite the number of my accusers in the imperial court.

> *Ind.* 50

---

15 Text here and throughout: *Galien. Ne pas se chagriner (περὶ ἀλυπίας).* Ed. V. Boudon-Millot and J. Jouanna, with A. Pietrobelli. Paris: Les Belles Lettres, 2010.

16 See Boudon-Millot and Jouanna *Galien*, 132. cf n.9 above and *Praen.* XIV.647–9 K. with Gleason, M. 'Shock and Awe: the performance dimension of Galen's Anatomy Demonstrations' in Gill, C., Whitmarsh, T., and Wilkins, J. eds., *Galen and the World of Knowledge*, 2009, 85–114, for Galen's reluctance to have his successes brought to the attention of Marcus Aurelius, for fear that he would be summoned to return to Rome when his desire was to go home to Pergamum.

This is not the only time that Galen mentions enemies and accusers, whether at court or elsewhere.[17] The effect here is to show that not only was Galen reluctant to join the court, but also that he was not a popular member once there: he was not, then, a creature of the regime, but a reluctant outsider, resentful of the poisonous environment he had been drawn into and (it is implied) not complicit in the emperor's crimes.

With Galen's reluctant presence established in the reader's mind, there follows the *PA*'s most explicit passage of criticism of Commodus:

> Πέπεισαι δ᾽οἶμαι καὶ αὐτὸς παρ᾽ὅλον τὸν χρόνον, ὡς τὰς ἱστορίας ἔγραψαν οἱ τοῦτ᾽ἔργο<ν> ἔχοντες, ἥττω γεγονέναι κακὰ τοῖς ἀνθρώποις ὧν νῦν ἔπραξεν Κόμοδος ὀλίγοις ἔτεσιν, ὥστε καθ᾽ἑκάστην ἡμέραν κἀγὼ θεώμενος ἕκαστον αὐτῶν ἐγύμνασά μου τὰς φαντασίας πρὸς ἀπώλειαν πάντων ὧν ἔχω, μετὰ τοῦ καὶ αὐτός τι κλασθῆναι προσδοκήσας, ὥσπερ ἄλλοι μηδὲ ἀδικήσαντες, εἰς νῆσον πεμφθῆναι ἔρημον.

> You are persuaded yourself, I believe, that in all of history, judging by the historical accounts written by those whose metier that is, fewer evils have befallen men than Commodus has recently committed in just a few years, such that I, who witnessed each of them daily, exercised my imagination against the loss of everything that I owned, expecting that I too would also be snapped off, so to speak, as had others who had done no wrong, and sent to a desert island.
>
> *Ind.* 54–55

Galen gives a damning verdict on the reign, and tells us that it is shared by his correspondent. The suggestion is that although Galen's position afforded a particularly close-up view of the horrors of Commodus' reign, they were by 192 generally known. There is a literary allusion in Galen's citation at *Ind.* 52 of lines from an unknown play of Euripides in which Theseus undergoes similar mental preparations for possible adversities, including exile and untimely deaths,[18] but it is the reference to previous writers of history that is particularly important here: Galen is claiming an acquaintance with historical writers and explicitly comparing (his account of) Commodus' reign to their historical accounts of other bad emperors. This is significant given the comparisons to

---

17   cf e.g. *Praen.* XIV.625 11–14 K. for accusations of φθόνος and criticisms from others at court; *Libr. Propr.* XIX.21 K. for numerous intellectual rivals at Rome.

18   See Kaufman, D. H., 'Galen on the Therapy of Distress and the Limits of Emotional Therapy', Oxford Studies in Ancient Philosophy 47, 2014, 275–296 (p. 281).

Nero which we will consider below, and it also implies Galen's awareness that he is creating a historical testimony of a sort.

There is no reason to doubt the tenor of what Galen says here. The prospect of banishment and/or confiscation of goods was real enough under Commodus, in the unanimous testimony of our sources. Execution, whether summary or judicial, seems to have been more common, or at least more commonly reported by authors with no shortage of grim material to choose from, but both the punishments mentioned here by Galen are attested fairly often in the principal surviving accounts of the reign.[19]

Galen returns to the idea of banishment and confiscation again at *Ind.* 71:

Ἐγὼ δὲ εἰ μέν τίς ἐστιν τοιοῦτος σοφὸς ὡς ἀπαθὴς εἶναι τὸ πᾶν, οὐκ ἔχω λέγειν, τοῦ δ᾽αὐτὸς εἶναι τοιοῦτος ἀκρίβη γνῶσιν ἔχω· χρημάτων μὲν γὰρ ἀπωλείας καταφ<ρ>ονῶ μέχρι τοῦ μὴ πάντων ἀποστερηθεὶς εἰς νῆσον ἐρήμην πεμφθῆναι, πόνου δὲ σωματικοῦ μέχρι τοῦ μὴ καταφρονεῖν ἐπαγγέλ<λ>εσθαι τοῦ Φαλά-ριδος ταύρου. Λυπῆσαι δέ με καὶ πατρὶς ἀνάστατος γενομένη καὶ φίλος ὑπὸ τυράννου κολαζόμενος ὅσα τ᾽ἄλλα τοιαῦτα. Καὶ θεοῖς εὔχομαι μηδέν μοι τούτων συμβῆναι ποτε· καὶ διότι μέχρι τοῦ δεῦρό μοι μηδὲν τοιοῦτον συνέβη, διὰ τοῦτο ἄλυπόν με τεθέασαι.

For my part, I cannot say whether there exists a man so wise that he is totally immune to suffering, but I have an accurate understanding of the sort of man I am: I can scorn the loss of money, until the point of being exiled to a desert island, deprived of everything, and physical suffering, until the point of declaring that I can hold the Bull of Phalaris in disdain. What will grieve me is my homeland ruined, a friend punished by a tyrant, and I pray the gods that none of these things will befall me. And since up until now none of those things has befallen me, you see me undistressed.

Ind. 71–72

---

19   Instances of confiscation and exile/banishment:
      SHA *Comm.*: 3.4 (actors), 4.4 (Paralius' mother and Lucilla); 4.11 (Aemilius Iuncus and Atilius Severus, the consuls); 5.7 (Commodus' sister, Lucilla, subsequently killed); 5.9 (his wife Crispina, subsequently killed); 5.13 (Perennis confiscates the wealth of provincials after false accusations); 6.9–10 (peculation of Cleander); 6.10 (recall of exiles at Cleander's whim); 7.8 (multiple murders for the sake of financial gain); 13.8 (ditto); 14.2 (ditto); 14.4 (substitution of punishments for financial gain).
      Dio: 73.4.6 (Lucilla and Crispina); 73.6 (flight into presumed self-imposed exile of Sextus Condianus); 73.12.3 (a joking reference to Julius Solon's 'banishment' to the senate at the cost of all of his property).
      Herodian: confiscation of property (8.2, 17.2), expulsion from the palace of men of intelligence (13.8).

Here Galen locates his tolerance on a scale of suffering, from mere confiscation of assets (bearable) to desert island exile (not bearable), and from physical punishment to roasting alive in the legendary bronze bull of the Sicilian
tyrant Phalaris.[20] The reintroduction of the themes of confiscation and exile,
heightened here by corporal and grotesque capital punishment, strengthens
by repetition the criticisms of Commodus made in the earlier passages.

Galen also adds something new in this passage, taking the time to remind
his correspondent and readership that his homeland, presumably Asia Minor,
has not suffered ruin, and his own friends have not been exiled. This small
addition, seeming almost an aside, serves several purposes. It sets up a pre-
emptive defence against accusations of betrayal from contacts at home in
Pergamum, and it also helps deflect any charge that Galen should have spoken
out: not only was he afraid for his own safety, but (and one must admit the
rather thin moral grounds of this argument) his own friends and countrymen
were not in danger. Moreover, it would insulate him against association with
those punished by the regime, should a pro-Commodus faction come to power
looking for revenge. Granted, Commodus was a tyrant; but, as his death eventually showed, he was right to suspect plots against him,[21] and Galen is keen
to let us know that he was not associated with those who were punished by
Commodus, whether deservedly or not. Given the uncertainty still in air when
Galen was writing, as discussed below, this series of statements adds up to a
calculated declaration of almost complete neutrality in Commodus' court: he
didn't want to be there, he was not party to any crimes, he feared for his own
safety, he was not friends with anyone who was punished, he did not stand idly
by while anyone or anywhere close to him suffered.

Galen's testimony, short as it is, is that of an eyewitness and is the closest
in date to the reign of any of our sources. It is undoubtedly valuable, but our
reading of it must be tempered, as we have started to see, by an understanding
of its limitations and context. We must first acknowledge that the new historical testimony offered by the passages of the PA discussed above, though an
important early witness to Commodus' brutality, is not particularly extensive
or dramatic.[22] Moreover, for all the relatively apolitical status he tries hard to

---

20   Cicero *Verr*. 4.73; Diodorus Siculus 9.19.1. cf. Rothschild 'Apocolocyntosis', 185–87, which
      suggests that the connection in AD 192/3 of a tyrannical ruler with a bull would have
      brought to mind Commodus (as Hercules).

21   cf. Suet. *Dom*. 21: "[Domitian] used to say that the lot of princes was most unhappy, since
      when they discovered a conspiracy, no one believed them unless they had been killed."

22   Rothschild 'Apocolocyntosis' combs the text for further implied criticisms of Commodus;
      of these the most convincing are an allusion at *Ind*. 76 to "τὴν Ἡρακλέους Ῥώμην" ("the
      strength (ῥώμη) of Heracles", but a play on Commodus' megalomaniac association with

establish, Galen cannot be thought of as a disinterested observer. His proximity to the discredited regime, a useful professional connection during the reigns of the Antonines, could have become dangerous for him in the aftermath of Commodus' fall. We have already begun to read the PA as an initial attempt to outline a defence against the multitude of intellectual and perhaps political enemies who often lurk at the margins of Galen's accounts of himself, or the accusations of whatever faction would eventually come to power:[23] his case here is that he had, like a Tacitus or a Pliny, been an unhappy bystander in a tyrant's court, and was now finally in a position to reveal Commodus' guilt, and his own innocence. In such a context, the brevity of these remarks compared to Galen's overall silence on politics might itself be eloquent, a claim to be absorbed in the life of letters that occupies much of the first part of the PA, rather than caught up in the extraordinary political dramas that were playing out in the year that Rome burned: dynasties might fall and rise, and the city is in ashes, but Galen presents himself as barely a participant, bookishly concerned instead with the loss of his glossaries of Attic old comedy and prose.[24]

Moreover, we might reasonably believe that Galen is hedging his bets. His distancing of himself from Commodus is cautious, and incidental to the purported substance of the PA. He was writing at an uncertain moment. Commodus was dead, but the next emperors Pertinax and Didius Julianus would follow him within a matter of months, with three more claimants still in play. It was not until 197 that Septimius Severus finally saw off the challenges to his reign. It is not surprising, then, if Galen, writing when the final outcome of the 'year of the five emperors' was far from clear, used the PA to put some distance between himself and Commodus without committing himself too far. Historical verdicts on emperors' reigns took some time to settle down, even if they came in hindsight to look immutable. The tussle over Nero's reputation in 68–9 and afterwards, with the emergence of false Neros as late as the reign of Domitian,[25] is an obvious case in point. There is some suggestion that an alternative historiographical tradition retained a measure of praise for Commodus, indicating that his negative reputation was not immediately established and may not (as with Nero) have been universally shared.[26] Hekster suggests that Commodus

---

Hercules and his attempts to refound Rome ('Ρώμη) in his own image), and at *Ind.* 62 a suggestion of Rome's (or Commodus') moral decline through sexual incontinence in the metaphor of breeding birds rented out to stud.

23   See *Ind.* 50a and n.17 above for enemies explicitly in the court and elsewhere

24   *Ind.* 20.

25   Suet. *Nero* 57.

26   e.g. the 5th C AD testimony of Dracontius *Satisfactio* 187–190, calling Commodus "*vir pietate boni*" (perhaps echoing the Pius legend added to his coinage from AD 182–3: Hekster

retained a greater measure of popularity among the army and in the provinces than with the later authors who shape our view.[27] Galen's anonymous correspondent, and his initial intended audience, may have been at home in Asia Minor, and we have seen that Galen takes care to point out that this homeland did not suffer: perhaps this was a nod to a sceptical provincial audience.

We must also, of course, remember that Septimius Severus, into whose service Galen passed,[28] reversed the senate's *damnatio memoriae* of Commodus, promulgated his deification, renamed his son Caracalla as Marcus Aurelius Antoninus, and included Divi Commodi Frater in his own titulature.[29] Evidently Septimius Severus prized an adoptive association with the Antonines, including their last emperor, above any negative memories of Commodus' recent reign. He also, of course, continued to claim a very strong association with Commodus' patron deity Hercules.[30]

There was still an audience, then, to whom the memory of Commodus was not entirely toxic in the 190s and the 200s; the Senate were clearly hostile to his memory, but Severus had other constituencies to consider. In this context Galen's restraint in his criticism of Commodus proved to have been wisely judged, allowing him to escape any fatal recrimination in the immediate aftermath of Commodus' fall, and to remain in imperial service once the new Severan regime (if not senatorial opinion, or the overall judgement of posterity) had decided that Commodus' reputation was to be rehabilitated for political reasons of its own.

With all these caveats in mind, the fact remains that the PA is far more politically engaged than the rest of Galen's work, strongly suggesting that part of its purpose was to place on record (muted, cautious) criticism of Commodus' reign.[31] Galen is protecting himself, distancing himself from a regime he had

---

       Commodus p. 92 for coin legend date). Although no modern author seeks to rehabilitate
       Commodus entirely, recent scholarship has tried to achieve a more balanced view. Olivier
       Hekster's *Commodus* applies a careful attention to image-making and self-presentation,
       reading the ideological implications of Commodus' *Bildprogramm* as expressed in visual media like coinage, architecture, sculpture, and spectacle. He finds some echoes of
       Commodus' self-presentation in contemporary art.

27   Hekster *Commodus*, 201.

28   Galen XIV.217f K.; Birley, A. (1971). *Septimius Severus, The African Emperor*, 286–87.

29   Dio 76.7.4; cf SHA *Sev.* 10.6, 11.4; Aurelius Victor 20.30. Hekster *Commodus*, 189ff.

30   cf Jordanes *Rom.* 372, Malalas 12.1; 283 and the neutral description of Commodus' association with Hercules by Athenaeus, whose patron Larensis was that emperor's *procurator patrimonii*: Ath. 12.537ff. and Hekster *Commodus*, 184 n.116–7.

31   Which does not rule out other aims – a genuine essay in philosophical consolation, for example; an announcement to his friends and supporters that he was alive and undaunted after the fire; and a warning against purported copies of works now irredeemably lost: the

every reason to have loathed but with which he was nonetheless associated; he was hedging because the position was still fluid and he knew he had enemies at court and elsewhere. For all these limitations – indeed, in a sense *because* of the fact that Galen is treading carefully, holding back – this immediate but carefully limited condemnation of the reign is a valuable addition to the historiographical record.

Galen was not the first author to wait until the fall of a regime to criticise it, and would not be the last: Tacitus earlier in the century, and Dio in the next, did the same. We have already seen that Galen was aware of historical and historiographical precedent. In *Ind.* 54 he compares Commodus' reign to what can be found in the accounts of historical writers and in doing so alludes to Commodus' place, and of his own brief account of it, in the historiographical record. With this in mind, I will spend the rest of this chapter looking at Galen's treatment of the fire of Rome in AD 192, which provides the backdrop for the whole of the περὶ ἀλυπίας, and suggest that it may be intended to evoke earlier disasters in Rome and particularly to invite comparisons with Nero.

The fire of 192 seems to have come in a period of growing tension, when Commodus' divinising self-aggrandisement was already causing, or responding to, faltering popularity and the alienation of the senatorial order. A riot in 190 at the fall of Commodus' freedman and Praetorian commander Cleander, linked to rising grain prices, seems to have alarmed the emperor or caused a change of tactics in his self-presentation.[32] His promotion of a 'Commodian' golden age and increasing self-presentation as Hercules had accelerated from around that time; Hercules-Commodus was celebrated in coin issues, going "well beyond what all but the most extravagant Roman emperors had put forward".[33]

At this critical juncture came the fire of 192. There are several points of connection between the accounts offered by Galen and Dio, who were contemporaries and both in or near Rome at the time. Dio, a senator under Commodus, may have been an eyewitness; Galen was away in Campania, but clearly returned to Rome shortly afterwards.[34] They may have had similar sources for their accounts of the fire and there is little reason to doubt the congruence in points of detail. For example, Dio (whose account of the fire is at 73.24) mentions dwelling houses as a starting point, and Galen stresses the understood

---

detail entered into suggests that Galen was trying to establish firmly what had been lost. He returns to his warning against plagiarized and fraudulent literary works in *Lib. Propr.*, XIV.8–48 K.

32   Dio 73.13.1; Herodian 1.13.7; SHA *Comm.* 14.1–3, cf Dio 73.15.6.

33   Hekster *Commodus*, 103.

34   *Ind.* 11.

risk of fire posed by proximity to dwelling houses (*Ind.* 8). The route of the fire and its path of destruction from the Templum Pacis across the Sacra Via to the Palatine is broadly similar in both authors (see map), and – the most telling point of detailed correspondence – both mention the destruction of state records, with Dio turning this loss into a portent of global misfortune.[35] If Dio was right that this destruction had been seen at the time as a portent of a more universal turmoil, then by the time of Galen's writing the following year, after Commodus' fall, it might have begun to acquire an air of retrospective confirmation: although, as we have seen, Commodus is absent from the PA until past the half-way point of the text, Galen flags up this ominous destruction of imperial records early on at *Ind.* 8.

Both authors, then, give the fire a similar treatment. It is not surprising that for Dio, writing with the benefit of hindsight, the fire acquired a teleological force, forming part of a crescendo of events that would sweep Commodus from power. He links the fire explicitly to the downfall of the emperor, placing it in a sentence that begins "before the death of Commodus the following portents occurred".[36] In fact, his account of Commodus' reign and the entire (excerpted) book ends with a sentence ostensibly describing the fire but clearly referring also to the emperor's career and death: "But when it had destroyed everything which it had seized, it spent its force and died out".[37] Herodian follows Dio in making it a portent of the end of the reign, with the blaze started either by a lightning bolt or an earthquake (either way, a sign of divine displeasure).[38] It is not unreasonable to suggest that this view of the fire was available immediately to contemporaries, including Galen who was writing, we should remember, when the fallout of the events of 192 was still occurring: he might well have intended the PA's account of the fire to point towards the fall of the emperor at whom the same work direct unprecedented criticism.

Moreover, since it is also possible to observe deliberate echoes of the Neronian fire in Dio's treatment of the fire under Commodus, this trope – which

---

35   Dio 73.24.2 (the text throughout is *Dio Cassius. Roman History. Ed. H. B. Foster. Cambridge, MA: Harvard University Press 1927*): "... ὥστε καὶ τὰ γράμματα τὰ τῇ ἀρχῇ προσήκοντα ὀλίγου δεῖν πάντα φθαρῆναι. ἀφ' οὗ δὴ καὶ τὰ μάλιστα δῆλον ἐγένετο ὅτι οὐκ ἐν τῇ πόλει τὸ δεινὸν στήσεται, ἀλλὰ καὶ ἐπὶ πᾶσαν τὴν οἰκουμένην αὐτῆς ἀφίξεται." "... so that almost all the records belonging to the state were destroyed. From this in particular it was clear that the evil would not stay within the city, but would spread to its whole empire." Galen *Ind.* 8: "τεττάρων ἐπιτρόπων Καίσαρος ἀποκεῖσθαι κατὰ τὸ χωρίον ἐκεῖνο γράμματα." "because of the presence in that place [the burned storehouse] of the archives of four imperial procurators." Cf Herodian 1.14.6.

36   Dio 73.24.1: "Πρὸ δὲ τῆς τοῦ Κομμόδου τελευτῆς σημεῖα τάδε ἐγένετο."

37   Dio 72.24.3: "ἀλλ' ἐπειδὴ πάντα ὅσα κατέσχε διέφθειρεν, ἐξαναλωθὲν ἐπαύσατο".

38   Herodian 1.14.2.

is, after all, a fairly obvious one – could also have been in Galen's mind as he described the devastation caused by the fire and more cautiously alluded to the tyrannical reign of the late emperor. We have already seen that Galen was able to connect Commodus' reign to the historiographical tradition of bad emperors. There was also a historiographical tradition of disaster-narrative, linking the ruination of cities across time both to make comparisons and to imply the cyclicality of human affairs. Thus Scipio wept for the future fall of Rome as he watched Carthage burn,[39] while Tacitus' account of the Neronian fire of 64 explicitly connects it in the Roman imagination with the sack of the city by the Gauls 418 years previously,[40] implying that disasters like the fire were understood through comparison to accounts of earlier catastrophes. In literary terms, the antecedents for Tacitus' fire narrative draw heavily on Livy's account of the Gallic sack and also on Virgil's account of the fall of Troy (while Scipio quoted Homer), depicting historical events through a series of literary references stretching all the way back to the founding story of Classical literature.[41]

Galen, and later Dio, placed their own accounts of the fire of 192 into this tradition. We would expect to find historiographical connections in the accounts left by the historians. We can certainly observe commonalities in Dio's and Tacitus' accounts; Dio explicitly follows Tacitus, for example, in claiming that as the Neronian fire advanced to consume the city as a whole, it was compared to national disasters like the Gallic sack.[42] Another theme shared by Tacitus and Dio's account of the earlier fire, which also emerges in Galen's account of the later one, is the self-defeating response of the overwhelmed citizens. Dio writes that "many, crazed by the disaster, were leaping into the flames".[43] Tacitus similarly reports irresolute and ill-advised conduct during the fire, and claims that some were engulfed by despair afterwards: "some who had lost their entire fortunes – including their daily bread – and others, through love for the relatives whom they had been unable to rescue, chose to die, though an escape route was open".[44] These reports of irrational, self-harming surrender to emotions of various sorts sound like the sort of conduct Galen warns against

---

39   Appian *Bellum Punicum* 19.132.

40   Tac. *Ann.* 15.41.

41   Livy 5.43–59 with Kraus, C., 'No second Troy: topoi and refoundation in Livy Book V', *Transactions of the American Philological Association* 124, 1994, 267–89 and Champlin, E. T., *Nero*, 2003, 178–209. For Tacitus and Virgil: Feeney, D., *Caesar's Calendar: Ancient Time and the Beginnings of History*, 2007, 107. Cf. Edwards, C. 'The City in Ruins' in Erdkamp, P., ed., *The Cambridge Companion to Ancient Rome*, 2013, 549–557.

42   Dio 62.17.3.

43   Dio 62.18.1: "καὶ πολλῶν καὶ ἐς αὐτὸ τὸ πῦρ ὑπὸ τοῦ πάθους ἐμπηδώντω."

44   Tac. *Ann.* 15.38: "*quidam amissis omnibus fortunis, diurni quoque victus, alii caritate suorum, quos eripere nequiverant, quamvis patente effugio interiere.*"

in the *PA*. In particular, the *PA's* account of Galen's own exemplary resistance to grief in the aftermath of the fire, placed in contrast with the conduct of the grammarian 'Philides' and unnamed others who suffered grief at their losses to the point of mourning or even death,[45] may itself have been patterned after these historical accounts of similar self-destructive grief of Romans and others after earlier disasters, and in particular the fire of AD 64, as well as by the parallel tradition of evoking city-ruins in consolation.[46]

Galen and Dio may therefore have had accounts of Nero's fire in mind when they wrote of the fire under Commodus. The parallels between Commodus' and Nero's involvement in and response to fires at Rome, and the ways in which Dio and (for Nero) earlier writers portrayed them, are therefore worth exploring.

Firstly, and most obviously, the Neronian fire of Rome in 64 seems to have been viewed in retrospect as one of the turning points in Nero's reign, just as we have seen for the fire of AD 192. Suetonius places the fire at the end of his account of Nero in a list of "disaster and abuses" which herald his downfall;[47] Tacitus includes it in a year which ends with "portents heralding disaster to come" and moves straight into the Pisonian conspiracy of 65.[48] Dio, who blames the fire squarely on Nero himself, gives some space to Corbulo's successful exploits in Armenia in the sort of chiaroscuro alternation that Tacitus also enjoyed, and then moves on to the conspiracy against Nero, whose repression marked a new low in the reign.[49]

The conduct attributed to each emperor during and after the fires was similar. Both were outside Rome when it broke and out, and both came into take (fairly ineffectual) measures against it. Nero, according to Tacitus, was staying at Antium and only returned to Rome when his Domus Transitoria was threatened. He then opened up the Campus Martius, the buildings of Agrippa, and his own Gardens to homeless refugees from the fire, and built shelters for them.[50] Though traces of a practical and humane response are evident in Suetonius and Tacitus' account, the fire is explicitly attributed to Nero (Suetonius *Nero* 38, Dio 62.16.2) or linked to his agency by strong and undenied rumour (Tacitus

---

45   *Ind.* 7.
46   E.g. Cicero *Fam.* 4.5.4 for Servius Sulpicius Rufus' famous evocation of the ruins of Aegina, Megara, Piraeus and Corinth to console Cicero on the death of his daughter Tullia.
47   Suet. *Nero* 38–9.
48   Fire: Tac. *Ann.* 15.38–44; portents ("*fine anni vulgantur prodigia, inminentium malorum nuntia*") listed at 47–8.
49   Fire: Dio 62.16–18. Corbulo and Armenia: 62.19–23. Plot against Nero and its repression: 62.24–28.
50   Tac. *Ann.* 15.39.

Ann. 15.38). Commodus, according to Dio, also travelled into Rome, from the suburbs, and encouraged ineffective military and civilian measures to extinguish the blaze.[51]

A more substantial correspondence between the emperors is found in their conduct after the fire. The reason for Nero's alleged culpability for the fire lay in his megalomaniac building ambitions, while Commodus' actions around the time of the fire and in the aftermath show similar vainglorious tendencies. Commodus is only blamed for the fire by the unreliable *Historia Augusta* ("He ordered the burning of the city, as if it were his private colony"),[52] but while we have no reason to believe this, the obvious patterning of the accusation after accounts of Nero's arsonism is illuminating in this context: while not explicitly blaming Commodus for the fire of 192, the more reputable sources do agree that both emperors allegedly wanted to rebuild Rome in their own image, renaming it and refashioning it to suit their own ends.

The evidence for Nero's architectural ambition and actual achievements is plentiful; multiple literary testimonies, the renaissance rediscovery of the Golden House, and more recent archaeological work shows a huge construction effort which reshaped parts of the Palatine, Esquiline, and Caelian hills and the low ground between them, where the Colosseum now sits, and the equally rapid effacement of these projects in the succeeding reigns.[53] The evidence for Commodus' ambitions, both literary and archaeological, is more slender, but the point here is that the way Dio, the SHA, and perhaps Galen viewed and wrote about the fire in his reign was shaped by the way that they and others had viewed Nero's.

For Tacitus, who professes to be uncertain on the question of whether Nero actually started the fire, "it seemed that Nero was seeking the glory of founding a new city and calling it by his own name".[54] The emperor "made use of the destruction of his fatherland by building a palace", which Tacitus called "hated and built of the spoils taken from citizens".[55] Particularly objectionable was

---

51 Dio 73.24.3.

52 SHA *Comm.* 15.7: *"urbem incendi iusserat, utpote coloniam suam."*

53 Domus Aurea: Suet. *Nero* 31, 39; Pliny *NH* 33.54, 36.111; Martial *Spect.* 2; Tacitus *Ann.*15.42. Champlin, *Nero*, 178–209. For the archaeology, see e.g. Steinby, E. M. ed., *Lexicon Topographicum Urbis Romae*, Vol. II, 1995, 49–64; Panella, C. et al. *Meta Sudans I: un area sacra in Palatio e la valle del Colosseo prima e dopo Nerone*, 1996.

54 Tac. *Ann.* 15.40: *"videbaturque Nero condendae urbis novae et cognomento suo appellandae gloriam quaerere."*

55 Tac *Ann* 15.42 (*"Nero usus est patriae ruinis exstruxitque domum"*), 15.52 (*"in illa invisa et spoliis civium extructa domo"*). *Ann.* 14.53 (cf Suet. *Nero* 16) does in fairness list a series of impressive and practical rebuilding measures taken by Nero after the fire with a view to preventing a recurrence, including regulations on building heights and materials and the

the Colossus, an enormous (120ft) bronze statue of Nero in the palace vestibule which – too impressive to go to waste after Nero's fall – was later remodelled as the sun god Helios, becoming the eponym of the nearby Colosseum.[56]

Nero's ambitions extended beyond the palace and over the entire city, which the palace was rapidly swallowing up, as the famous pasquinade related by Suetonius complains.[57] Suetonius claims that he wanted to rename the city Neropolis, deftly signaling both the emperor's megalomania and his unseemly philhellenism; the same passage reports that the emperor also wanted to rename the month of April 'Neroneus'.[58] Tacitus also reports the emperor's purported ambition to rename Rome after himself, linking it to his widely believed responsibility for the fire.[59]

We can now turn to what Dio tells us about Commodus' conduct around the time of the fire of 192. He posed as the founder of a renascent Rome, to be renamed after himself: Colonia Antoniniana Commodiana.[60] The Colossus near the Colosseum was, according to Dio, remodelled in his likeness, its head replaced with Commodus', a lion skin and club added to evoke his patron deity, and a bathetic list of the gladiator-emperor's arena victories added to the base.[61] Commodus' onomastic vainglory extended to the months of the year, all twelve of which he intended to name after himself.[62]

This sequence, linking fire and megalomaniac rebuilding with the renaming of the months and the remodelling of the Colossus, sounds suspiciously familiar: Dio surely has Nero in mind. His portrayal of the stagey, degenerate emperor whose reign ended in a conflagration naturally looked back to his and others' accounts of Nero, adding or emphasising those elements – renaming the city and the months, representing himself in the giant Colossus – that would remind his readers of that proverbially disastrous reign. A sense of crisis mounts as the emperor's deeds and ambitions spiral out of any semblance of

---

provision of fire-fighting equipment, but only after strongly implying Nero's involvement in firing the city for his own gain, and mentioning the Gallic sack again.

56   Suet. *Nero* 31, Pliny *NH* 34.45, Dio 65.15. For the remodelling, Pliny loc. cit., Suet. *Vesp.* 18, Martial 1.70.7 and *Spect.* 2.1.

57   "The whole of Rome's becoming a single house! Move to Veii, citizens, unless that house doesn't spread to Veii as well". Suet. *Nero* 39.

58   Suet. *Nero* 55.

59   Tac. *Ann.* 15.40.

60   Dio 73.15.2; cf SHA *Com.* 8.6–9, 15.7. RIC 3, 247, 629.

61   Dio 73.22.3, SHA *Com.* 17.9–10; Herodian 1.15.9; Hekster *Commodus*, 123–4; Bergman, M., *Der Koloß Neros, die Domus Aurea und der Mentalitätswandel im Rom der frühen Kaiserzeit*, 1994, 12. For Nero's own disreputable career as a performer and its pseudo-triumphal commemoration in Rome, see e.g. Suet. *Nero* 1–14, 20–25.

62   Dio 73.15.3–4; Herodian 1.14.9.

rational control, and the fire is used as the final point of correspondence with Nero, and the harbinger of Commodus' downfall.

Galen, though not a historian and writing much closer in time to these events, uncertain of their final outcome, was nonetheless able to see Commodus' reign in both a historical and a historiographical context. He seems to have been aware of previous accounts of bad emperors, and of the way previous urban catastrophes at Rome had been written about and linked to these reigns. Connections between Galen's treatment of Commodus' reign and the fire and those of later authors suggest a degree of similarity in their respective approaches. The comparison with Nero, which is so strongly evident in Dio's account, would have been available to Galen as well, and earlier accounts of Nero's fire may have shaped his thinking and writing in the immediate aftermath of Commodus' downfall. In the context of what is by far the most politicised treatment of Commodus that Galen gives us, these connections help show us how immediate contemporaries thought about the terrible events of 192, and point the way forward to what would become the conventional historiographical verdict on Commodus and his reign.

References

Alföldy, G. 'Bellum Desertorum.' *Bonner Jahrbuch*, 171 (1971): 367–76.

Bergman, M. *Der Koloß Neros, die Domus Aurea und der Mentalitätswandel im Rom der frühen Kaiserzeit*. Mainz: Trierer Winckelmannprogramm, 1994.

Birley, A. *Septimius Severus, The African Emperor*. London: Eyre and Spottiswoode, 1971.

Champlin, E. T. *Nero*. Cambridge, Mass and London: Harvard, 2003

Edwards, C. 'The City in Ruins' in *The Cambridge Companion to Ancient Rome*, ed. Erdkamp, P., 541–57. Cambridge, 2013.

Feeney, D. *Caesar's Calendar: Ancient Time and the Beginnings of History*. Berkeley: University of California Press, 2007.

Gleason, M. 'Shock and Awe: the performance dimension of Galen's Anatomy Demonstrations' in *Galen and the World of Knowledge*, edd. Gill, C., Whitmarsh, T., and Wilkins, J., 85–114. Cambridge: 2009.

Hankinson, R. J. 'The Man and his work' in *The Cambridge Companion to Galen*, ed. id. 1–33. Cambridge: 2008.

Hekster, O. *Commodus: An Emperor at the Crossroads*. Amsterdam: J. C. Gieben, 2002.

Kaufman, D. H. 'Galen on the Therapy of Distress and the Limits of Emotional Therapy', *Oxford Studies in Ancient Philosophy* 47 (2014), 275–96.

Kolb, F. *Literarische Beziehungen zwischen Cassius Dio, Herodian, under der Historia Augusta*. Bonn: *Antiquitas* Reihe 4.9, 1972.

Kraus, C. 'No second Troy: topoi and refoundation in Livy Book V', *Transactions of the American Philological Association* 124 (1994), 267–89.

Nutton, V. 'The Chronology of Galen's Career', *Classical Quarterly* 23 no. 1, (1973): 158–71.

Nutton, V. *Ancient Medicine*. 2nd ed., London: Routledge, 2012.

Panella, C. (ed.). *Meta Sudans I: un area sacra in Palatio e la valle del Colosseo prima e dopo Nerone*. Rome: IPZS, 1996.

Rothschild, C. K. 'The Apocolocyntosis of Commodus' in *Galen's* De Indolentia, ed. ead. and T. W. Thompson, 175–202. Tübingen: Mohr Siebeck, Studien und Texte zu Antike und Christentum 88: 2014.

Steinby, E. M. (ed.). *Lexicon Topographicum Urbis Romae*, Vol. II, D–G. Rome: Edizioni Quasar, 1995.

Texts Used

Dio Cassius. Roman History. Ed. H. B. Foster. Cambridge, MA: Harvard University Press 1927.

Historia Augusta, Commodus. Ed. D. Magie. Cambridge, MA: Harvard University Press, 1921.

Galien. Ne pas se chagriner (περὶ ἀλυπίας). Ed. V. Boudon-Millot and J. Jouanna, with A. Pietrobelli. Paris: Les Belles Lettres, 2010.

Tacitus. Annals. Ed. J. Jackson. Cambridge, MA: Harvard University Press, 1937.

EPILOGUE

The Lost Readership of Galen's Περὶ Ἀλυπίας

CHAPTER 11

Arabic Περὶ Ἀλυπίας: Did al-Kindî and Râzî Read Galen?

Antoine Pietrobelli

The starting point of my question is a previous inquiry I made some years ago about two chapters of Oribasius' *Medical collections* on sexual pleasures (*Peri aphrodisiôn*). In a paper published in 2011,[1] I showed that both of the small chapters of *excerpta* drawn by Oribasius from Rufus and Galen were considered by Arabic scholars as independent short treatises written by two Greek authorities. They imitated them, giving birth to a specific literary genre *On coitus* (*Kitâb al-bâh*). We may count up to one hundred Arabic medical texts on that topic. Letters, short treatises, dialogues *On coitus* were produced by famous Arabic thinkers such as al-Jâḥiz, Ḥunayn ibn Isḥâq, al-Kindî, Râzî, Avicenna or Maimonides, each of them taking up, developing and amplifying every single remark or idea held *in nuce* in Oribasius' *excerpta*.

Considering the numerous Arabic texts dealing with the topic of dispelling sorrow or avoiding grief, I wondered if a similar relationship could be established between Galen's περὶ ἀλυπίας and the later Arabic production. We have a letter of Al-Kindî (*ca* 800–873) *On dispelling Sorrow*.[2] A chapter of Râzî (865–925) is devoted to this topic in his *Spiritual Medicine*.[3] The physician

---

1 Pietrobelli, A., "La *scientia sexualis* des médecins grecs: histoire et enjeux du corpus *Peri aphrodisiôn*", *Mètis* n. s. 9, 2011, pp. 309–338.

2 For the Arabic text, see Ritter, H./Walzer, R., "Uno scritto morale inedito di al-Kindî (Temestio Περὶ ἀλυπίας ?)», *Atti della R. Accademia nazionale dei Lincei, Memorie della classe di scienze morali, storiche e filologiche*, serie VI, vol. 8, 1938–39, pp. 3–63 or better Badawi, A., *Traités philosophiques par al-Kindî, al-Fârâbî, Ibn Bajjah, Ibn 'Adyy*, Beirut, 1983³, pp. 6–32; for the English translation, see Adamson, P./Pormann, P., *The Philosophical Works of Al-Kindî*, Oxford, 2012, pp. 245–266). On this text, see also Adamson, P., *Al-Kindî*, Oxford, 2007, pp. 150–156; Butterworth, C. E., "Al-Kindî and the Beginnings of Islamic Political Philosophy", in *eiusd.* (ed.), *The Political Aspects of Islamic Philosophy. Essays in Honor of Muhsin S. Mahdi*, Cambridge Mass., 1992 pp. 11–60; Druart, Th. -A., "Al-Kindi's Ethics", *The Review of Metaphysics. A Philosophical Quarterly* 47, 1, n° 185, 1993, pp. 329–357 and "Philosophical Consolation in Christianity and Islam: Boethius and al-Kindi", *Topoi* 19, 2000, pp. 25–34; Mestiri, S./Dye, G., *Al-Kindî, Le moyen de chasser les tristesses et autres textes éthiques*, Paris, 2004.

3 Chapter 12. For the Arabic text, see Kraus, P. *Abi Bakr Mohammadi Filii Zachariae Raghensis (Razis) Opera Philosophica fragmentae quae supersunt*, Cairo, 1939, pp. 15–96; for an English

---

Miskawayh (932–1030), in a section of his *Refinement of Character*,[4] includes a discussion of how to prevent and cure grief. Such reflections can also be found in Ibn Gabirol's *Ethics*[5] (xɪth century) or Maimonides *Regimen of health*[6] (xɪɪth century). Even in Christian Arabic literature the topic is well represented. The Copt Elias al-Jawharî (fl. late ɪxth century), Severus ibn al Muqaffaʻ (xth century), and Elias bar Shinâya of Nisibis (975–*ca* 1050) wrote specific treatises on the dissipation of sorrows.[7] Could Galen's περὶ ἀλυπίας underlie this flourishing literature, as Oribasius' chapters did for writing *De coitu*?

The problem is that the basis of sources among which the Arabs could pick is much wider than two small chapters. Galen, in his περὶ ἀλυπίας, gives an autobiographical adaptation of a prevalent philosophical genre. The story of this genre starts, as far as we know, with Antiphon the Sophist's περὶ ἀλυπίας[8] (5th century BC). Among the lost ones, two are attested by authors living in the Hellenistic period (3rd–2nd century BC): one is by the famous Eratosthenes of Cyrene,[9] the other by the Epicurean Diogenes of Seleucia, better known as Diogenes of Babylon.[10] There is also a papyrological testimony mentioning a περὶ ἀλυπίας by an obscure Aristophanes the Peripatetic.[11] The only one preserved in Greek is by Maximus of Tyre.[12] Apart from these texts with the same title, there are many others dealing with the same issue: book three of Cicero's *Tusculan Disputations*[13] or Plutarch's *On Tranquility of Mind*, developing the

---

translation, see Arberry, A.J., *The Spiritual Physick of Rhazes*, London 1950. On this text, see also Brague, R., *Razi, La Médecine spirituelle*, Paris, 2003.

4   For the Arabic text, see Zurayk (1967:217–222); for the English translation, see Zurayk (1967: 192–196).

5   Wise, S. S., *The Improvement of Moral Qualities. An Ethical Treatise of the Eleventh Century by Solomon Ibn Gabirol* ..., New York, 1902, pp. 78–81.

6   Bar-Sela, A./Hoff, H. E./Faris, E., 'Moses Maimonides' Two Treatises on the Regimen of Health *Fî Tadbîr al-Sihhah* and *Maqâlah fi Bayân Baʻd al-ʻrâd wa-al Jawâb ʻanhâ*,' *Transactions of the American Philosophical Society* 54, 4, 1964, pp. 26–27.

7   Griffith, S. H., "The Muslim Philosopher al-Kindi and his Christian Readers: Three Arab Christian Texts on the "The Dissipation of Sorrow"", *Bulletin of the John Rylands University Library of Manchester* 78, 1996, pp. 111–127.

8   Ps.-Plutarch, *Lifes of the Ten Orators*, 833c–d, see below n. 21.

9   *Suda* E 2898.

10   Goulet, R. (ed.), *Dictionnaire des philosophes antiques*, t. ɪɪ, Paris, 1994, p. 810.

11   *P. Oxy.* 3656, l. 12–15; see Goulet, R., *Dictionnaire*, tome ɪ, 1989, p. 406.

12   See *oratio* 28 in Trapp, M. B., *Maximus of Tyre, The Philosophical Orations*, Oxford, 1997, pp. 231–236.

13   Graver, M., *Cicero on the Emotions. Tusculan Disputations 3 and 4*, Chicago-London, 2002, and D'Jeranian, O., *Cicéron. Du chagrin*, Paris, 2014.

genre of consolation.[14] Consequently, we have to be more cautious in crediting Galen with a seminal influence on Arabic authors.

2. Many Orientalists (Bar-Asher,[15] Druart[16] or more recently Adamson[17]) who have worked on Arabic ethics have underlined that Galen was extremely influential in this field. P. Adamson[18] stressed that Galen was "a direct source for much of al-Râzî's *Spiritual Medicine*" and more generally, he attributes to Galen the introduction of a medical pattern to speak about the soul. The soul has to be cured from its illness or passions (fear, sorrow, anger, greed, etc.) by philosophy as well as the body has to be freed from pain, suffering and illness by medicine. According to Adamson,[19] this medical view of Arabic ethics goes back to Galen. But it must be also specified that such an analogy is very ancient. It can be found for example in Cicero's *Tusculan Disputations*,[20] in Epicurus' metaphor of the *tetrapharmakon* or even earlier in Antiphon the Sophist, who erected a little house in the agora of Corinth to practice the art of *alupia*.[21]

---

14   Boudon-Millot, V., "Un traité perdu miraculeusement retrouvé, le *Sur l'inutilité de se chagriner*: texte grec et traduction française", in Boudon-Millot, V./Guardasole, A./Magdelaine, C. (ed.), 2007, pp. 72–123; and Nutton, V, "Avoiding Distress", in Singer, P. (ed), *Galen. Psychological Writings*, 2013, pp. 45–106.

15   Bar-Asher, M. M., "Quelques aspects de l'éthique d'Abû-Bakr al-Râzî et ses origines dans l'œuvre de Galien", *Studia islamica* 69, 1989, pp. 5–38 et 119–147.

16   Druart, Th. -A., "Al-Razi's Conception of the Soul: Psychological Background to his Ethics", *Medieval Philosophy and Theology* 5, 1996, pp. 245–263 (p. 246, 248); Druart, Th. -A., "Philosophical Consolation in Christianity and Islam: Boethius and al-Kindi", *Topoi* 19, 2000, pp. 25–34 (p. 25).

17   Adamson, P., "The Arabic Tradition", in Skorupski, J. (ed.), *The Routledge Companion to Ethics*, London-New York, 2012, pp. 63–75, (p. 64–65); Adamson, P., "Arabic Ethics and the Limits of Philosophical Consolation", in Baltussen, H. (ed), 2013, pp. 177–96, (p. 177). More generally on Arabic ethics, see Gutas, D., "Ethische Schriften im Islam", in Heinrichs, W. (ed.), *Orientalisches Mittelalter*, Wiesbaden, 1990, pp. 346–365.

18   Adamson, P., "The Arabic Tradition", 2012, p. 69.

19   Adamson, P., *ibid.* p. 69: "Again, there is Greek precedent for this "medical" way of seeing ethics. [...] But the chief Greek model for this approach is Galen".

20   Cicero, *Tusculan Disputations*, III, 3–5 (5–11).

21   Ps.-Plutarch, *Life of the Ten Orators*, 833c–d: [...] τέχνην ἀλυπίας συνεστήσατο, ὥσπερ τοῖς νοσοῦσιν ἡ παρὰ τῶν ἰατρῶν θεραπεία ὑπάρχει· ἐν Κορίνθῳ τε κατεσκευασμένος οἴκημά τι παρὰ τὴν ἀγορὰν προέγραψεν, δύναται τοὺς λυπουμένους διὰ λόγων θεραπεύειν "he invented a method of curing distress, just as physicians have a treatment for those who are ill; and at Corinth, fitting up a room near the market-place, he wrote on the door that he could cure by words those who were in distress" (ed. and trans. by Fowler, p. 350). On the medical model applied to ethics in Greek philosophy, see Nussbaum, M., *The Therapy of Desire*, Princeton, 1994.

On the other hand, before the discovery of Galen's περὶ ἀλυπίας, some editors or translators of the Arabic texts of al-Kindî[22] and Râzî,[23] as well as M. Zonta[24] editing the Hebrew text of Ibn Falaquera, used to reckon in their prefaces or footnotes that Galen's περὶ ἀλυπίας was a source for the Oriental authors. If the editors[25] of περὶ ἀλυπίας have clarified the links between the fragment of Ibn Falaquera and the Galenic text, they have not shown any interest in al-Kindî and Râzî. Now that the περὶ ἀλυπίας has been discovered, edited and translated several times, these issues need a reappraisal. I would like to deepen the question: Are there hints of Galen's περὶ ἀλυπίας in al-Kindî and Râzî's texts? P. Adamson[26] has supposed that both authors had common sources they reworked. Could Galen be one of them? If so, what are the ressemblances and the differences in the literary form used by our three authors? Do they prescribe the same remedies to cope with sadness and sorrow? What are their respective *technai alupias*? How did the Arabs adapt the Galenic ethics to their monotheist and Islamic context?

I will first briefly recall the evidence of the Arabic translation of the περὶ ἀλυπίας. Secondly, I will try to show the influence of Galen on the literary form of the ethical works of Al-Kindî and Râzî. Finally I would like to emphasize the inheritance or the rejection of the Galenic model by both Islamic authors.

1   The Arabic Tradition of περὶ ἀλυπίας

3. It cannot be denied that the περὶ ἀλυπίας was translated into Arabic and thus well-known and widespread in the Islamic world since Ḥunayn's translation. In his *Risala*[27] (n°120) first written in 855 and completed in 863, Ḥunayn asserts that there were two Syriac translations of Galen's booklet: one by Ayyub al-Ruhâwî or Job of Edessa, the other by Ḥunayn himself. Ḥunayn's translation

---

22   Mestiri, S./Dye, G., *Al-Kindî, Le moyen de chasser les tristesses et autres textes éthiques*, Paris, 2004, p. 28.

23   Brague, R., *Razi, La Médecine spirituelle*, Paris, 2003, p. 113, n.1.

24   Zonta, M., *Un interprete ebreo della filosofia di Galeno*, Torino, 1995, pp. 18–20.

25   Boudon-Millot, V., "Un traité perdu miraculeusement retrouvé, le *Sur l'inutilité de se chagriner*: texte grec et traduction française", in Boudon-Millot, V./Guardasole, A./Magdelaine, C. (ed.), 2008, pp. 72–123, (p. 86 n. 42); Boudon-Millot, V. /Jouanna, J./Pietrobelli, A., Galien, *Ne pas se chagriner*, Paris, 2010, LXXIII, n. 76; see also Davis, D., "Some Quotations from Galen's *De indolentia*", in Rothschild, C. K./Thompson, T. W. (ed.), 2014, pp. 57–61.

26   Adamson, P., "Arabic ethics", 2013, p. 183.

27   Bergstässer, G., "Ḥunain ibn Isḥāq, Über die syrischen und arabischen Galen-Übersetzungen", *Abhandlungen für die Kunde des Morgenlandes*, XVII, 2, 1925, p. 40, n°120.

was made for Dâ'ûd al-Mutaṭabbib,[28] who was probably a physician working for the caliph Hârûn al-Rashîd and his wife Zubayda. One of Ḥunayn's pupil, his nephew Ḥubaysh, translated the περὶ ἀλυπίας from Syriac to Arabic for Muḥammad ibn Mûsâ,[29] the eldest of the three famous Mûsâ brothers, fond of mathematics, astronomy and mechanics, who sponsored Ḥunayn's activities.

But Ḥubaish's translation did not remain only in the Banû Mûsâ's private library. Both Mubashshir Ibn Fâtik from Cairo in the xith century and Ibn ʿAbî Uṣaybiʿa, a physician who lived between Damascus and Cairo in the xiiith century, could provide a more or less accurate summary of Galen's booklet.[30] Maimonides's disciple, the Jewish writer Ibn ʿAknîn,[31] settled in Fez (Morocco), could quote Galen's treatise in Hebrew at the end of the xiith or at the beginning of the xiiith century. So we may think that Ḥunayn's translation was available in Baghdad in the second half of the ixth century and that al-Kindî and Râzî could read it. Can we trace signs of Galen's Περὶ ἀλυπίας in their respective texts?

2   Formal Connections

4. There are *prima facie* noteworthy formal coincidences between Galen and both Arabic writers' text. In one of his paper on Arabic ethics, P. Adamson[32] has stated that the literary form of Arabic ethical works often follows that used by Galen, but this statement was based on Galen's *On Character Traits* and *On the Error and Passions of the Soul* which were models for Râzî, Miskaway or al-Fârâbî. What about the περὶ ἀλυπίας?

The most obvious formal parallel is between Galen and Al-Kindî. περὶ ἀλυπίας and *On Dispelling Sorrows* are both short treatises in the shape of an epistle, whereas Râzî's *Spiritual Medicine* is a much longer and systematic essay. Unlike Galen's letter, Al-Kindî's does not rely on his own misfortune. We know

---

28   Micheau, F., "Mécènes et médecins à Bagdad au IIIᵉ/IXᵉ siècle. Les commanditaires des traductions de Galien par Ḥunain ibn Isḥāq», in D. Jacquart (ed.), *Les Voies de la science grecque*, Paris-Genève, 1997, pp. 147–179, (p. 159–161).

29   Micheau, F., *ibid.* pp. 167–169.

30   On these passages, see Meyerhof M., "Autobiographische Bruchstücke Galena us arabischen Quellen", *Archiv für Geschichte der Medizin* 22, 1929, pp. 72–86 (p. 85); Boudon-Millot, V., "Un traité perdu", 2007, pp. 84–85; and Boudon-Millot, V. /Jouanna, J./Pietrobelli, A., *Ne pas se chagriner*, 2010, pp. LXXI–LXXIII.

31   Halkin, A, S., "Classical and Arabic Material in Ibn ʿAknin's "Hygiene of the Soul"", *Proceedings of the American Academy for Jewish Research* 14, 1944, pp. 25–147, (p. 60–65 and 110–115).

32   Adamson, P., "Arabic ethics", 2013, p. 177.

that the Banû Mûsâ brothers had developed a real hostility to al-Kindî and that they managed to get him beaten and maybe also jailed.[33] This allowed them to sequestrate his comprehensive library. We could have expected al-Kindî's epistle to start with a complaint about the loss of his books, but it did not. Like Galen's letter however, al-Kindî's is addressed to a good friend, "a beloved brother". Both Galen and al-Kindî wrote to fulfill the request of a friend:

> Gal.: I have received your letter in which you invite me to show you what kind of training, what arguments or what considerations had prepared me never to be distressed.[34]
>
> Al-K.: May God keep you, beloved brother, from all vileness [...]. I understand that you ask me to put down in writing arguments which counteract sadness, show its weak spots, and fortify one, by possessing them, against pain.[35]

And at the end of their letters both authors express in a similar way that they hope to have carried out their friend's request:

> Gal.: Finally, while I believe I have responded completely to the question you raised about avoiding distress, I do hold the view, nevertheless, that this requires a further definition.[36]
>
> Al-K.: This is sufficient for what you asked me, even if there are many [other] possible points one could make on the subject. If the proposed aim has been achieved, we have arrived at the end of what was wanted, even if there are many [other] ways to reach the goal, ways which are nearly endless.[37]

Furthermore both recipients are well-educated and persons with high moral standards:

> Gal.: In writing for others on avoiding distress I have given you some advice that is superfluous for you, for I have been aware from the start that, both by nature and by education, you always prefer simple food and dress, and are most restrained in sexual matters.[38]

---

33   Adamson, P./Pormann, P., *The Philosophical Works of Al-Kindî*, 2012, pp. XXII–XXIII.

34   Gal., *Ind.*, 1; tr. Nutton, 2013, p. 77.

35   Al-Kindî, *On Dispelling Sorrows*, prol.; tr. Adamson/Pormann, 2012, p. 249.

36   Gal., *Ind.*, 69; tr. Nutton, 2013, p. 95.

37   Al-Kindî, *On Dispelling Sorrows*, 13, 4; tr. Adamson/Pormann, 2012, p. 266.

38   Gal., *Ind.*, 79; tr. Nutton, 2013, p. 98.

>   Al-K.: An excellent soul and a just character like yours recoil from pos-
>   sessing vices and strive fortify themselves against the pains which they
>   bring and against the tyranny of their rule.[39]

Nevertheless these similarities make it hard to argue that al-Kindî read Galen.
Most of al-Kindî's works are epistles addressed to members of the political
elite. And the coincidence between the two recipients is to linked far more
with the aristocratic status of writers and readers in Antiquity and Middle
Ages than to a formal filiation. The fact remains that Galen's and Al-Kindî's letters are exceptions in their respective corpus: on the one hand Galen's letter is
much more autobiographical, historical and philosophical than the rest of his
surviving corpus; on the other hand, al-Kindî's epistle polishes a literary style,
which stands out from the usual prose of "the Philosopher of the Arabs".

Galen, al-Kindî and Râzî use anecdotes in their demonstrations. From § 39
to § 45, Galen recalls two stories about of Aristippus of Cyrene: Aristippus' bag
full of gold and Aristippus' lost field. In section 6 and 9, al-Kindî relates many
different anecdotes, each one borrowed from Greco-Roman Antiquity: one in-
vokes the last letter written by Alexander the Great to his mother Olympias;[40]
another is about Emperor Nero's disappointment with the destruction of his
crystal pavilion; a third story is about a Cynic Socrates, content with very little,
if not with nothing. Râzî resorts also to some anecdotes about a childless philosopher or a woman afraid of giving birth. The topic of the loss of a child is
also present in section 6 of al-Kindî. But none of these anecdotes is identical. None of the Arabic authors borrows his stories from Galen. Nevertheless
Galen, al-Kindî and Râzî's anecdotes have parallels in Plutarch.[41] It seems that
they draw to a same common stock, conveyed from Hellenistic period up to
Late Antiquity and Islamic world. All three texts also exhibit a gallery of philosophers, who are summoned for their exemplary conduct. Galen (§ 45) takes
Crates and Diogenes as paragons of poverty, while al-Kindî (§ 9) chooses a

---

39   Al-Kindî, *On Dispelling Sorrows*, prol.; tr. Adamson/Pormann, 2012, p. 249.
40   This letter belongs to the extensive apocryphal literature about Alexander the Great. It de-
      rives from one of the numerous versions of the *Alexander Romance*, wrongly attributed to
      Callisthenes. This letter of consolation can also be found in Ḥunayn's *Nawâdir al-Falâsifa*,
      in al-Masʿûdi, al-Yaʿqûbî or Mubashshir Ibn Fâtik; see Badawi, A., *Histoire de la philosophie
      en islam*, Paris, 1972, pp. 471–473. On *Alexander Magnus Arabicus*, see Doufikar-Aerts, F.,
      *Alexander Magnus Arabicus. A Survey of the Alexander Tradition through Seven Centuries:
      from Pseudo-Callisthenes to Ṣûrî*, Paris-Leuven-Walpole MA., 2010.
41   Galen's anecdote about Aristippus and his lost field is also related in Plutarch's *On
      Tranquillity of Mind* (469c–d). Razi's brief anecdote about the childless philosopher has
      a parallel in Plutarch's *Life of Solon* (6). The story of Nero and his crystal pavilion told by
      Al-Kindî can be found in Plutarch's *De cohibenda ira* (13).

Cynic Socrates living in a barrel. These common features did not prove a direct borrowing, since they are *topoi* of the ethical literature.

5. A more striking stylistic similarity appears between Galen and Râzî. Twice Galen quotes six verses pronounced by Theseus from a lost tragedy of Euripides to illustrate the exercise of *praemeditatio malorum*, which Galen says he used to practice every day:

> As I once learned from a wise man,
> I fell to considering disasters constantly,
> Adding for myself exile from my native land,
> Untimely deaths and other ways of misfortune,
> So that, should I ever suffer any of what I was imagining,
> It might not gnaw at my soul because it was a novel arrival.[42]

Strangely enough, when Râzî mentions the same technique, he also quotes six verses, attributing them to an anonymous poet:

> The wise man pictures in his soul,
> The disasters before they fall on him
> So, if they fall on him suddenly, he is not afraid,
> Since he copied them into his soul,
> He sees what is the latest end,
> And make of this end a beginning (my transl.[43]).

None of the editors[44] of *Spiritual Physicks* could identify the Arabic poet who composed those verses. Both poems express the same idea, even if the final message seems a bit different. It is really puzzling to see that the method of *praemeditatio malorum* is highlighted by some poetry in Râzî's text as it was in Galen with the words of Theseus. These verses could have been forged by Râzî himself but they are more likely Ḥunayn's translation of the Galenic quotation of Euripides. Such a hypothesis must be backed up, because the initial

---

42   Gal., *Ind.*, 52 and 77, tr. Nutton, 2013, p. 93 and 97.

43   For the Arabic text, see Kraus, P., *Abi Bakr Mohammadi Filii Zachariae Raghensis (Razis) Opera Philosophica fragmentae quae supersunt*, Cairo, 1939, p. 68, 8–10. I give here a new translation of these verses, the previous versified translation by Arberry (*The Spiritual Physick of Rhazes*, 1950, p. 71) is the following: "The man of prudence pictures in his soul/ Ere they descend, what mishaps may befall/ So, come they sudden, he is not dismayed, / Having within his soul their image laid. / He views the matter reaching to its worst, / And what must hap at last, faces at first".

44   Brague, R., *Razi*, 2003, p. 138, n. 161.

Greek text is quite different from the Arabic version. The context of enouncia-
tion is modified: the pagan figure of Theseus is not mentioned and the master/
disciple relationship is obliterated. All misfortune's examples (exile, untimely
deaths) are omitted and the discourse is more general. If the idea of anticipation of a future pain is preserved in the first four verses, the two last express
a slightly different teaching. It seems that the translator rewrites the idea of
not being chocked by a sudden misfortune in a exquisitely crafted sentence
based on an antithesis between end and beginning.[45] Such a divergent translation is neither very helpful for editing the Greek Galenic text nor for choosing
between the variants of the Euripides' fragment.[46] Ḥunayn's testimony is not
as faithful as it is for medical texts. How to explain, if Ḥunayn is the translator,
such differences in his translation of poetry?

First of all, it is a *topos* of Arabic literature that poetry is untranslatable.[47]
The six verses given as an equivalent of Euripides's could in such a context
illustrate Ḥunayn's virtuosity. The fourteenth-century historian al-Ṣafadî describes the translation technique of Ḥunayn in a famous passage:

> The translators use two methods of translation. One of them is that of
> Yuḥannâ ibn al-Biṭrîq, Ibn al-Nâʾimah al-Ḥimsî and others. According to
> this method, the translator studies each individual Greek word and its
> meaning, chooses an Arabic word of corresponding meaning and uses it.
> Then he turns to the next word and proceeds in the same manner until in
> the end he has rendered into Arabic the text he wishes to translate. This
> method is bad [...]
>
> The second method is that of Ḥunayn ibn Isḥâq, al-Jawharî and others.
> Here the translator considers a whole sentence, ascertains its full mean-
> ing and then expresses it in Arabic with a sentence identical in meaning,
> without concern for the correspondence of individual words. This

---

45   Remi Brague (*ibid.*) wants to recognize a sentence attributed to Aristoteles in the last
      verses; he refers to Stern M. S., "The first in thought is the last in action. The history of a
      Saying attributed to Aristotle", *Journal of Semitic Studies* 7, 1962, pp. 234–252. But this *coda*
      could also be interpreted as a Christian rewriting.

46   On this problem, see Boudon-Millot/Jouanna/Pietrobelli, *Ne pas se chagriner*, 2010,
      pp. 139–142; and Lami, A., "Il nuovo Galeno e il fr. 964 di Euripide", *Galenos* 3, 2009,
      pp. 11–19.

47   Al-Jâḥiẓ, in *The Book of Animals* (*Kitâb al-Ḥayawân*, ed. Cairo, I, 75), could write: "If one
      were to transpose the wisdom of the Arabs [into another tongue], however, then the won-
      derful splendour of the meter would be lost, and those attempting to do so would not
      comprehend the meaning"; this translation is given by Pormann, P. E./Savage-Smith, E.,
      Medieval Islamic Medicine, Washington D. C., 2007, p. 23 and p. 39, n. 29.

method is superior, and hence there is no need to improve the works of Ḥunayn ibn Isḥâq.[48]

Al-Ṣafadî refers to an old debate, as ancient as the translation itself, between the word-for-word (*verbum de verbo*) and the meaning-by-meaning (*sensum de sensu*) methods,[49] to praise the superiority of Ḥunayn over his colleagues and competitors. If such an assertion about the progress of Ḥunayn's method has to be tempered[50] and if Ḥunayn seems to endorse a much more literal technique in translating medical texts,[51] these verses could offer a new aspect of Ḥunayn's philological talent. Ḥunayn is said to have known his Homer by heart[52] and to have undertaken, during his imprisonment, a translation of the Bible in Arabic, which the historian and geographer al-Masʿûdî[53] considered the best one available. If this translation is Ḥunayn's work, these Arabic verses provide new evidence of his multifaceted art of translation and we should considerer it as a sign of Galen's influence upon Râzî.

6. As far as the literary form is concerned, we must also stress the differences between Galen and the others. Galen's περὶ ἀλυπίας is autobiographical and based on his personal experience, whereas al-Kindî and Râzî's texts are more general and neutral. At the end of his epistle (§ 11), al-Kindî offers a marvellous parable. Al-Kindî starts a long simile in which he compares our life in this world to a sea travel interrupted by a landing on an island. Some of the passengers stay in the ship when it drops anchor at the island, whereas others are distracted by the island's beauties, collecting stones, sea-shells and flowers. Some of these lovers of pleasures and distractions will miss the call of

48   This translation is borrowed from Rosenthal, F., *The Classical Heritage in Islam*, Berkeley-Los Angeles, 1965, p. 17 and Pormann/Savage-Smith, *Medieval Islamic Medicine*, 2007, p. 27 and p. 39, n. 34.

49   The opposition between *verbum de verbo* and *sensum de sensu* translations is formulated by Cicero, *De optimo genere oratorum* (14) or Jerome, *Letters* (57). On this topic, see Brock S., "Aspects of Translation Technique in Antiquity", *Greek, Roman and Byzantine Studies* 20, 1979, pp. 69–87.

50   See Gutas, D., *Greek Thought, Arabic Culture. The graeco-Arabic Translation Movement in Baghdad and Early ʿAbbâsid Society (2nd–4th/8th–10th centuries)*, London-New York, 1998, pp. 142–143.

51   For some examples of Ḥunayn's technique in translating Galen, see Overwien in Gundert 2009, pp. 131–138; *eiusd.* "The Art of the Translator, or: How did Ḥunayn ibn 'Isḥâq and his School Translate", in Pormann, P. E. (ed.), *Epidemics in Context. Greek Commentaries on Hippocrates in the Arabic Tradition*, Berlin-Boston, 2012, pp. 151–169.

52   According to Yûsuf ibn Ibrâhîm, quoted by Ibn Abî Uṣaybiʿa; see Strohmaier, G., "Homer in Bagdad", *Byzantinoslavica* 41, 1980, 196–200.

53   Strohmaier, G., *s. v.* "Ḥunayn b. Isḥâq al-ʿIbâdî", in *Encyclopédie de l'Islam*, t. III, Leiden-Paris, 1971, pp. 598–601, (p. 599).

the captain and remain on the island for ever, without coming back to their homeland. Others will come back to the ship with their burden, getting the worst places to sit and being annoyed by the putridness of the flowers and sea-shells. Al-Kindî explains the parable: the ship is our life, the destination is the next world, afterlife, and one should not be attached to material and transitory goods. This parable does not come from Galen, but we find it in Epictetus' *Enchiridion* (§ 7).[54]

These remarks show a variety of literary models interacting in al-Kindî's *On Dispelling Sorrows*. It is well admitted that the Arabs did not translate Greek literary texts such as theatre, novels or rhetoric to focus their interests and efforts on scientific texts, which were available.[55] But we have noticed here that philosophical and medical texts could be vectors for literary forms and not only for ideas. Except perhaps for Râzî, there is however no cogent proofs of the use of Galen's περὶ ἀλυπίας, as if the two Arabic authors had wanted to mask their debt towards Galen.[56]

3   *Technai alupias*

7. Let us now consider more precisely the content of the texts and especially their τέχνη ἀλυπίας, the way they prescribe how to alleviate and dispell sorrow. As Adamson[57] noticed, the medical pattern is a *topos* of every περὶ ἀλυπίας: sorrow is a pain of the soul. Just as the body has to be cured from its pains by drugs, surgery or dietetics, the περὶ ἀλυπίας treatises display themselves as remedies for the soul. This analogy between the illness of the body and the passions of the soul, between the remedies of medicine and the consolation of philosophy is obvious in Râzî's title, *Spiritual Medicine*. Al-Kindî also endorses this analogy, but claims the superiority of the soul over the body, to defend

---

54   See Pohlenz M., "Die Araber und die griechische Kultur", *Göttingen Gelehrte Anzeigen*, 200, 10, 1938, pp. 409–416. It is not so surprising to find the Stoic Epictetus as a formal model of al-Kindî's epistle. Epictetus' *Enchiridion* has been commented by Simplicius (VIth century) and it was part of the basic Neoplatonic curriculum; see Hadot, I., *Le néoplatonicien Simplicius à la lumière des recherches contemporaines. Un bilan critique*, Sankt Augustin, 2014, pp. 149–152.

55   For a revision of the misconceptions about the Greco-Arabic translation movement, see Pormann/Savage-Smith, *Medieval Islamic Medicine*, 2007, pp. 27–29.

56   It is worth noting that al-Kindî tells the story of Nero and his crystal pavilion without mentioning his sources and omitting the name of the philosopher Seneca who was in discussion with Nero in Plutarch's account; see Badawî, *Histoire de la philosophie en islam*, 1972, pp. 469–471.

57   Cf. *supra* n. 18.

the preeminence of the soul's care over bodily cure and thus the primacy of philosophy over medicine:

> Since sorrow is caused by pains of the soul; since it is incumbent upon us to remove pains of the body from ourselves by way of nasty drugs, cauterization, bandaging, abstinence and similar things which cure the body, and to bear the great expense consisting of the moneys owed to the person who cured the illness; and since the welfare of the soul and curing it from its diseases is superior to the welfare of the body and curing it from its diseases in the same way as the soul is superior to the body – for the soul rules and the body is ruled, and the soul remains while the body is obliterated ... Therefore it is much more incumbent upon us to improve the soul and cure it from its ailments than it is that we improve the body.[58]

I would not, with Adamson, interpret this analogy as Galen's inheritance, because it is also, for example, the main point of Maximus of Tyre's περὶ ἀλυπίας, and because we can date it back at least from Antiphon (5th century BC). But another idea seems more Galenic.

The trigger of Galen's περὶ ἀλυπίας is, of course, the fire of 192 and the loss of his goods and books. Al-Kindî and Râzi and both give a first definition of sorrow in relation to the loss of beloved persons or objects:

> Al-K.: Every pain for which one does not know the causes is incurable. We therefore ought to set out both what sadness is and what causes it in order to find a cure and to apply it with ease. Hence we say that sadness is a psychic pain occurring because one loses what one loves or is frustrate in obtaining what one seeks. Therefore, the causes of sadness are already apparent from what has just been said: it occurs because one loses what one loves or is frustrated in obtaining what one seeks.[59]

> Râz.: When the passion through the reason pictures the loss of a beloved associate, grief thereby follows ... Since the substance out of which sorrows are generated is simply and solely the loss of one's loved ones, and since it is impossible that these loved ones should not be lost because men have their turns with them and by reason of the fact that they are subject to the succession of generation and corruption, it follows that the man most severely afflicted by grief must be he who has the greatest

---

58   Al-Kindî, *On Dispelling Sorrows*, 4, 1; tr. Adamson/Pormann, 2012, p. 252.
59   Al-Kindî, *On Dispelling Sorrows*, 1, 1; tr. Adamson/Pormann, 2012, p. 247.

number of loved ones and whose love is the most ardent, while the man least affected by grief is he whose circumstances are the reverse.[60]

In his *On the Errors and Passions of the Soul* and περὶ ἀλυπίας, Galen methodically seeks the causes of distress and his principal explanation is cupidity (φιλοχρηματία) and insatiability (ἀπληστία).[61] Râzî is likely to have made his own this Galenic idea, including it in his very first definition of sorrow and Al-Kindî also points out frustration in obtaining sought after objects as a major cause of sadness.

Such an analysis leads to a similar set of advice. Through the example of Aristippus, Galen calls on us to forget what is lost and to focus on what is left. He exhorts readers to limit themselves to the necessary and to despise the superfluous. This precept that Galen inherited from his father can be found at the very beginning of Râzî's discourse. Râzî emphasizes that one should draw away from material and transient things or at least limit ones attachment to them:

> It would therefore seem that the intelligent man ought to cut away from himself the substance of his griefs, by making himself independent of the things whose loss involves him in grief.[62]

Al-Kindî gives a more Platonic and religious emphasis to this idea repeating that one must focus on the psychic goods and the immortal soul. He illustrates the notion of autarky through the zoological models of the "great whale and the marvellously created elephant", which only need food and a shelter to have a good life without lacking anything (§ 10).

8. We can draw other parallels between the three *technai* against sadness. Galen, after his addressee, mentions as a counterexample the case of Philistides the grammarian, his companion of misfortune, who died of depression and distress after the loss of his books in the fire. According to al-Kindî, since the wise man yearns for happiness, it is a sign of ignorance and lack of intellect to be sad. Both Arabic authors recommend us to remember how limited past sorrows were and how they could turn to happiness again. They exhort readers

---

60 Râzî, *Spiritual Medicine*, 12; tr. Arberry, 1950, pp. 68–69.

61 Becchi, F., "La psicopatologia di Galeno: il *Περὶ ἀλυπίας*", in Manetti, D (ed.), 2012, pp. 23–31; *eiusd.* "Dalla τέχνη ἀλυπίας di Antifonte al περὶ ἀλυπίας di Plutarco e di Galeno: evoluzione storica di un ideale di vita", *Studi italiani di filologia classica*, n. s. 10, 2012, pp. 88–99; Kotzia, P., «Galen, *De indolentia*: Commonplaces, Traditions and Contexts», in Rotschild, C. K./Thompson, T. W. (ed.), 2014, pp. 91–126.

62 Râzî, *Spiritual Medicine*, 12; tr. Arberry, 1950, p. 69.

to keep in mind examples of the numerous sufferers of misfortune who have overcome pain and sorrow:

> Al-K.: A nice method for this is to remember the things which made us sad in the past, and from which we were consoled, as well as the things which made other people sad, whose sadness and consolation we have witnessed.[63]
>
> Râz.: Moreover the loss of those things that are not necessary to the continuance of life does not call for everlasting grief and sorrow; they are soon replaced and made good, and this leads on to consolation and oblivion; gaiety returns, and things come back to what they were before the misfortune happened. How many men we have seen struck down by a terrible and shocking calamity, and presently pick themselves the blow fell, enjoying life to the full and entirely content with their circumstances![64]

Such advice could echo back to the reminder, at the beginning of Galen's letter, of the loss of his slaves during a major attack of the plague. Putting the present loss into perspective, all of the three authors intend to moderate the sadness, following the Aristotelian way of metriopathy.

When Galen reveals the secrets of his *alupia*, he enumerates his natural talent and his education, but as an example for others, he mentions his daily spiritual exercise of *praemeditatio malorum*.[65] Râzî also lists this training in his collection of remedies against sorrow:

> After this it follows that a man should picture and represent to himself the loss of his loved ones, and keep this constantly in his mind and imagination, knowing that it is impossible for them to continue unchanged forever. He should never for a moment give up remembering this and putting it into his thoughts, strengthening his resolve and fortifying his endurance against the day when the calamity happens. That is the way to train and gradually to discipline and strengthen the soul, so that it will protest little when misfortunes occur.[66]

If al-Kindî praises the power of habituation in ethical behaviour, he does not explicitly mention this method, he goes further in criticizing the process:

---

63   Al-Kindî, *On Dispelling Sorrows*, 6, 1; tr. Adamson/Pormann, 2012, p. 254.
64   Râzî, *Spiritual Medicine*, 12; tr. Arberry, 1950, p. 72.
65   See above n. 42.
66   Râzî, *Spiritual Medicine*, 12; tr. Arberry, 1950, p. 71.

For if we are sad before that which causes sadness occurs, then we impart to ourselves a sadness which might not occur because that which was going to cause sadness desists from doing so. Then we impart to ourselves a sadness which nothing else imparts to us.[67]

Such a polemic can be traced back to a Hellenistic context. Al-Kindî's position was also Epicurus' feeling: Cicero[68] reports that the philosopher considered it pure madness to envision bad things that will probably never happen. According to Cicero, Epicurus was reacting against the teaching of the Cyrenaean school, which recommended the practise of *praemeditatio malorum*, considering the element of surprise as the major cause of distress. Râzî also adopts some Epicurian precepts when he offers distraction or prescribes non-exclusive attachment to fight against distress.

Reading those three texts, we can understand that all authors are attentive to the need to draw an eclectic panel of remedies or a spectrum of doxographical positions, in which they select examples and ideas to express a personal thought. In a doxographical sequence, Râzî juxtaposes the ways to protect from sadness before it happens and the means to repel it when it is happening. Some of his techniques are borrowed from Galen, Epicurus or Aristippus. P. Adamson has tried to identify every argument of al-Kindî's demonstration with Hellenistic references. Describing *On Dispelling Sorrows*, Adamson writes: "It blends together arguments, themes and gnomological materials beholden to several ethical traditions – Stoicism, Cynism (we find Socrates conflated with Diogenes) and Aristotelianism".[69] Already Galen defined his own position against the rigorism of the Stoic to endorse a more Cyrenaic inspiration. The material gathered by Cicero in the *Tusculan Disputations* links the *praemeditatio malorum*, as well as the examples of Socrates and Diogenes to the Cyrenaic school.[70] Galen twice mentions its founder Aristippus and he might have borrowed his diagnosis of insatiability ($\dot{\alpha}\pi\lambda\eta\sigma\tau\acute{\iota}\alpha$) and his ideal of autarky from Aristippus as well.[71]

The major difference between Galen and the two Arabic authors is, however, that the physician of Pergamon gives a personal and self-centred version

---

67   Al-Kindî, *On Dispelling Sorrows*, 5, 3; tr. Adamson/Pormann, 2012, p. 253.

68   Cicero, *Tusculan Disputations*, III, 15 (31–33).

69   Adamson, P., *Al-Kindî*, p. 155.

70   Zilioli, U., *The Cyrenaics*, Durham, 2012, sp. 157–164.

71   Kotzia, P., "Galen, *De indolentia*: Commonplaces, Traditions and Contexts" (2014) in a brilliant paper has rendered the doxographical background of Galen's περὶ ἀλυπίας in connecting it with a Cynic, Cyrenaic and Stoic tradition. Kotzia attributes rightly the technique of *praemeditatio malorum* to the Presocratic Anaxagoras.

of the philosophical genre, whereas Râzî and al-Kindî's discourses are more universal. Râzî calls for common sense and stresses the notion of pleasure as the criterion of human existence to avoid sadness. Al-Kindî believes in the all-mighty reason. He delights in providing an irrefutable, mathematical demonstration and resorts heavily to his favourite technique of *reductio ad absurdum* to show that every distressful thought is a sign of lack of intellect. He displays a rigourous logic and rationalism, considering that the rational and immortal soul is the main essence of the person.

9. Let us turn back to our initial question: are there hints of περὶ ἀλυπίας in al-Kindi and Râzî's writings? I would say that Râzî had read and imitated the Galenic περὶ ἀλυπίας. The formal and thematic coincidences should not be fortuitous from such a connoisseur of Galen like Râzî. In Al-Kindî's *On Dispelling Sorrows*, there are no patent traces of any interest for the Galenic περὶ ἀλυπίας neither of a tribute to Galen. We could recall the fact that the Arabic translation of the treatise was sponsored by one of the Banû Mûsâ, Al-Kindî's enemies, and that the Nestorian school of Ḥunayn, specializing in the translation of medical texts, was in rivalry with al-Kindî's own circle,[72] which translated mostly philosophical texts. Galen and Râzî are physicians who acknowledged a strong interaction between body and soul in the analysis and therapy of distress, whereas Al-Kindî did not care at all about physical health but praised a "thoroughly intellectualist ethics".[73] In his undertaking to reunite the Platonic demiurge and the God of the Muslims, he sometimes seems to borrow from the Galenic *De usu partium*. But his *On Dispelling Sorrows* betrays a rejection of the Galenic medical approach. Above all, he adapted the Greek philosophical tradition to the Islamic context in which he wrote.

Beyond the influence of Galen's περὶ ἀλυπίας on Al-Kindî and Râzî, I would like to conclude with another question: How could Presocratic, Cynic, Cyrenaean, Epicurean or Stoic materials reach Râzî and al-Kindî, since no translations of the Hellenistic authors are preserved in Arabic[74]? What access did they have to a knowledge that we can nowadays only reach through Cicero or Plutarch? Questioning Galen's περὶ ἀλυπίας through the filter of the Arabic

---

72   Endress, G., "The Circle of al-Kindî. Early Arabic Translations from the Greek and the Rise of Islamic Philosophy", in Endress, G./Kurk, R. (ed.), *The Ancient Tradition in Christian and Islamic Hellenism*, 1997, pp. 43–76.

73   Adamson, P., *Al-Kindî*, 2007, p. 150.

74   The Aetius Arabus, a Greek doxographical collection translated by Quṣṭâ ibn Lûqâ in the IXth century, provided the Arabic thinkers with access to Presocratic and Hellenistic philosophy, see Daiber, H., *Aetius Arabus. Die Vorsokratiker in arabischer Überlieferung*, Wiesbaden, 1980. But another way of access to this ancient doxography was Aristotle's neoplatonic commentators; see above n. 55.

authors seems to bring a new light to understand how each one, at a different level, inherited a doxographical set from the Hellenistic period and made
it vivid, centuries later, to fit to their own context. Seven centuries separate
Al-Kindî and Galen, the same time period as between Galen and Antiphon or
Anaxagoras, and we should not forget that the Abbasid renaissance was the
first to translate and assimilate the Greek pagan inheritance in a monotheistic
context, long before the European Renaissance.

Acknowledgements

Thanks go to Caroline Petit for her invitation at the Warwick conference and
to all the participants for their useful advice; to Evelyne Samama and Xavier
Giudicelli for taking time to correct my English and to Simon Swain who has
revised this paper extensively.

Bibliography

Adamson, P., *Al-Kindî*, Oxford, 2007, pp. 150–156.

Adamson, P., "The Arabic Tradition", in Skorupski, J. (ed.), 2012, pp. 63–75.

Adamson, P./Pormann, P., *The Philosophical Works of Al-Kindî*, 2012, Oxford.

Adamson, P., "Arabic Ethics and the Limits of Philosophical Consolation", in
    Baltussen, H. (ed), 2013, pp. 177–96.

Adamson, P., "The Arabic Reception of Greek Philosophy" in Sheffield, F./Warren, J.
    (ed.), 2013, pp. 672–88.

Arberry, A. J., *The Spiritual Physick of Rhazes*, 1950, London.

Arkoun, M., *Miskawayh, Traité d'éthique*, 1969, Damas.

Badawi, A., *Histoire de la philosophie en islam*, Paris, 1972.

Badawi, A., *Traités philosophiques par al-Kindî, al-Fârâbî, Ibn Bajjah, Ibn 'Adyy*, Beirut,
    1983[3].

Baltussen, H. (ed), *Greek and Roman Consolations: Eight Studies of a Tradition and its
    Afterlife*, Swansea, 2013.

Bar-Asher, M. M., "Quelques aspects de l'éthique d'Abû-Bakr al – Râzî et ses origines
    dans l'œuvre de Galien", *Studia islamica* 69, 1989, pp. 5–38 et 119–147.

Bar-Sela, A./Hoff, H. E./Faris, E., 'Moses Maimonides' Two Treatises on the Regimen
    of Health *Fî Tadbîr al-Sihhah* and *Maqâlah fi Bayân Ba'd al-'râd wa-al Jawâb 'anhâ*,
    Transactions of the American Philosophical Society 54, 4, 1964, p. 26–27.

Becchi, F., "La psicopatologia di Galeno: il *Περì ἀλυπίας*", in Manetti, D (ed.), 2012,
    pp. 23–31.

Becchi, F., "Dalla τέχνη ἀλυπίας di Antifonte al περὶ ἀλυπίας di Plutarco e di Galeno: evoluzione storica di un ideale di vita", *Studi italiani di filologia classica*, n. s. 10, 2012, pp. 88–99.

Bergsträsser, G., "Ḥunain ibn Isḥāq, Über die syrischen und arabischen Galen-Übersetzungen", *Abhandlungen für die Kunde des Morgenlandes*, XVII, 2, 1925.

Bergsträsser, G., "Neue Materialien zu Ḥunain ibn Isḥāq's Galen-Bibliographie", *Abhandlungen für die Kunde des Morgenlandes*, XIX, 2, 1932.

Boileau D. A./Dick, J. A. (ed.), *Tradition and Renewal. The Centennial of Louvain Institute of Philosophy*, Louvain, 2 vol., 1993.

Boudon-Millot, V., "Un traité perdu miraculeusement retrouvé, le *Sur l'inutilité de se chagriner*: texte grec et traduction française", in Boudon-Millot, V./Guardasole, A./ Magdelaine, C. (ed.), 2007, pp. 72–123.

Boudon-Millot, V./Guardasole, A. /Magdelaine, C. (ed.), *La Science médicale antique. Nouveaux regards, études réunies en l'honneur de Jacques Jouanna*, 2008, Paris.

Boudon-Millot, V. /Jouanna, J./Pietrobelli, A., Galien, *Ne pas se chagriner*, Paris, 2010.

Brague, R., *Razi, La Médecine spirituelle*, Paris, 2003.

Brock S., "Aspects of Translation Technique in Antiquity", *Greek, Roman and Byzantine Studies* 20, 1979, pp. 69–87.

Butterworth, C. E., "Al-Kindî and the Beginnings of Islamic Political Philosophy", in Butterworth, C. E. (ed.), 1992, pp. 11–60.

Butterworth, C. E. (ed.), *The Political Aspects of Islamic Philosophy. Essays in Honor of Muhsin S. Mahdi*, Cambridge Mass., 1992.

D'Jeranian, O., *Cicéron. Du chagrin*, Paris, 2014.

Daiber, H., *Aetius Arabus. Die Vorsokratiker in arabischer Überlieferung*, Wiesbaden, 1980.

Davis, D., "Some Quotations from Galen's *De indolentia*", in Rothschild, C. K./ Thompson, T. W. (ed.), 2014, pp. 57–61.

Doufikar-Aerts, F., *Alexander Magnus Arabicus. A Survey of the Alexander Tradition through Seven Centuries: from Pseudo-Callisthenes to Ṣūrî*, Paris-Leuven-Walpole MA., 2010.

Druart, Th. -A., "Al-Kindi's Ethics", *The Review of Metaphysics. A Philosophical Quarterly* 47, 1, n° 185, 1993, pp. 329–357.

Druart, Th. -A., "Al-Razi (Rhazes) and Normative Ethics", in Boileau D. A./Dick, J. A. (ed.), vol. 2, 1993, pp. 167–181.

Druart, Th. -A., "Al-Razi's Conception of the Soul: Psychological Background to his Ethics", *Medieval Philosophy and Theology* 5, 1996, pp. 245–263.

Druart, Th. -A., "Philosophical Consolation in Christianity and Islam: Boethius and al-Kindi", *Topoi* 19, 2000, pp. 25–34.

Endress, G., "The Circle of al-Kindî. Early Arabic Translations from the Greek and the Rise of Islamic Philosophy", in Endress, G./ Kurk, R. (ed.), 1997, pp. 43–76.

Endress, G./Kurk, R. (ed.), *The Ancient Tradition in Christian and Islamic Hellenism*, Leyde.

Fowler, H. N. (1936), *Plutarch, Moralia X*, London, 1997.

Garofalo, I/Lami, A., *Galeno, L'Anima e il dolore, De indolentia, De propriis placitis*, Milan, 2012.

Goulet, R. (ed.), *Dictionnaire des philosophes antiques*, t. I-vb, Paris, 1989–2012.

Graver, M., *Cicero on the Emotions. Tusculan Disputations 3 and 4*, Chicago-London, 2002.

Gundert, B., *Galeni De symptomatum differentiis*, in *Corpus Medicorum Graecorum* V 5, 1, Berlin, 2009.

Griffith, S. H., "The Muslim Philosopher al-Kindi and his Christian Readers: Three Arab Christian Texts on the "The Dissipation of Sorrow"", *Bulletin of the John Rylands University Library of Manchester* 78, 1996, pp. 111–127.

Gutas, D., "Ethische Schriften im Islam", in Heinrichs, W. (ed.), *Orientalisches Mittelalter*, Wiesbaden, 1990, pp. 346–365.

Gutas, D., *Greek Thought, Arabic Culture. The graeco-Arabic Translation Movement in Baghdad and Early 'Abbâsid Society (2nd–4th/8th–10th centuries)*, London-New York, 1998.

Hadot, I., *Le Néoplatonicien Simplicius à la lumière des recherches contemporaines. Un bilan critique*, Sankt Augustin, 2014.

Halkin, A, S., "Classical and Arabic Material in Ibn 'Aknin's 'Hygiene of the Soul'", *Proceedings of the American Academy for Jewish Research* 14, 1944, pp. 25–147.

Heinrichs, W. (ed.), *Orientalisches Mittelalter*, Wiesbaden, 1990.

Jacquart, D. (ed.), *Les Voies de la science grecque*, Paris-Genève, 1997.

Kotzia, P./ Sotiroudis, P., "Γαληνοῦ Περὶ ἀλυπίας", *Hellenica* 60, 1, 2010, pp. 63–150.

Kotzia, P., "Galen, *De indolentia*: Commonplaces, Traditions and Contexts", in Rotschild, C. K./Thompson, T. W. (ed.), 2014, pp. 91–126.

Kraus, P., *Abi Bakr Mohammadi Filii Zachariae Raghensis (Razis) Opera Philosophica fragmentae quae supersunt*, Cairo, 1939.

Lami, A., "Il nuovo Galeno e il fr. 964 di Euripide", *Galenos* 3, 2009, pp. 11–19.

Manetti, D. (ed.), *Studi sul «de indolentia» di Galeno*, Atti del seminario fiorentino (22 novembre 2010), Pise-Rome (Biblioteca di "Galenos" 4), 2012.

Mestiri, S./Dye, G., *Al-Kindî, Le moyen de chasser les tristesses et autres textes éthiques*, Paris, 2004.

Meyerhof, M., "Autobiographische Bruchstücke Galen aus arabischen Quellen", *Archiv für Geschichte der Medizin* 22, 1929, pp. 72–86.

Micheau, F., "Mécènes et médecins à Bagdad au IIIe/IXe siècle. Les commanditaires des traductions de Galien par Ḥunain ibn Isḥāq", in D. Jacquart (ed.), *Les Voies de la science grecque*, Paris-Genève, 1997, pp. 147–179.

Nussbaum, M., *The Therapy of Desire*, Princeton, 1994.

Nutton, V, "Avoiding Distress", in Singer, P. (ed), 2013, pp. 45–106.

Overwien, O., "Die orientalische Überlieferung", in Gundert (2009), pp. 103–152.

Overwien, O. (2012), "The Art of the Translator, or: How did Ḥunayn ibn 'Isḥâq and his School Translate", in Pormann, P. E. (ed.), *Epidemics in Context. Greek Commentaries on Hippocrates in the Arabic Tradition*, Berlin-Boston, 2012, pp. 151–169.

Pietrobelli, A., "La *scientia sexualis* des médecins grecs: histoire et enjeux du corpus *Peri aphrodisiôn*", *Mètis* n. s. 9, 2011, pp. 309–338.

Pietrobelli, A., "*Ne pas se chagriner*: quelques apports du nouveau Galien", *Actes de la journée académique des langues anciennes 2013-Arelacler-Cnarela*, Clermont-Ferrand, 2013, pp. 5–19.

Pohlenz M., "Die Araber und die griechische Kultur", *Göttingen Gelehrte Anzeigen*, 200, 10, 1938, pp. 409–416.

Pormann, P. E./Savage-Smith, E., *Medieval Islamic Medicine*, Washington D. C., 2007.

Pormann, P. E. (ed), *Epidemics in Context. Greek Commentaries on Hippocrates in the Arabic Tradition*, Berlin-Boston, 2012.

Ritter, H./Walzer, R., "Uno scritto morale inedito di al-Kindî (Temestio Περὶ ἀλυπίας ?)", *Atti della R. Accademia nazionale dei Lincei, Memorie della classe di scienze morali, storiche e filologiche*, serie VI, vol. 8, 1938–1939, pp. 3–63.

Rosenthal, F., *The Classical Heritage in Islam*, Berkeley-Los Angeles, 1965.

Rotschild, C. K./Thompson, T. W. (ed.), *Galen's De indolentia*, Tübingen, 2014.

Sheffield F./Warren J. (ed.), *The Routledge Companion to Ancient Philosophy*, London, 2013.

Singer, P. (ed), *Galen: Psychological Writings*, Cambridge, 2013.

Skorupski, J. (ed.), *The Routledge Companion to Ethics*, London-New York, 2012.

Stern M. S., "The first in thought is the last in action. The history of a Saying attributed to Aristotle", *Journal of Semitic Studies* 7, 1962, pp. 234–252.

Strohmaier, G., *s. v.* "Ḥunayn b. Isḥâq al-'Ibâdî", in *Encyclopédie de l'Islam*, t. III, Leiden-Paris, 1971, pp. 598–601.

Strohmaier, G., "Homer in Bagdad", *Byzantinoslavica* 41, 1980, 196–200.

Wise, S. S., *The Improvement of Moral Qualities. An Ethical Treatise of the Eleventh Century by Solomon Ibn Gabirol …*, New York, 1902.

Trapp, M. B., *Maximus of Tyre, The Philosophical Orations*, Oxford, 1997.

Zilioli, U., *The Cyrenaics*, Durham, 2012.

Zonta, M., *Un interprete ebreo della filosofia di Galeno*, Torino, 1995.

Zurayk C. K., *Tahdhîb al-Akhlâq. The Refinement of Character by Abu 'Ali Ahmad Ibn Muhammad Miskawayh*, Beirout, 1967.

Index Locorum

General Index